"This is an important book, which will become required reading for scholars and students of pandemic lockdowns. It is the first volume to offer a genuinely inter-disciplinary approach from the humanities and social sciences which addresses as a totality the humanistic and social costs of lockdowns. By the end of the book, the reader is in no doubt that, had perspectives from the humanities and social sciences been incorporated into the pandemic response, the response would have been materially different – and this shift in perspective is a huge achievement."

Toby Green, *King's College London, UK*

"This is an important contribution to issues which are being swept under the carpet – an impressive demolition of the social and moral case for lockdowns and a reminder of their devastating collateral consequences."

Lord Jonathan Sumption, *former judge of the Supreme Court of the UK*

"Social scientists were not just ignored during the COVID-19 pandemic but typ-ically silent or even supportive of measures that inflicted enormous harm. This important volume starts to correct this tragedy, ranging widely across disciplines and societies to explore questions of scientism, moralism, freedom, harm, and more. Essential reading for anyone longing for critical perspectives on the disasters that unfolded after March 2020."

Lee Jones, *Professor of Political Economy and International Relations, Queen Mary University of London, UK*

"A thought-provoking set of essays which go well beyond standard criticisms of the pandemic response, investigating the deeper harms and questioning our understanding of concepts such as health and immunity, as well as being one of the rare texts to document the effects of pandemic policies on the Global South."

Sunetra Gupta, *Professor of Theoretical Epidemiology in the Department of Zoology, University of Oxford, UK*

PANDEMIC RESPONSE AND THE COST OF LOCKDOWNS

Pandemic Response and the Cost of Lockdowns brings the vast analytical apparatus of the humanities and social sciences to the task of critically analysing the political decisions taken in 2020–21.

The global response to the COVID-19 pandemic left little time for critical debate about the impact of lockdowns. Across the world, governments claimed to "follow the science", but they rarely paid attention to the humanities and social sciences. Indeed, the absence of these perspectives is symptomatic of a longer-term trend in the marginalisation of the humanities and social sciences in policymaking and public debate. This book exposes the tragic consequences of this omission in 2020–21 and demonstrates the potential for a different path in the future – a path in which we pay attention to power, complexity, and our biases. The authors establish what these disciplines have to offer in a global emergency and how we can ensure they help us avoid the mistakes of 2020–21 in the future.

This original and interdisciplinary book will be of great interest to students, scholars, and researchers throughout the humanities and social sciences, including the fields of philosophy, sociology, anthropology, law, political science, and history, as well as relevant policymakers.

Peter Sutoris is Assistant Professor in Education at the University of York, UK, and Honorary Senior Research Associate at University College London, UK. He is an environmental anthropologist.

Sinéad Murphy is an Associate Researcher in Philosophy at Newcastle University, UK.

Aleida Mendes Borges is a Research Associate at the Global Institute for Women's Leadership at King's College London, UK, where she leads the Women Grassroots Leaders research stream. She is a jurist, specialising in International Public Law (Human Rights).

Yossi Nehushtan is Professor of Law and Philosophy, Founder and General Editor of the *Keele Law Review*, and Co-Director of the MA in Human Rights at Keele University, UK.

THE POLITICS OF PANDEMICS

Understanding the Politics of Pandemic Emergencies in the time of COVID-19
An Introduction to Global Politosomatics
Mika Aaltola

Pandemic Response and the Cost of Lockdowns
Global Debates from Humanities and Social Sciences
Edited by Peter Sutoris, Sinéad Murphy, Aleida Mendes Borges, and Yossi Nehushtan

The COVID-19 Pandemic in the Middle East and North Africa
Public Policy Responses
Edited by Anis Ben Brik

For more information see https://www.routledge.com/The-Politics-of-Pandemics/book-series/TPOP

PANDEMIC RESPONSE AND THE COST OF LOCKDOWNS

Global Debates from Humanities and Social Sciences

Edited by Peter Sutoris, Sinéad Murphy,
Aleida Mendes Borges, and Yossi Nehushtan

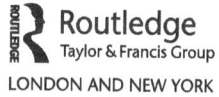

Routledge
Taylor & Francis Group

LONDON AND NEW YORK

Cover image: © Getty Images; Maria Ponomariova

First published 2023
by Routledge
4 Park Square, Milton Park, Abingdon, Oxon OX14 4RN

and by Routledge
605 Third Avenue, New York, NY 10158

Routledge is an imprint of the Taylor & Francis Group, an informa business

British Library Cataloguing-in-Publication Data
A catalogue record for this book is available from the British Library

Library of Congress Cataloging-in-Publication Data
Names: Sutoris, Peter, editor. | Murphy, Sinéad, editor. |
Mendes Borges, Aleida, editor. | Nehushtan, Yossi, 1971– editor.
Title: Pandemic response and the cost of lockdowns : global debates from humanities and social sciences / edited by Peter Sutoris, Sinéad Murphy, Aleida Mendes Borges and Yossi Nehushtan.
Description: Abingdon, Oxon ; New York, NY : Routledge, 2023. |
Series: Politics of pandemics | Includes bibliographical references and index.
Identifiers: LCCN 2022019941 (print) | LCCN 2022019942 (ebook) |
ISBN 9781032194714 (hardback) | ISBN 9781032193892 (paperback) |
ISBN 9781003259336 (ebook)
Subjects: LCSH: COVID-19 Pandemic, 2020–Social aspects. |
COVID-19 Pandemic, 2020–Government policy. | Quarantine–Social aspects. |
Health planning–Social aspects. | Emergency management–Social aspects.
Classification: LCC RA644.C67 P3678 2023 (print) | LCC RA644.C67 (ebook) |
DDC 362.1962/414–dc23/eng/20220805
LC record available at https://lccn.loc.gov/2022019941
LC ebook record available at https://lccn.loc.gov/2022019942

ISBN: 978-1-032-19471-4 (hbk)
ISBN: 978-1-032-19389-2 (pbk)
ISBN: 978-1-003-25933-6 (ebk)

DOI: 10.4324/9781003259336

Typeset in Bembo
by Newgen Publishing UK

CONTENTS

CONTRIBUTORS

Samuel Adu-Gyamfi is an Applied Historian at the Kwame Nkrumah University of Science and Technology (KNUST), Ghana. His research focus is applied history including the social studies of health and medicine in Africa. His current interests are in applied history of epidemics, pandemics, education, and politics in Ghana.

Roxana Baiasu is Lecturer in Philosophy at Stanford University in Oxford, Associate Member of the Philosophy Faculty at the University of Oxford, and Wellcome Trust Research Fellow at Birmingham University. She writes in the areas of Post-Kantian metaphysics and epistemology, philosophy of illness and wellbeing, philosophy of religion, and feminist philosophy.

Aleida Mendes Borges is a Research Associate at the Global Institute for Women's Leadership at King's College London, UK, where she leads the Women Grassroots Leaders research stream. She is a jurist, specialising in International Public Law (Human Rights), and her research focuses on grassroots politics. Building on her interdisciplinary background, she has worked on several international research projects in the Global South, mainly in Africa and Latin America.

Maddalena Cevese is an Independent Researcher in Political Economy. Her main fields of research deal with urban development, corruption, and regional economy.

Rose Cook is a Senior Research Fellow at the Global Institute for Women's Leadership (GIWL) at King's College London, UK, where she leads on GIWL's research stream examining gender equality at work. Recent work includes a project seeking to examine whether the UK's social policy response to COVID-19 is gender sensitive, gender blind, or gender neutral in its design, access, and impacts.

Michael Lewis is Senior Lecturer in Philosophy at the University of Newcastle upon Tyne, UK. He co-founded the Faculty Research Group in Critical Theory and Practice.

Anthony Mckeown is a Lecturer in International Relations at Staffordshire University, UK. He teaches modules related to international relations, international security, and international political economy.

Kai Möller is Professor of Law at the London School of Economics and Political Science (LSE), UK. His work in human and constitutional rights law and theory attempts to specify the moral, legal, constitutional, and institutional implications of a commitment to human dignity, freedom, and equality.

Sinéad Murphy is an Associate Researcher in Philosophy at Newcastle University, UK.

Yossi Nehushtan is Professor of Law and Philosophy, Founder and General Editor of the *Keele Law Review*, and Co-Director of the MA in Human Rights at Keele University, UK. His areas of research are legal and political theory, public law, human rights law, and law and religion.

Llanos Ortiz-Montero is a Public Health postgraduate nurse who has been working on front-line humanitarian health programmes since 1998, most recently as the Deputy Head of the Emergency Unit for the Spanish branch of Medicins Sans Frontieres from 2013 to 2020. She has completed her MSc in Medical Anthropology at the Universidad Rovira i Virgili, Spain.

Kunal R. Purohit is an award-winning Indian independent journalist. He has reported across India, the UK, and Hong Kong on issues of development, social justice, and right-wing politics and the author of an upcoming non-fiction book on the modus operandi driving the rising popularity of the Hindu right-wing in India.

Matthew Ratcliffe is Professor of Philosophy at the University of York, UK. His research topics include emotions, feelings and moods, perception, belief, the structure of intentionality, the sense of reality, intersubjectivity and empathy, delusions, hallucinations, certainty and trust, and the nature of grief.

Peter Sutoris is Assistant Professor in Education at the University of York, UK, and Honorary Senior Research Associate at University College London, UK. He is an environmental anthropologist.

Fernandes Wanda is a political economist. He is the Coordinator of CISE (the Centre for Social and Economic Research) in the Faculty of Economics at the

Universidade Agostinho Neto, Angola. He has published on foreign direct investment and employment patterns in Angola.

Mark Wong is a Senior Lecturer in Public Policy and Research Methods at the University of Glasgow, UK. His research focuses on digital society, inequalities and precarity, and AI and data. He is the Principal/Co-Investigator of multiple UKRI-funded research projects on inclusive and equitable AI. He served as a policy advisor for the Scottish Government and Public Health Scotland on the ethical collection of ethnicity data during the COVID-19 pandemic response.

ACKNOWLEDGEMENTS

Thanks are due to Faye Thomas and Isobel Horsley for creating the index and editing the proofs.

INTRODUCTION

The Role of Humanities and Social Sciences at a Time of Crisis

Peter Sutoris and Sinéad Murphy

In the wake of the global spread of SARS-CoV-2, governments across the world claimed to "follow the science" as they put in place unprecedented public health measures, including countrywide lockdowns that affected billions of people. While such policies had been implemented on a smaller scale in localised outbreaks of diseases, 2020 was the first time in human history that we could speak of a "world under lockdown". The "science" that policymakers relied on for guidance rarely encompassed humanities and social science knowledge, and the world's response to the virus was shaped almost exclusively by emergent findings of researchers within narrowly defined fields of the natural sciences, such as computational epidemiology. As the world tries to make sense of the last two years, questions are being asked about the appropriateness of this response, the collateral damage caused by these public health policies, and the lessons that we can learn for future crises. This book brings together a collection of 15 essays by humanists and social scientists who contribute to this important debate by voicing perspectives that were largely ignored and marginalised by policy elites in 2020–22 as the "Covid consensus" (Green, 2021) became the dominant narrative around the world.

Why did the humanities and social sciences not play a bigger role? On the one hand, their near absence was symptomatic of a longer-term trend toward the marginalisation of the social sciences and humanities in policymaking and public debate. This is at least in part due to a false dichotomy between "pure" and "applied" knowledge and the systemic headwinds faced by scholars who seek to tackle "controversial" subjects as they unfold. It is also likely the result of the humanities and social sciences producing more "messy" findings than their STEM (science, engineering, technology, and maths) counterparts, and humanists and social scientists being less successful at "selling" their findings to policymakers.

But there was more to this omission than the politics of knowledge production and consumption. The magnitude of the threat posed by the SARS-CoV-2 virus,

DOI: 10.4324/9781003259336-1

as presented in media and public discourse, afforded little time and space for a considered debate about how society ought to respond. As the year 2020 dawned, two words began to loom on the UK horizon as well as over most other countries in the world: "pandemic" and "lockdown". Through an unrelenting broadcast of these two words, the pandemic quickly became the enemy in public consciousness, and lockdowns became the only solution. The first casualty in a war is the truth, or so the saying goes; in the war on COVID-19, attention to nuance and complexity—the hallmark of the humanities and social sciences—became one of the first casualties, contributing to a collective intellectual paralysis.

In a newspaper article from 1786, the German philosopher Immanuel Kant anticipated such paralysis and set about describing how it is to be prevented, how to hold our course of reason and humanity in the face of ideas which are in danger of getting out of control. What we require in dealing with such ideas, Kant (1786) wrote, is a sense of direction, an *orientation*. The ability to orientate ourselves in thought is crucial, Kant insisted, for it ensures the proper regulation of our moral and intellectual faculties when they are confronted with ideas that are beyond the bounds of experience. We would usually express Kant's insight nowadays as the advice that we "keep some perspective" even in the throes of a novel threat.

We may, therefore, hazard the claim that, as 2020 unfolded, the stunning presentation of the sublime threat of a pandemic and its sublime mitigation by lockdowns obscured our usual landmarks, scrambled our moral and intellectual compass, and left us without our bearings. What might have prevented this disorientation? What might redress it now? Fortunately, Kant clearly named the one thing that can orientate us in the face of destabilising experiences and ideas: what he called "the public use of reason". On this crucial possibility, it is worth quoting him in full:

> Opposition to freedom of thought comes firstly from *civil coercion*. We do admittedly say that, whereas a higher authority may deprive us of freedom of *speech* or of *writing*, it cannot deprive us of freedom of *thought*. But how much and how accurately would we *think* if we did not think, so to speak, in community with others to whom we *communicate* our thoughts and who communicate their thoughts to us! We may therefore conclude that the same external constraint which deprives people of the freedom to *communicate* their thoughts in public also removes their freedom of *thought*, the one treasure which remains to us amidst all the burdens of civil life, and which alone offers us a means of overcoming all the evils of this condition.
>
> *Kant, 1786: 247*

As several of the essays in this volume attest, the freedom to speak and write in public has, in the UK and worldwide, been drastically reduced under the aegis of COVID-19 containment: eminent scientists have found their arguments rejected outright by unqualified journalists; on-the-ground testimony of healthcare workers has been summarily deleted by social media companies; restatements of government data have been labelled "misinformation"; and hundreds of thousands of protesters have gathered, sometimes without attracting so much as a sentence of reporting on the information and insights that they strove to disseminate.

In this context of the drastic suppression of our freedom to speak and write in public, and in accordance with Kant's heartfelt statement from 1786, we can only acknowledge that our freedom to think – the one treasure which ought to remain to us amid all the burdens of civil life – has been attenuated, at least since March 2020 in the case of the UK. Robbed of the grounding effect of open and energetic public discourse, our thinking has come unmoored from its vital reference points. We have been disorientated.

Humanities, social sciences, and public policy

Insofar as there has been discussion about the reasonableness of governments' responses to COVID-19, it has been conducted around the relative merit of aspects of new and unprecedented policies. What has been almost wholly missing is consideration of the *principles* at stake in these policies. Abstract concepts such as "human", "health", "life", and "death" have been thrown into public discourse with little hesitation about their basic philosophical implications.

It is time to examine these concepts and their place in public debate in greater depth. The essays in this book are motivated by questions such as: What is at stake in the distinction between life and bare-life? Has death become an unacceptable or unusable limit in our society? Can human health be administered as a public phenomenon? Who have been the winners and the losers of lockdowns? What does the response to COVID-19 tell us about the strengths and limitations of positivist science as a tool for policymaking? What have lockdowns and their consequences revealed about the symbols, rituals, and myths driving civilisation? To what extent were lockdowns and strict social-distancing rules based on valid moral grounds? To what extent were they constitutional? What can we learn from 2020–22 about the geopolitics of global emergencies and about the relationship between the Global North and the Global South? Why have the voices of social scientists and humanists been muted in most countries throughout the crisis? What do the social sciences and humanities have to offer in a global emergency, and how can we ensure that these fields of scholarship help us avoid repeating the mistakes of 2020–22 in the future?

The relative lack of participation by humanists and social scientists in shaping governments' pandemic responses is, in part, an expression of the fault line in academia between "pure" and "applied" knowledge. At its most extreme, this fault line divides "pure" scholars – who are viewed as being concerned with pushing the boundaries of knowledge and advancing their disciplines through "timeless", theoretical contributions to academic discourse – and "applied" scholars, who are seen as simply applying "pure" ideas in real-world situations, piggybacking on the ingeniousness of the theories developed by their colleagues.

This pure/applied dichotomy is a false one. Some of the longest-lasting intellectual contributions by humanists and social scientists have historically come through direct engagement with pressing societal challenges. Hannah Arendt's insights into human nature in *The Human Condition* built on her work on totalitarianism, trying to understand what enabled the evils of Nazism and Stalinism (Arendt, 1998). The exploitation of colonies by European empires inspired generations of intellectuals, from Aimé Césaire to Frantz Fanon. The "real world" outside the ivory tower is not the enemy of good scholarship; it is its closest ally.

But the false dichotomy between pure and applied scholarship is far from the only reason that the "hard" sciences tend to have a greater impact on policy. STEM disciplines have a long history of collaborative work on "real-world" problems, whereas in the humanities and social sciences academics often work solo, trying to prove as individual thinkers that their ideas make meaningful contributions to knowledge – a mode of work often less conducive to generating policy impacts. Much research funding in the hard sciences revolves around impacting the world in material ways – finding a cure to a disease, discovering a new material – which is perhaps less frequently the case in the humanities and social sciences.

Furthermore, because the humanities and social sciences deal with subjects that are often politically polarising – such as power, justice or bias – humanists and social scientists might choose not to address the "big issues" of the day in their work to avoid confrontation, even if their contributions might have been a vital form of "positive contestation" of public policy and debate. In the context of the neo-liberal university – an institution designed to reproduce the status quo rather than to challenge it – holding a mirror to the powers that be often means swimming against the stream in ways potentially detrimental to career progression (compare Morrissey, 2015). This is especially so for the many under-employed academics on temporary, precarious contracts who might rightly see engaging in political con-testation as a threat to their job security (compare Courtois and O'Keefe, 2015).

But many of the giants on whose shoulders the humanities and social sciences stand in fact engaged in work intended to be applicable to the big challenges of the time. The sociologist Michael Burawoy captured this "applied" spirit of his discip-line when he talked about Walter Benjamin's idea of the "angel of history" – a tragic figure battling society's self-destructive forces – in his 2004 address to the American Sociological Association, which is worth quoting at length:

> In its beginning sociology aspired to be such an angel of history, searching for order in the broken fragments of modernity, seeking to salvage the promise of progress. Thus, Karl Marx recovered socialism from alienation; Emile Durkheim redeemed organic solidarity from anomie and egoism....On this side of the Atlantic W. E. B. Du Bois pioneered pan-Africanism in reaction to racism and imperialism, while Jane Addams tried to snatch peace and inter-nationalism from the jaws of war. But then the storm of progress got caught in sociology's wings. If our predecessors set out to change the world we have too often ended up conserving it. Fighting for a place in the academic sun, sociology developed its own specialized knowledge[.]
>
> *Burawoy, 2005: 5*

Perhaps the muted response of humanists and social scientists in the wake of the spread of COVID-19 is one indication that, today, too many scholars focus on their "place in the academic sun" over engaging with controversial, messy issues – a trend that this volume hopes to help challenge.

We are not suggesting that the humanities and social sciences should abandon any of the rigour that we typically associate with "pure" research. Doing so would hamper our ability to deal with the complexities of the realities that we study. Commenting on the relationship between poverty, the "applied" field of development studies and the "pure" field of post-colonial studies, the political scientist Christine Sylvester (1999: 703) observed: "Development studies does not tend to listen to subalterns and postcolonial studies does not tend to concern itself with whether the subaltern is eating". It is fair to assume that subalterns – the marginalised populations of (former) colonies – want to both eat and be heard, and as scholars we ought to keep both these realities in mind. Similarly, coming up with a response to the spread of the SARS-CoV-2 virus means recognising that people do not just wish to be safe from the dangers posed by the virus, they also wish to have their rights respected, to not have their economic futures destroyed, to lead lives that they "have a reason to value", in the words of Amartya Sen (1999:18). This is the spirit that led to the creation of this book.

"The Science"

Aside from the marginalisation of perspectives from the humanities and the social sciences, governments' responses to COVID-19 have also marginalised many perspectives from within the "harder" sciences. The claim made by the UK government – and many other governments around the world – to be following "the science" is by now revealed as hollow; bewildering U-turns in government policy over the COVID-19 months have long belied the implication that scientific expertise is sufficiently in accord to merit the singular designator "the science".

We ought not to be surprised by this. Not even the "hardest" sciences would purport for a moment to arrive at conclusions so definitive as to justify the implicit exclusion of alternative opinions and future discoveries. As pathologist Dr. Claire Craig (2021) reminded us, the three achievements essential to science are: the recognition that we do not know everything yet; the ability to admit that some previously held beliefs were wrong; and – most vitally – an openness to new ideas. Breakthroughs in science happen "only when there is freedom to include all comers", she wrote, echoing Kant's insistence that it is only in community that we are truly free to think.

Appeals to "the science" are undoubtedly not scientific. Rather, they are *scientistic*, mistaking empirical research for the assurance of certainty and collaborative enterprise for the guarantee of univocity. Nothing could be further from the truth for science, which trades in hypotheses, thrives on dispute, and never lays claim to having found a final solution.

If scientism thus mistakes the essentially hypothetical, disputational, and provisional character of science, then one of its regrettable effects is the sidelining of just those disciplines in the humanities and social sciences that frame and regulate hypothetical, disputational, and provisional debate – fields of study that can police the grey zones of scientific theories and practices, their inevitable uncertainties, gaps, contradictions, and hesitations. Far from being irrelevant to the successes of the natural and mathematical sciences, the humanities and social sciences are their vital companions, furnishing the ethical and intellectual guidance necessary to negotiate the difficult tasks of applying general maxims to particular cases, identifying the proper course of action in the face of contradictions in available data, establishing in-principle agreement between divergent views, and determining the nature and significance of the vastly different social, cultural, economic, and political environments in which different populations, and different cohorts within populations, live – in short, judging what we ought to think and do in the context of the inevitable shortage of evidence for what to think and do, a shortage that arises from the finitude of all of human effort, including all scientific endeavour.

This collection of essays features examples of the many arguments, methods, devices, principles, and concepts with which the humanities and social sciences might have accompanied contributions from the life and mathematical sciences to provide essential regulation of debate and of policy during the COVID-19 crisis. We must begin at last and in earnest to rebuild our moral and intellectual community to which we can communicate our thoughts and which can communicate its thoughts to us.

Intellectual diversity, interdisciplinarity, geographical inclusion, and timeliness

It is in the spirit of this rebuilding project that the present volume has been put together. In compiling this book, the editors sought to avoid some of the stumbling blocks that we believe often get in the way of humanists and social scientists having a meaningful influence on public policy.

The ability of the social sciences and humanities to have an impact is often hampered by their getting stuck in an echo chamber. Writing for a limited audience of fellow scholars with similar analytical perspectives rarely leads to the wider world paying attention. To minimise the likelihood of such a scenario, we aimed to ensure that the essays represented intellectually diverse perspectives. We approached a wide range of scholars across many disciplines. Each of the four editors comes from a different disciplinary background, allowing this project to become an intersection of networks of scholars who, in the normal course of things, rarely interact with each other.

The often convoluted language and unnecessary length of publications by humanists and those in social sciences can make it difficult for policymakers to pay attention. We challenged each of the contributors to write in an accessible style, open to non-specialist readers, almost like a newspaper op-ed, but maintaining a high level of scholarly rigour and analysis, and to keep their contributions as succinct as possible.

Another factor that often gets in the way of impact is the extent of geographical relevance. Scholarship that speaks to realities within a particular nation state rarely appeals to audiences outside that state. Here, the humanities and social sciences can make a real contribution. The phenomena that they deal with often transcend the boundaries of individual countries, and the response to COVID-19 is no exception. Indeed, many of the gravest consequences of the policy choices made in the Global North were felt in the Global South. While most of our contributors are based in the United Kingdom, we made sure to include several perspectives from African, Asian, and Latin American countries in this volume to provide a more complete picture of the global nature of the consequences of COVID-19-related public health policies enacted during the last two years.

Humanists and social scientists often take a long time to respond to events unfolding around them. By the time it gets published, the subject of much humanities and social sciences scholarship is long in the past. To counter this, we aimed to bring this book to print as quickly as possible, and asked our contributors to work on very tight timelines. We owe a debt of gratitude to our publisher for agreeing to a very speedy production timeline for this book, which allowed us to publish before the COVID-19 crisis is in the rear-view mirror and while the perspectives contained in the book still speak to what we are experiencing in the here and now. We believe that an approach to creating and disseminating knowledge that stresses intellectual diversity, interdisciplinarity, geographical inclusion, and timeliness can help increase humanists' and social scientists' chances of meaningfully impacting public policy by drawing attention to the complexity of the underlying issues through diverse perspectives and analytic lenses.

Alternative perspectives

That there can only be – that there could only ever have been – *perspectives* on the issue of management of the spread of the SARS-CoV-2 virus is a founding premise of this project. No viewpoint is ever definitive and no conclusion ever final; all we have are perspectives. As Hans-Georg Gadamer put it:

> We are always affected, in hope and fear, by what is nearest to us....It determines in advance both what seems to us worth inquiring about and what will appear as an object of investigation, and we more or less forget half of what is really there – in fact, we miss the whole truth of the phenomenon – when we take its immediate appearance as the whole truth.
>
> *Gadamer, 2003: 305*

The motivation for this collection was to provide a platform for a range of perspectives that utilise the analytic lenses of the social sciences and humanities, and thereby both to demonstrate that alternative perspectives are possible and available and to encourage other qualified commentators to contribute more.

In accordance with this goal, the collection is divided into three sections. Each section highlights one of the significant ways in which alternative perspectives arise and are justified: by the multiplicity of plausible *interpretations* of key concepts; by the variety of geographical and cultural *contexts*; and by the profound constitutive influence wrought by different *paradigms* of thought and action. This mode of organisation requires a caveat. By their nature, the horizons of human efforts comprise a complex intersection of operative factors – to attempt to separate them out and to emphasise three of them is an inevitably artificial and partial project. Nonetheless, isolating different ways in which human thought and action are perspectival has the double merit of helping us understand the different mechanisms through which the "Covid consensus" arose and of illustrating the ways in which any policy, no matter how vital, is shaped by a particular horizon of knowledge and therefore subject to constant review.

The first section considers the key COVID-19 concepts of consensus, health, care, data and immunity and their use in the justification of governments' responses to COVID-19, as well as in the media and public discourse. The chapters in this part show that the use of these concepts was often truncated or quite simply erroneous, and that it was not just worth considering their alternative interpretations but in fact vital to do so. Mckeown's essay (Chapter 1) argues that, far from being a genuine consensus about the inevitability of lockdowns, the so-called "lockdown consensus" operated as a "regime of truth", to use Foucault's language. Performative scientism and moralism fostered this regime and stifled meaningful debate about what the response to the spread of the virus should be. Murphy (Chapter 2) goes on to show that the concept of health is open to an alternative interpretation that sees it as travelling along precisely the channels of human contact that a respiratory virus spreads in; according to this interpretation, viral infection and human health are not mutually exclusive but must coexist if health is to be genuinely promoted. Sutoris's contribution (Chapter 3) offers an interpretation of what may be the most important Covid concept of them all, the concept of care, arguing that the "caring society" is in fact a Western myth. This helps explain the ritualistic nature of many efforts to mitigate the spread of the SARS-CoV-2 virus, and strongly suggests that, until the concept of care is defetishised, it is unlikely that it can be rationally linked to policy. Wong's chapter (Chapter 4) provides a new perspective on the harms and exploitative processes hidden in digital platforms and algorithms, which have been more frequently used and adopted in 2020–22. Wong uses the concept of "algorithmic harm" to illustrate how biases in data and algorithmic processes adversely affect marginalised communities – a trend that was amplified due to the accelerated ubiquity of these technologies at the time of COVID-19. Finally in this first section, Lewis (Chapter 5) offers a re-examination of the very concepts of "pandemic" and "lockdown," subjecting them to the most fundamental philosophical questions of "quid" (what is it?) and "quod" (did it happen?); emerging from his analysis is the importance of a reinterpretation of the logic of immunisation as possibly inherently irrational and exclusive.

Essays in the second section of this volume offer accounts of the significance of governments' pandemic responses in the Global South, far from the locations that largely defined the global COVID-19 agenda. These essays illustrate that any assessment of the unprecedented policies adopted by governments in the Global North must include the underreported effects that those policies have had on populations in the Global South. Purohit (Chapter 6) addresses the outrage around COVID-19 mitigation measures in India, where 1.3 billion people were placed into lockdown with only four hours' notice, detailing the human cost of such a shocking government policy among the 400 million informally employed in India whose precarious existence was put immediately at extreme risk. Wanda's chapter (Chapter 7), which outlines aspects of the pandemic response in Angola, identifies the dangers of lockdown policies rolled out in highly militarised contexts. The co-opting of the issue of viral infection by other agendas is also discussed in Cevese's chapter (Chapter 8), which describes the manner in which financial restructuring and state-indebtedness in Argentina have been drastically intensified under the aegis of the emergence of COVID-19, effectively weaponising financial arrangements deemed necessary to facilitate appropriate management of the disease and reinforcing pre-existing social and economic inequalities. Adu-Gyamfi's contribution (Chapter 9) provides an account of the effects of pandemic policy in Ghana, detailing aspects of what a response tailored to the local context might have looked like and the advantages of such a response over the blanket imposition of Chinese-style measures as promoted by the Global North. The final chapter (Chapter 10) in this section, by Ortiz-Montero, details the lessons that might have been learned very early in the emergence of COVID-19 from the management and mismanagement of Ebola in countries in Africa; in this context, Ortiz-Montero's title, "One Size Does Not Fit All", succinctly captures the vital importance of taking account of highly diverse social, cultural, economic, and historical contexts when designing and implementing (public health) policy.

Essays in the third and final section of this collection present alternative lenses through which we can analyse the global response to the spread of SARS-CoV-2. Möller's contribution (Chapter 11) sets out how the paradigm of proportionality, when applied to lockdowns of entire populations, throws serious doubt on the legal and moral justifiability of much of the official COVID-19 response; in particular, this chapter points to the bias of public discourse in favour of lockdowns that resulted from the quickly established taboo on discussing the relative age of those affected or potentially affected by the disease. The pernicious effects of this taboo are also central to Nehushtan's essay (Chapter 12), which considers government public-health policies through the lens of intergenerational justice. Much was made in 2020–22 of the necessity of developing and implementing policies in spite of inevitable partial ignorance with respect to the virus and its mitigation. Nehushtan turns this potential excuse for the failures of government policy on its head by showing that reasonable application of the established philosophical device of "the veil of ignorance" could have corrected from the outset many of the most damaging errors. Baiasu's chapter (Chapter 13) employs the practical paradigm of phenomenology in its discussion of the lived experiences of those in lockdowns, so many of which were obscured by the notion of "being in this together" promoted by governments and the media. Baiasu also shows how genealogy can be used to illuminate power relations embedded from the outset in the structures of government decision-making that were devastating to many of the under-represented and disenfranchised groups in society. Ratcliffe's chapter (Chapter 14) introduces the paradigm of "potential" as a defining but almost wholly overlooked framework for understanding the nature of people's COVID-19-crisis experiences. This essay argues that due to the unprecedented life-limitations imposed by lockdowns, people lost whole swathes of potentialities that are integral to who they are and what they seek to become and which cannot, by definition, be reinstated or recaptured once freedoms are restored. Any analysis of the harms caused by government lockdowns must incorporate the life possibilities of which so many were irrevocably deprived. The final essay (Chapter 15), by Cook and Mendes-Borges, employs the framework of gender to give an account of the justifiability and effectiveness of government pandemic responses. Given that women are disproportionately represented among "key workers", as well as among precarious workers and the poor worldwide, this chapter's analysis of the gendered impact of lockdowns helps to address a significant oversight implied by the proclaimed "in this together" spirit of government policy response.

Meaningful debate can only take place with the acceptance that other parties to the debate might be right, that alternative perspectives to those that are accepted or prioritised might in the end prove more credible. Given the intellectual paralysis and the political hurry that prevailed during the first phase of COVID-19, this willingness was in abeyance. Looking forward, it is reasonable to hope that it will return. The purpose of this volume is to exemplify and encourage the willingness to debate issues that have been considered immune to critical discussion.

References

Arendt, Hannah. 1998. *The Human Condition*. Chicago and London: University of Chicago Press.

Burawoy, Michael. 2005. "For Public Sociology". *American Sociological Review* 70 (1): 4–28.

Courtois, A.D.M., and Theresa O'Keefe. 2015. "Precarity in the Ivory Cage: Neoliberalism and Casualisation of Work in the Irish Higher Education Sector". *Journal for Critical Education Policy Studies* 13 (1): 43–66.

Craig, Clare. 2021. Twitter, 13 November, 10:15 a.m., https://twitter.com/ClareCraigPath/status/1459465021596045317

Gadamer, Hans-Georg. 2003. *Truth and Method* (2nd edn.). Translated and revised by Joel Weinsheimer and Donald. G. Marshall. New York and London: Continuum.

Green, Toby. 2021. *The Covid Consensus: The New Politics of Global Inequality*. New York: Hurst & Co.

Kant, Immanuel. 1786. "What is Orientation in Thinking?" In *Kant: Political Writings* (2nd edn.). Edited by Hans Reiss. Cambridge: Cambridge University Press, 1991.

Morrissey, John. 2015. "Regimes of Performance: Practices of the Normalised Self in the Neoliberal University". *British Journal of Sociology of Education* 36 (4): 614–34.

Purcell, Trevor W. 2000. "Public Anthropology: An Idea Searching for a Reality" / *Transforming Anthropology* 9 (2).

Sen, Amartya. 1999. *Development as Freedom*. Oxford: Oxford University Press.

Sylvester, Christine. 1999. "Development Studies and Postcolonial Studies: Disparate Tales of the 'Third World'". *Third World Quarterly* 20 (4): 703–21.

SECTION 1

Key Covid Concepts Re-examined

Human efforts – experiences, decisions, policies, and laws – are perspectival in nature. This is because the concepts that capture and inform them, however familiar or fundamental, are open to interpretation. Different interpretations of these concepts can generate and justify significantly different efforts. During 2020–22, a number of abstract concepts were abroad as never before – including "life", "death", and "health" – and were far too quickly bandied about as having self-evident implications. It might be argued that a time of crisis is a time to deploy basic concepts without considering the finer points of their meaning. But a time of crisis is also a time when the definition of such concepts is likely to have immediate and profound practical effects that make their careful discussion even more vital than it usually is. It is such discussion that the chapters in this section seek to contribute towards.

DOI: 10.4324/9781003259336-2

1

THE "LOCKDOWN CONSENSUS" IN THE UK AND THE DANGERS OF PERFORMATIVE SCIENTISM

Anthony Mckeown

Introduction: The birth of the lockdown consensus

The object of discussion in this chapter is the "lockdown consensus". This consensus is unified around three essential claims. The first is that lockdowns work in achieving their aim of reducing virus transmission. The second is that lockdowns are incontestably the most ethical response to the pandemic among a range of feasible alternatives. And the third is that experts almost universally support lockdowns. These claims are addressed with reference to literature on lockdowns. However, the argument of the chapter is that "lockdown science" has a weak evidence base, is contested by many epistemic authorities, and that lockdowns have been enacted with little concern for their social costs.

The lockdown consensus pivots around the idea that "zero-Covid" responses in Australia, New Zealand, Taiwan, and Vietnam can be replicated elsewhere to mitigate or even, in some accounts, suppress virus spread (Galway, 2021). By now, however, many of the zero-Covid countries have experienced large rises in cases and deaths, and New Zealand has abandoned its own zero-Covid strategy (Frost, 2021). Prior to COVID-19, all significant pandemic-response guidance either ruled out lockdowns or did not even mention them (World Health Organisation, 2019). Given that their implementation had no prior historical precedent, the lockdown consensus "contradict[s] all previous research into the best ways to mitigate outbreaks of new infectious diseases" (Bell and Green, 2021: 21).

Pandemic planning orthodoxy, which had previously focused only on quarantining the sick, among other measures, was transformed almost overnight by what occurred in China. Professor Neil Ferguson, whose modelling formed the basis for lockdown measures, is clear that he and other influential experts initially did not think they could "get away with" implementing lockdowns in Europe (Sayers, 2020). Once Italy had done so with little resistance, though, it became an option

DOI: 10.4324/9781003259336-3

(Sayers, 2020). The decision to lockdown in the UK was made, Ferguson concedes, despite there being "an enormous cost associated with it" (Whipple, 2020). However, these costs appear never to have been factored into the UK's response, and the government has instead been monomaniacally committed to "defeating the virus" (Telegraph, 2020).

Today, despite emerging evidence of their potential inefficacy, lockdowns continue to be part of the pandemic planning calculi of states. In what follows, the ways in which lockdown arguments have been insulated from critique is the object of analysis. The chapter is structured as follows. First, the following section draws on Michel Foucault to frame the lockdown consensus as a "regime of truth". The second section deepens this analysis by arguing that pandemic response discourse is divided into spheres of "consensus, legitimate criticism, and deviance", through which non-lockdown approaches are cast as "deviant".

In section three, it is shown that the lockdown consensus is also perpetuated through the mechanism of "performative scientism", which, as outlined below, enables policymakers, scientists (including social scientists), and other pro-lockdown advocates to claim to be operating on the basis of conclusive science while marginalising those whose readings of the data differ. The final section briefly touches upon how such scientism has enabled performative moralism, manifest through journalistic and left-activist endeavours to act on an assumed moral basis to campaign for lockdowns, powered by scientism. Through these mechanisms, adherents to the consensus have been just as successful in shutting down debates on lockdowns as lockdowns have been in shutting down whole societies. The conclusion brings together these ideas and calls for a widening discourse on the UK's pandemic response.

The lockdown consensus as a regime of truth

In *Truth and Power*, Michel Foucault made the case that what is perceived as truth does not exist outside of power relations. "Truth", he argued, is not the product of the interplay of free-wielding communicative interaction but is instead produced within the context of "multiple forms of constraint". These constraints are social, cultural, political, and scientific, and together they produce emergent and historically specific understandings of "truth" in any given domain. Moreover, these truth/power relations induce "regular effects of power", making "true" particular claims about the nature of reality and suppressing other forms of thought (Foucault and Faubion, 2002: 131). According to Foucault,

> Each society has its regime of truth, its "general politics" of truth – that is, the types of discourse it accepts and makes function as true; the mechanisms and instances that enable one to distinguish true and false statements; the means by which each is sanctioned; the techniques and procedures accorded value in the acquisition of truth; the status of those who are charged with saying what counts as true.
>
> *Foucault and Faubion, 2002: 131*

In Foucault's understanding, though, knowledge does not necessarily steadily accumulate over time, "getting closer and closer to the truth", and the process of science itself is not seen as "guided by any underlying principle which remains fixed and constant while all around it changes" (McHoul, McHoul, and Grace, 2015: 4). One need not adopt the extreme epistemology often attributed to Foucault – that "truth" itself refers to little more than a play of discourses – to see that truth-claims are usually connected to wider political circuits. This position is outlined by Seamus Miller, who notes that it is "naïve and implausible" to suggest that "(a) everything is discourse; (b) that anything discursive in nature is by definition fictive or without foundation; and (c) that, therefore, everything is fictive and without foundation" (Miller, 1990: 115). Adopting this view of epistemology would result in the denial of "any independently existing reality or world", involving the dual assertions that scientific claims can never accurately correspond to the world and that "we cannot get 'outside' of discourse to gain access to anything beyond it" (Miller, 1990: 116). This approach is categorically not what is intended in this chapter.

Instead, I am making the simpler claim that truth claims are always made in political contexts, and that there is always a "process of appropriation" of scientific claims, as Foucault reminds us (Foucault, 2002: 77). This appropriation process draws our attention to the "ensemble of relations" which constitute the "non-discursive context" in which scientific claims are made (McHoul, McHoul, and Grace, 2015: 44).

There are differences of scientific opinion about whether lockdowns minimise virus transmission and ultimately reduce deaths caused by COVID-19, and yet these differences rarely make their way into public discourse. Foucault's framework can help us to ground our own thinking on what has become known as "the science" in a politically informed way. Some, for instance, argue that lockdowns have been an overwhelming success. Seth Flaxman et al. argue that the first lockdowns worldwide "had a large effect on reducing transmission", ultimately averting between 2.8 and 3 million deaths (Flaxman et al., 2020: 260). This conclusion, however, assumes that these effects were "an immediate response to [lockdown] interventions rather than gradual changes in behaviour" (Flaxman et al., 2020: 257).

As Douglas W. Allen and others suggest (Allen, 2021), pro-lockdown claims in this regard have generally been predicated on sets of questionable assumptions. Consider, for instance, the claim made by Neil Ferguson et al. in March 2020 that an "unmitigated epidemic" would have resulted in "approximately 510 000 deaths in GB and 2.2 million in the US, not accounting for the potential negative effects of health systems being overwhelmed on mortality" (Ferguson et al., 2020: 7). This claim appears to be predicated on the assumption that there would have been no "control measures or spontaneous changes in individual behaviour" by people in the UK or the US in conditions where people were told that a deadly pandemic was about to decimate their population. Ferguson et al. themselves concede that this assumption was "unlikely" to be accurate (Ferguson et al., 2020: 6). Yet this predicate has not been subject to the interrogation it arguably deserves, especially at the political level, where wider concerns about the collateral damages of lockdowns have been largely absent from policy discussion, at least in the UK.

This is all the more surprising when we read in a paper by Douglas W. Allen that several academic studies find there is "strong evidence that changes in human behavior significantly affected the progression of the virus, and that this channel was more important than mandated lockdowns for altering the number of cases, transmission rates, and deaths" (for a list of references on this, see Allen, 2021). In fact, according to Allen, up to April 2021 there were "close to twenty studies that distinguish between voluntary and mandated lockdown effects ... find[ing] that mandated lockdowns have only marginal effects and that voluntary changes in behavior explain large parts of the changes in cases, transmissions, and deaths" (Allen, 2021: 21). This appears to bring into question Ferguson et al.'s claim "that epidemic suppression [was] the only viable strategy" at the outset of the pandemic (Ferguson et al., 2020: 16).

The certainty of the lockdown scientists is made all the more remarkable by the fact that the Imperial College report acknowledges that "[t]he social and economic effects of the measures" would "be profound" (Ferguson et al., 2020: 16). From the early days of the pandemic, then, it appears with hindsight that the UK's COVID-19 response was hardening into a regime of truth that accorded some scientific claims value on questions of virus suppression, while failing to adequately take into account medical ethics animated by the commitment to first do no harm, including harms to the structure of society and culture.

Jonas Herby argues that Flaxman et al. "do not contribute to answering the central question of whether it is the governmental economic lockdown or the voluntary behavior of the citizens that is most important to the growth rate of the pandemic" (Herby, 2021: 5). It should be noted, though, that, *pace* Herby, this need not be an "either/or" question. However, the possibility of recognising the potential that lockdowns may not be as efficacious as often assumed is negated by a discursive environment in which lockdown efficacy is seen as something of an incontrovertible fact, supported by a regime of thinking that reproduces this idea. In the UK, for example, the government has consistently claimed to be "following the science", but alternative scientific claims that people's voluntary behaviour might have been key to reducing transmission appear to have been largely ignored. This is despite real-world evidence of the efficacy of more voluntaristic approaches. For example, in Sweden, where voluntary measures predominated, comparable results to the rest of Europe were achieved in the absence of a lockdown.

A study cited by Reuters on 24 March 2021, for example, found that 21 of 30 EU countries with available statistics had higher rates of excess mortality than Sweden (Ahlander, 2021), suggesting that social distancing (both voluntary and mandated) may have been more effective than is accepted in pro-lockdown science (UK Government, 2021). Lockdown advocates often point to differences in population density between countries to argue that Sweden has a low population density and therefore cannot be compared to countries such as the UK. However, according to Statista, 87.9 percent of Sweden's population lives in an urban area (Statista,

2021a), compared to 83.9 percent in the UK (Statista, 2021b). Thus, this factor's value as an explanatory variable seems to be overstated.

The problem is that science has been treated as an institution of selected experts. Alternative understandings, as is demonstrated below, have been deemed not just "wrong" but beyond the boundaries of acceptable discourse. Hence the idea that the lockdown consensus is more akin to a regime of truth than to a process of open scientific enquiry. As the philosopher Susan Haack argues, even if a body of knowledge seems to be well warranted, science by definition involves counter-arguments, even "speculative conjectures, most of which come to nothing". A flow of claims and counter-claims indicates healthy debate, and sound science is "bound to be obscured if", as Haack explains, "we use 'scientific' more or less interchangeably with 'reliable, established, solid', and so forth" (Haack, 2012: 80). Yet the lockdown consensus has rendered uncertain claims "reliable, established, and solid", being seemingly committed to defending lockdowns at all costs.

The lockdown consensus's internal regime of power and the spheres of consensus, controversy, and deviance

A framework for understanding how this "internal regime of power" works in practice can be further concretised by drawing on the work of Daniel C. Hallin, professor of communication at the University of California, San Diego (Hallin, 1989). Hallin is not utilising a Foucauldian framework and does not use the term "regime of truth", but his understanding of how inconvenient ideas are censored in media representations of the world is instructive and can be rendered, for the purposes of the present argument, consistent with the elements of Foucault being drawn on in this chapter. Hallin argues that media representations of reality are divided into "spheres" of consensus, controversy, and deviance (Hallin, 1989: 116–118). As he explains, the sphere of consensus "encompasses those social objects not regarded by…journalists and most of…society as controversial. Within this region journalists do not feel compelled either to present opposing views or to remain disinterested observers" (Hallin, 1989: 116–17). Instead, "the journalist's role is to serve as an advocate or celebrant of consensus values" (Hallin, 1989: 117), and this has certainly been a feature of how the lockdown consensus has been represented in the UK media.

Journalists working in major established news outlets (the BBC, AFP, *Financial Times*, and "big-tech" companies) have worked as part of the Trusted News Initiative (TNI) to censor what they regard as "disinformation". In this role, the aforementioned news outlets are "trusted brands" (Newman, 2021), and all have taken a consistent line on the "truth" of the pandemic response. As AFP puts it, through the TNI, "alerts…flag up content that undermines trust in partner news providers by identifying imposter content which claims to come from trusted brand identities or sources" (AFP, 2020). Exactly what constitutes "imposter content", though, should be subject to wide debate rather than left to the singular collective agency of a media oligopoly. This oligopoly broadly adopts, in the UK, the general position of the government-linked Scientific Advisory Group for Emergencies (SAGE) (SAGE, 2021), thus helping to generate the discursive bedrock for lockdown's "sphere of consensus".

In Hallin's model there is also a "sphere of legitimate controversy". This relates to claims that are deemed to be "legitimate" by "major established actors" (Hallin, 1989: 116), where the latter are understood in the present context to refer to actors including the World Health Organisation, the World Economic Forum, the state managers of national governments, and assorted mainstream international organisations such as the United Nations (UN). With respect to the sphere of legitimate controversy in the UK, Independent SAGE, who advocate a zero-Covid strategy that aims to "suppress" or near "eliminate" the virus (Independent SAGE, 2021), occupy this sphere of legitimate controversy. They are highly critical of government claims (and of SAGE), but while they differ in terms of thinking on pandemic management, they have never systematically interrogated the idea that lockdowns are the most effective form of pandemic management. They have regularly appeared in UK media advocating a zero-Covid approach, but non-lockdown approaches are seen as beyond the pale. The zero-Covid approach has also enjoyed support from the British left, which has tended to frame it as the left-wing alternative to the UK government's approach, widely derided, erroneously, as a "herd immunity" strategy.[1] For example, the Zero Covid Campaign in the UK was heavily supported by British trade unions (Zero Covid Campaign, 2020).

Outside the spheres of consensus and legitimate controversy lie those scientists occupying the sphere of deviance. Reframing Hallin, scientists occupying this sphere are "reject[ed] as unworthy of being heard" (Hallin, 1989: 117). The authors of the "Great Barrington Declaration" (GBD), for example, rejected the idea of blanket lockdowns and instead advocated a more differentiated "focused protection" strategy aimed at "minimiz[ing] overall mortality from both COVID-19 and other diseases by balancing the need to protect high-risk individuals from COVID-19 while reducing the harm that lockdowns have had on other aspects of medical care and public health" (Kulldorff, Sunetra, and Bhattacharya, 2020). Scientists occupying this sphere – such as Martin Kulldorff, Jay Bhattacharya, and Sunetra Gupta – have been largely excluded from mainstream pandemic debates. In the following section, I outline, in brief, how the lockdown consensus is maintained, focusing on how it has served to marginalise those lying within the sphere of deviance in a way which props up the lockdown regime of truth.

Performative scientism as a disciplinary apparatus for the lockdown consensus' regime of truth

A basic definition of scientism is "a belief that science, especially natural science, is much the most valuable part of human learning…because it is…the most authoritative, or serious, or beneficial" mode of enquiring about the world (Sorell, 2013: 1). The concept is complex, and a discussion of these complexities is beyond the scope of this chapter. Suffice it to say, though, that the basic idea is that scientism involves an unquestioned belief that science alone has the answers to complex problems. The aim in this section is to elaborate on the claim that the lockdown consensus is performatively scientistic, a concept which, as used here, denotes two sets of phenomena. The first is that political decision makers have sought credibility for the lockdown approach "by performing excessive deference to what they believe to be 'science'" (Muller, 2021: 139), or at least what they present to the public as what they believe to be "the science". The second claim is that pro-lockdown scientists themselves engage in performative scientism by utilising unscientific techniques to marginalise those arguing against lockdowns.

The "performative" aspect of the concept refers to the idea that claims to be "following the science" grant policymakers, scientists, and other adherents to the consensus the power to (re-)produce and regulate pandemic discourse while marginalising those in the sphere of deviance (Butler, 2011: 3). In what follows, I will address two mechanisms that contribute to the regime's performative scientism. The first is the drawing of a false demarcation between "science" and "pseudoscience", and the second is the privileging of epidemiology over other disciplines and forms of knowledge, which leads to an excessive focus on the precautionary principle at the expense of any engagement with the proportionality principle. The two mechanisms are addressed in turn.

Mechanism I: Drawing a false line of demarcation between "science" and "pseudoscience"

Pro-lockdown scientists have contributed to lockdowns as an internally consistent regime of truth by helping to generate a false demarcation between "science", framed as the certainty that lockdowns have worked, and "pseudoscience", attributed to those scientists, including social scientists and humanities scholars, who beg to differ. For example, some lockdown-consensus scientists openly called for scientists dissenting from the lockdown consensus to be "deplatformed" by the social media oligopoly (Gurdasani, 2020). Not only does this false demarcation between science and pseudoscience shield "consensus" scientists from scrutiny (Muller, 2021: 1), it also limits the capacity of science as a whole to "encourage good, honest, thorough work, and [to] discourage cheating" (Haack, 2012: 88–89). As Sunetra Gupta, a scientist who has been subject to ridicule from those working within the lockdown consensus, argues, deriding dissenting scientists as "fringe" and "dangerous" (that is, in Hallin's framework, "deviant") is "ridiculous" because it implies "that only mainstream science matters". If this was true, Gupta points out, science itself would "stagnate". Moreover, the use of emotionally charged, inflammatory terms like "pseudoscientist" is a "toxic" form of decidedly *unscientific* discourse (Gupta, 2020). The fact is that the GDB, whatever its (de)merits, was authored by credible scholars in their respective fields. Consequently, this kind of dogmatic labelling uses science honorifically because it dismisses out of hand non-orthodox scientific claims on COVID-19 (on the honorific use of the word "science", see Haack, 2012: 78–80).

This dimension of performative scientism is insidious because it also involves scientists using their influence to create and propagate smear tactics. For example, leaked emails from the pro-lockdown, zero-Covid group the Independent Scientific Advisory Group in Ireland (ISAG) purport to show how some of its members have recommended "go[ing] after people and not institutions because 'people hurt faster than institutions'" (McConnell, 2021). This argument is straight from the playbook of Saul Alinsky's *Rules for Radicals*, and has little to do with scientific discourse (Alinsky, 1989). Instead, it functions as a means of silencing those who hold different scientific views on the pandemic. In other words, it helps to render some scientific views irredeemably "deviant", but without going to the trouble of engaging their ideas in the spirit of open enquiry.

Furthermore, leaked emails purportedly show that Susan Michie, a behavioural psychologist working for both SAGE and Independent SAGE in the UK, and Dr Michael Head, a research fellow in global health at the University of Southampton, worked covertly to smear dissenting scientists as "anti-vaxxers" (Maddox, 2021). The scientists being attacked include Carl Heneghan, the director of Oxford University's Centre for Evidence-Based Medicine. As one of the smeared scientists, professor Peter C. Gøtzsche, points out (cited in Maddox, 2021), this kind of behaviour is more akin to "religious dogma" than to, as Hayek astutely put it, "the general spirit of disinterested inquiry" that informs science understood philosophically as the pursuit of truth outside of political influence (Hayek, quoted in Haack, 2012: 86). It is, instead, science overtly politicised.

Mechanism II: An excessive focus on the precautionary principle at the expense of any engagement with the proportionality principle

The lockdown regime of truth has functioned in part by insisting on a one-sided reliance on the precautionary principle at the expense of considering the proportionality principle.[2] As defined by Martin Blank and Reba Goodman, the precautionary principle denotes "a proactive policy for regulatory agencies when information about risk is inconclusive, but where there is a reasonable possibility that the public may be harmed if no action is taken" (Blank and Goodman, 2007: 242). This principle was the dominant logic underpinning lockdowns in March 2020, premised on the WHO's initial prediction that COVID-19 had an infection fatality rate (IFR) of 3.4 percent (Adhanom, 2020). In this situation, it made sense, as Silvia Camporesi, associate professor in bioethics at King's College London argues, to be "better safe than sorry" (Camporesi, 2020). Even here, though, one would have assumed that some attempt would have been made to balance the costs and benefits of lockdowns, no matter the uncertainties involved in doing so. There was no balancing, at least in the UK (Green, 2021).

What is odd, though, is that while uncertainties over the IFR were subsequently reduced as more became known about the disease, the principle of precaution has remained dominant. This continued primacy is even more surprising when it is now known that the age stratification of COVID-19 fatalities differs more than one-thousand-fold between the young and the old. The more general problem, as John Ioannidis points out, is that whole-of-society lockdowns make no distinction between different social groups, with the result that lockdowns unrealistically distribute risks equally between teenagers (who are at very little risk to the disease) and the elderly and the clinically vulnerable (who are at much higher risk) (Ioannidis, cited in Neil, 2020).

Under these conditions, blanket lockdowns are "neither scientific nor safe", Ioannidis argues, because they scatter scarce resources inequitably, reducing resource-generating economic activity while failing to protect the truly vulnerable (cited in Neil, 2020). Therefore, an effort is needed to balance epidemiological concerns and public health measures against the negative consequences of lockdowns (Muller, 2021: 139). Such an approach requires a clear-sighted consideration of the longer-term impacts of precautionary measures, not just on mortality and morbidity but also on the health and well-being of societies as a whole (Wise, 2020). By necessity, then, the social costs of lockdowns must be part of any reasoned calculation regarding pandemic responses. Yet the lockdown regime of truth, by pushing ideas regarding proportionality out into the sphere of deviance, negates such efforts.

A shift toward a more proportionate response would attempt to deal with a broader set of factors than is possible under precaution's guiding logic. Drawing on Göran Hermerén (2012), four conditions would enter into COVID-19 discourse if proportionality were adequately considered. First, the intended goal of reducing COVID-19 transmission would be recognised as necessary, but the efficacy of lockdowns would be addressed by drawing on a broader range of epistemic authorities to develop a more rounded understanding of the disease's real risks (Hermerén, 2012: 374–375). Second, lockdowns would be more seriously assessed with respect to the question of whether they "bring about" or "help to bring about" the intended effects of reduced virus transmission (Hermerén, 2012: 375), rather than this being a position asserted by some scientists and subsequently reproduced within a regime of truth that serves to render other scientific authorities "deviant".

Opening up the field of enquiry beyond experts within the lockdown regime of truth is more consistent with a communitarian approach to pandemic management because, as Henry Tam argues, one principle of communitarianism is co-operative enquiry. This principle states that any truth claim "may be judged to be valid only if informed participants deliberating together under conditions of co-operative enquiry would accept that claim" (Tam, 1998: 13). No individual or group can "legitimately declare any claim to be indisputably true" when working in accordance with this principle (Tam, 1998: 13). Unfortunately, though, the tendency within the lockdown regime of truth has been to draw on highly selective groups of experts and to ignore all others. Whether lockdowns are effective is a judgement that can only be arrived at via "open communication between people engaged in a common enquiry", with any "provisional consensus" necessarily open to revision through open and honest enquiry (Tam, 1998: 13). The spirit of open and honest enquiry has, though, been dealt a blow since March 2020. Lockdown-consensus scientists have been bolstered by media giants who have, as Pankaj Mehta, associate professor of physics at Boston University, puts it, "engaged in multiple acts of censorship against scientists holding a range of views on COVID-19 and the public health response to it" (Mehta, 2021).

Ultimately, any claim to the truth of lockdowns rests not with scientists discursively insulated from competing truth claims but within a more critical set of "deliberations of ever-expanding circles of co-operative enquirers" (Tam, 1998: 13). The lockdown regime of truth negates this principle because it entails a top-down technocratic approach. Moreover, the negation of co-operative enquiry automatically undermines two other fundamental principles of genuine communitarianism, namely, mutual responsibility, which "requires all members of any community to take responsibility for enabling each other to pursue common values" (Tam, 1998: 14), and citizen participation, which "requires that all those affected by any given power structure are able to participate as equal citizens in determining how the power in question is to be exercised" (Tam, 1998: 16–17).

Martin Kulldorff, a professor at Harvard Medical School and Katherine Yih, a biologist and epidemiologist at Harvard University who "is also a long-time activist in farm labor and anti-imperialist struggles" (Yih, 2020), make the case that a sustainable communitarian approach is one which minimises harms to the vulnerable while also recognising the "harm[s] caused by crude across-the-board lockdowns and their disproportionate impact on workers and people of color" (Yih and Kulldorff, 2020). As they argue, "The pandemic has laid bare the glaring and growing inequalities in our societ[ies]" (Yih and Kulldorff, 2020), and these must be addressed. However, this is not the same as campaigning for lockdowns that have drastically increased inequality and ramped up poverty, especially in the developing world.[3] In short, the discursive regime upholding "lockdown truth" has tended to use the language of community while systematically denying the possibility of a genuinely communitarian response.

Third, under the guiding logic of proportionality, the option chosen to tackle the pandemic must be arrived at through genuinely wide-ranging discourse, in the manner outlined above. Whatever option chosen would be the agreed-upon *most favourable option* to reduce transmission, a position arrived at through a genuine consensus that there are "no less controversial or risky means to achieve the goal" (Hermerén, 2012: 374–375). This condition demands open debate, not just among scientists but among broader groups of people affected by lockdowns. As with the second condition of proportionality, it would by necessity require the use of genuinely public reason, freed from the tyranny of designated experts. Considerations beyond transmission must be addressed, including the political, cultural, and economic fallout of different means-end packages. This condition also has an inescapable temporal dimension because lockdowns generate consequences far beyond their immediate effects. Hermerén puts this kind of issue schematically in the following way:

> Sometimes temporal aspects can be essential in discussing applications of the principle of proportionality. In general terms, first only method M_1 is

believed to bring about the intended goal X [in the present context, imposing lockdowns to reduce transmission], or make X possible. Then it becomes clear that this is not so, since also method M_2 appears as a possible – and less controversial – method to bring about X [this might be, for example, social distancing without lockdowns, as in Sweden]. Finally the picture may change due to discoveries of new problems with M_2. Both M_1 and M_2 may lead to X, but under different conditions, each raising partly separate problems. A further possible complication is this: suppose that M_1 and M_2 both lead to X. So does the combination of M_1 and M_2. However, it is later discovered that M_1 and M_2 combined will lead to X more quickly but with bigger risks.

Hermerén, 2012: 375

These are, of course, complex issues, and they require reasoning of a type that cannot be achieved under the precautionary principle, let alone through the performative scientism of lockdown dogma or the misplaced moralism of those representing "the science" in crudely one-sided ways. Again, this points to the need to enable a more communitarian approach to discourse on pandemic management to emerge, moving away from the lockdown regime of truth towards something more intellectually and practically democratic.

The fourth condition of proportionality states that the agreed-upon policy for addressing any future waves of COVID-19 "should not be excessive in relation to the intended goal" (Hermerén, 2012: 377). Experts alone cannot decide which values to privilege in a pandemic response strategy. As Haack points out, while medical science might be able to tell us "at what stage a fetus becomes viable", it cannot "tell us whether abortion is morally acceptable (nor, of course, whether it should be legally permitted)" (Haack, 2012: 90). Likewise, while epidemiologists and virologists can inform us about virus transmission dynamics (albeit with little evident certainty), they are not qualified, any more than the layman, to tell us whether their control recommendations are suitable candidates for being made policy. Expert knowledge can provide information about the relations between means and ends but it cannot determine what means or ends are desirable (Haack, 2012: 90). To claim otherwise is to subscribe to technocracy, or "rule by experts".

Hannah Arendt long ago warned of the dangers of according too much power to experts, who, convinced of their own mastery, can end up incorrectly "unify[ing] the most disparate phenomena with which reality present[s] them" (Arendt, 1972). While Arendt was writing about experts related to US defence policy, those studying natural phenomena are also prone to problems of overconfidence. In a paper titled "Forecasting for Covid has Failed", John Ioannidis, Sally Cripps, and Martin A. Tanner refer to "groupthink and bandwagon effects" among groups of scientists. As they put it, the danger is that

models can be tuned to get desirable results and predictions; e.g. by changing the input of what are deemed to be plausible values for key variables. This is especially true for models that depend on theory and speculation, but even data-driven forecasting can do the same, depending on how the modeling is performed. In the presence of strong groupthink and bandwagon effects, modelers may consciously fit their predictions to what is the dominant thinking and expectations – or they may be forced to do so.

Ioannidis, Cripps, and Tanner, 2020: 6

There have been many occasions in which this kind of problem has been evidenced in the UK's response to COVID-19. One example is when, in September 2020, Chris Whitty and Sir Patrick Vallance claimed that "coronavirus cases could reach 50,000 a day by mid-October if the numbers double every seven days, with deaths growing past 200 a day" (BBC, 2020). The claim was made on outdated information. Carl Heneghan, professor of evidence-based medicine at the University of Oxford, then pointed out that the "job [of] scientists is to reflect [on] the evidence and the uncertainties and to provide the latest estimates", not to present the worst possible scenario as if it is the likeliest one (Donnelly, 2020). Ultimately, the one-sidedness of the UK's COVID-19 response highlights the dangers of according too much deference to some scientists at the expense of others.

Performative moralism as an unwanted product of performative scientism

Performative scientism has enabled performative moralism in COVID-19 discourse, since the latter is predicated on the assumption that lockdown-consensus views are firmly rooted in "the science". Thus, we see the assertion that "every disaster movie starts with the government ignoring a scientist". Even the astrophysicist Neil deGrasse Tyson has tweeted it (deGrasse Tyson, 2020): "You know it's true…. Every disaster movie begins with a scientist being ignored."

This claim glibly ignores the fact that many disasters are directly associated with deference to expert authority. Two significant examples from history include the emergence of Nazism, as outlined so evocatively by Zygmunt Bauman in *Modernity and the Holocaust* (Bauman, 2000), and Lysenkoism, an approach to agriculture in the Soviet Union in the middle of the twentieth century that demanded "either censure or faith in agrobiology" (Joravsky, 2005: 1321). As David Joravsky puts it, Lysenkoism "defie[d] efforts to disentangle claims of scientific knowledge from assertions of practical authority and from the use of state power to achieve progress" (Joravsky, 2005: 1321). Both examples resulted in atrocities. We should be mindful of these historical references today, as the lockdown regime of truth's deference to some scientists and the silencing of others serves to transform "science" into a set of institutional demands rather than a mode of open enquiry. This should not be mistaken as a claim that the COVID-19 response is the same as historical atrocities in qualitative terms; this indeed would be absurd. The point is that scientific discourse is not neutral, not infallible, and never should be referred to as if it alone has the answers to any given problem.

Rule by experts, as the radical philosopher Paul Feyerabend famously argued, is undesirable. In *Knowledge, Science, and Relativism*, he argued that experts "are excellent, useful, irreplaceable, but mostly nasty, competitive, ungenerous slaves, slaves both in mentality, speech, and in social position" (Feyerabend, 1999: 118). While this might be ungenerous as a universal proposition, it does describe some of the central dynamics of the lockdown consensus. The scientific experts in SAGE and Independent SAGE have combined with the cultural experts in politics and the media to perform a regime of truth that negates efforts to subject the UK's pandemic response to vigorous questioning. Prominent UK left-wing journalist Paul Mason, for example, confidently asserts that

> the first lockdown worked, despite its late imposition, because schools and colleges were closed. The second lockdown in November [of 2020], during which schools and colleges remained open, managed only to stabilise the death rate. The outcome of the third lockdown depends on compliance, which the lockdown sceptics are helping to undermine with their arguments.
>
> *Mason, 2021*

Sonia Sodha, writing in the *Guardian*, goes as far as to claim that world-renowned scientists such as Sunetra Gupta and Carl Heneghan, both of whom hold prominent positions at the University of Oxford, are part of a "disinformation ecosystem". They are, she claims, engaged in "magical thinking", which is "len[ding] a sheen of legitimacy to those who wish to corrupt the legitimate debate about social restrictions with the assertion that they are not needed" (Sodha, 2020). Ash Sarkar, a self-proclaimed communist radical, has openly called for the deplatforming of scientists such as Carl Heneghan and Sunetra Gupta (Sarkar, 2021). In short, these are dangerous times, with performative moralism also shading into smear tactics.

Utilising Feyerabend once more, we might say that "the peculiar situation in which we find ourselves today is that these…slavish minds have convinced almost everyone that they have the knowledge and the insight not only to run their own playpens, *but [also] large parts of society as well*" (Feyerabend, 1999: 118, emphasis in original). Ultimately, as Susan Haack reminds us, there is a fine line between legitimate respect for science and illegitimate deference to it (Haack, 2012: 93). As the philosopher of science Karl Popper insisted, science is "always fallible, subject to error", and all must be humbly "aware of the severe limitations of all our contributions". Moreover, "science and rationality", Popper continues, "have really very little to do with specialization and the appeal to expert authority" (Popper, 1994: iv). Left-wing critics need to be reminded that their job is to interrogate scientific claims, not to render invisible "marginalized view[s] that violate the acceptable mainstream orthodoxy" (Parenti, 1999: 12). It is to be hoped that scientists, politicians, and media personalities heed these lessons and act with more prudence whenever panic sets in again. Only time will tell if these lessons will be recognised, let alone heeded.

Conclusion

In this chapter, I have argued that the lockdown consensus on how to address the COVID-19 pandemic rests on shaky grounds. First, the consensus itself can be understood as a regime of truth that discursively limits the boundaries of acceptable scientific thought, such that in the UK the only "legitimate" form of criticism of the government's approach is one which calls for earlier and harder lockdowns (for example, zero Covid). Scientists who stray beyond the boundaries of "acceptable" thought – such as Sunetra Gupta and Carl Heneghan – are cast as deviants whose views lie outside the lockdown status quo's sphere of consensus and legitimate controversy. Uncertain science has become a closed circuit, a regime of truth, and this has permeated the cultural sphere, with chilling effects on the relation between science and society.

Second, this approach to tackling the pandemic is perpetuated via performative scientism, which functions to discipline those outside the boundaries of "acceptable" criticism of the government's approach to tackling the pandemic. Performative scientism in the case of COVID-19 has systematically ignored proportionality in favour of a precautionary approach which is itself of dubious efficacy. The result is that in the UK, as in many other parts of the world, thinking on how to tackle pandemics has become constrained by a new orthodoxy that is impervious to critique. Not only does this not bode well for science and its role in society, it also does a disservice to populations who together must find a way of dealing with a disease that either is or will become endemic.

Third, emergent from such scientism is performative moralism, a disciplinary mechanism that functions to shut down ideas outside the spheres of consensus and heavily constrained "legitimate criticism". By underpinning their representations of the pandemic response with the claim that they are "rooted in science", journalists and even those on the radical left of politics objectively contribute to the lockdown regime of truth. Ultimately, if the UK is going to move beyond lockdowns as the primary means of disease control when winter next arrives, the lockdown consensus's internal regime of power must give way to more expansive forms of scientific and public reasoning.

Notes

1 As pointed out in a FAQ on the "Great Barrington Declaration", "All strategies lead to herd immunity, making it nonsensical to denote one specific approach as a herd immunity strategy just as it does not make sense for airplane pilots to talk about a 'gravity strategy' for safely landing a plane" (Bhattacharya, Gupta, and Kullforff, 2020).

2 Here we will put aside the contention that the lockdown strategy itself arguably violates the principle of precaution by ignoring decades of pandemic planning in order to implement a relatively unique strategy the harms of which were unknown but predicted to be "profound" (Ferguson et al., 2020: 16).

3 For an overview of this issue, see Green (2021) pp. 129–168.

References

Adhanom, Tedros. 2020. "WHO Director-General's opening remarks at the media briefing on COVID-19 - 3 March 2020'. *World Health Organisation*, 3 March. www.who.int/direc tor-general/speeches/detail/who-director-general-s-opening-remarks-at-the-media-briefing-on-covid-19---3-march-2020

AFP. 2020. "AFP joins Trusted News Initiative plans to tackle harmful Coronavirus disinformation". *AFP*, 27 March, www.afp.com/en/inside-afp/afp-joins-trusted-news-initiat ive-plans-tackle-harmful-coronavirus-disinformation

Ahlander, Johan. 2021. "Sweden saw lower 2020 death spike than much of Europe – data". *Reuters*, 24 March, www.reuters.com/business/healthcare-pharmaceuticals/sweden-saw-lower-2020-death-spike-than-much-europe-data-2021-03-24/

Alinsky, Saul David. 1989. *Rules for Radicals: A practical primer for realistic radicals.* New York: Vintage.

Allen, Douglas W. 2021. "Covid Lockdown Cost/Benefits: A Critical Assessment of the Literature". *International Journal of the Economics of Business* 22 (1): 1–32.

Arendt, Hannah. 1972. "Washington's problem-solvers: Where they went wrong". *New York Times*, 5 April.

Bauman, Zygmunt. 2000. *Modernity and the Holocaust.* Cambridge: Polity Press.

BBC. 2020. "COVID-19: UK could face 50,000 cases a day by October without action – Vallance". *BBC*, 1 September. www.bbc.co.uk/news/uk-54234084

Bell, David, and Toby Green. 2021. "The World Health Organization and COVID-19: Re-establishing Colonialism in Public Health". *Pandata*, 5 July. www.pandata.org/who-and-covid-19-re-establishing-colonialism-in-public-health/

Bhattacharya, Jayanti, Sunetra Gupta, and Martin Kullforff. 2020. "Frequently asked questions: lockdowns and collateral damage". *Great Barrington Declaration.* https://gbdecl aration.org/frequently-asked-questions/

Blank, Martin, and Reba Goodman. 2007. "BEMS, WHO, and the Precautionary Principle". *Bioelectromagnetics* 28: 242.

Butler, Judith. 2011. *Bodies That Matter: On the discursive limits of sex.* New York and London: Routledge.

Camporesi, Silvia. 2020. "It didn't have to be this way". *Aeon*, 27 April. https://aeon.co/ess ays/a-bioethicist-on-the-hidden-costs-of-lockdown-in-italy

deGrasse Tyson, Neil. 2020. Twitter, 25 April, 3:05 p.m.: https://twitter.com/neiltyson/sta tus/1254048358366416896?lang=en.

Donnelly, Laura. 2020. "Death scenarios used to justify second lockdown 'could be four times too high'". *Telegraph*, 1 November, www.telegraph.co.uk/news/2020/11/01/death-scenarios-used-government-justify-second-national-lockdown/

Ferguson, Neil M., Daniel Laydon, Gemma Nedjati-Gilani, Natsuko Imai, Kylie Ainslie, Marc Baguelin, Sangeeta Bhatia, Adhiratha Boonyasiri, Zulma Cucunubá, and Gina Cuomo-Dannenburg. 2020. "Impact of non-pharmaceutical interventions (NPIs) to reduce COVID-19 mortality and healthcare demand". Imperial College COVID-19 Response Team', *Imperial College COVID-19 Response Team.* www.imperial.ac.uk/mrc-global-infectious-disease-analysis/covid-19/report-9-impact-of-npis-on-covid-19/

Feyerabend, Paul K. 1999. *Knowledge, Science and Relativism.* New York: Cambridge University Press.

Flaxman, Seth, Swapnil Mishra, Axel Gandy, H, Juliette T, Unwin, Thomas A. Mellan, Helen Coupland, Charles Whittaker, Harrison Zhu, Tresnia Berah, and Jeffrey W. Eaton. 2020. "Estimating the effects of non-pharmaceutical interventions on COVID-19 in Europe". *Nature* 584: 257–261.

Foucault, Michel. 2002. "The Archaeology of Knowledge: Routledge Classics". London and New York: Routledge.

Foucault, Michel, and James D. Faubion. 2002. *The Essential Works of Foucault 1954– 1984: Power*. New York: The New Press..

Frost, Natasha. 2021. "Battling Delta, New Zealand Abandons Its Zero-Covid Ambitions". *New York Times*, 4 October, www.nytimes.com/2021/10/04/world/australia/new-zeal and-covid-zero.html

Galway, Ciarán. 2021. "Gabriel Scally: Get it down. Keep it down. Keep it out". *Agenda NI*, March. www.agendani.com/gabriel-scally-get-it-down-keep-it-down-keep-it-out/

Green, Toby. 2021. *The Covid Consensus: The new politics of global inequality*. London: Hurst and Company.

Gupta, Sunetra. 2020. "A contagion of hatred and hysteria: Oxford epidemiologist Professor Sunetra Gupta tells how she has been intimidated and shamed for backing shielding instead of lockdown". *Daily Mail*, 30 October, www.dailymail.co.uk/debate/article-8899 277/Professor-Sunetra-Gupta-reveals-crisis-ruthlessly-weaponised.html

Gurdasani, Deepti. 2020. Twitter, 6 October, 7:49 p.m.: https://twitter.com/dgurdasani1/sta tus/1313552043806687232

Haack, Susan. 2012. "Six signs of scientism". *Logos & Episteme*, 3: 75–95.

Hallin, Daniel C. 1989. *The Uncensored War: The Media and Vietnam*, London and New York: Oxford University Press.

Herby, Jonas. 2021. "A first literature review: Lockdowns only had a small effect on COVID-19". https://europepmc.org/article/ppr/ppr274020. doi: 10.2139/ssrn.3764553

Hermerén, Göran. 2012. "The principle of proportionality revisited: interpretations and applications". *Medicine, Health Care and Philosophy* 15: 373–382.

Independent SAGE. 2021. "Independent SAGE website". *Independent SAGE*, www.independ entsage.org/

Ioannidis, John P.A., Sally Cripps, and Martin A. Tanner. 2020. "Forecasting for COVID-19 has failed". *International Journal of Forecasting*, 38(2): 423–438.

Joravsky, David. 2005. "Lysenkoism". In *New Dictionary of the History of Ideas*, edited by Maryanne Cline Horowitz. New York: Charles Scribner's Sons.

Kulldorff, Martin, Sunetra Gupta, and Jayanti Bhattacharya. 2020. "Focused protection". *Great Barrington Declaration*, 25 November, https://gbdeclaration.org/focused-protection/

Maddox, David. 2021. "Pro-mask and lockdown government advisor sent email which 'smeared' fellow scientists". *Express*, 12 July, www.express.co.uk/news/politics/ 1461706/Independent-Sage-email-scientists-advisors-government-boris-john son-covid-anti-vax

Mason, Paul. 2021. "The Covid deniers have been humiliated but they are still dangerous". *New Statesman*, 6 January, www.newstatesman.com/politics/2021/01/covid-deniers- have-been-humiliated-they-are-still-dangerous

McConnell, Daniel. 2021. "Zero-Covid group rejects accusations of scaremongering". *Irish Examiner*, 12 March, www.irishexaminer.com/news/politics/arid-40243364.html

McHoul, Alec, and Wendy Grace. 2015. A Foucault Primer: Discourse, power and the subject. London and New York: Routledge.

Mehta, Pankaj. 2021. "Big Tech's Censors Come for Science". Jacobin, 7 May. https://jacobin mag.com/2021/05/big-tech-censorship-science-covid-19-debate

Miller, Seumas. 1990. "Foucault on discourse and power". *Theoria: A Journal of Social and Political Theory* 76: 115–125.

Muller, Seán M. 2021. "The dangers of performative scientism as the alternative to anti-scientific policymaking: A critical, preliminary assessment of South Africa's COVID-19 response and its consequences". *World Development* 140: 105290.

Neil, Floyd. 2020. "A Conversation with John Ioannidis". *Floyd Neill Techno* [blog], 9 July,. https://floydneilltechnoblog.wordpress.com/2020/07/09/a-conversation-with-john-ioannidis/

Newman, Nic. 2021. "COVID-19 is prompting more people to head to trusted mainstream news sites for information – new research". *The Conversation*, 13 July, https://theconversation.com/covid-19-is-prompting-more-people-to-head-to-trusted-mainstream-news-sites-for-information-new-research-164278

Parenti, Michael. 1999. *History as Mystery.* San Francicso: City Lights Books.

Popper, Karl R. 1994. *The Myth of the Framework.* London and New York: Routledge.

SAGE. 2021. "Scientific Advisory Group for Emergencies (SAGE)". *Gov.uk*, www.gov.uk/government/organisations/scientific-advisory-group-for-emergencies

Sarkar, Ash. 2021. Twitter. https://twitter.com/citizenjournos_/status/1419112047204347904?fbclid=IwAR23Sb5pENm1oDvgFVBGqNCInRb-yeM-JwSQ8OPNqby4iuzuRGvW4aBkXEg. Accessed 25 July 2021.

Sayers, Freddie. 2020. "Neil Ferguson interview: China changed what was possible". *Unherd*, 26 December, https://unherd.com/thepost/neil-ferguson-interview-china-changed-what-was-possible/

Sodha, Sonia. 2020. "We need scientists to quiz Covid consensus, not act as agents of disinformation". *The Guardian*, 22 November.

Sorell, Tom. 2013. *Scientism: Philosophy and the infatuation with science.* London and New York: Routledge.

Statista. 2021a. "Sweden: Urbanization from 2010 to 2020". *Statista*, December, www.statista.com/statistics/455935/urbanization-in-sweden/

Statista. 2021b. "United Kingdom: Degree of urbanization from 2010 to 2020", *Statista*, December, www.statista.com/statistics/270369/urbanization-in-the-united-kingdom/#:~:text=The%20degree%20of%20urbanization%20in,to%2083.4%20percent%20in%202018

Tam, Henry. 1998. *Communitarianism: A new agenda for politics and citizenship.* London: Macmillan.

Telegraph. 2020. "Boris Johnson claims nation will 'defeat' coronavirus by spring 2021". *The Telegraph.*

UK Government. 2021. "Living safely with respiratory infections, including COVID-19". *UK.gov*, 1 April, www.gov.uk/guidance/covid-19-coronavirus-restrictions-what-you-can-and-cannot-do

Whipple, Tom. 2020. "Professor Neil Ferguson: People don't agree with lockdown and try to undermine the scientists". *The Times*, 25 December, www.thetimes.co.uk/article/people-don-t-agree-with-lockdown-and-try-to-undermine-the-scientists-gnms7mp98

Wise, Jacqui. 2020. "COVID-19: Experts divide into two camps of action—shielding versus blanket policies". *BMJ* 370:3702.

World Health Organisation. 2019. "Non-pharmaceutical public health measures for mitigating the risk and impact of epidemic and pandemic influenza: annex: report of systematic literature reviews", *World Health Organisation*, https://apps.who.int/iris/handle/10665/329439

Yih, Katerhine. 2020. "Katherine Yih". *Jacobin*, https://jacobinmag.com/author/katherine-yih

Yih, Katerhine, and Martin Kulldorff. 2020. "We Need a Radically Different Approach to the Pandemic and Our Economy as a Whole", *Jacobin*, 10 September, https://jacobinmag.com/2020/09/covid-19-pandemic-economy-us-response-inequality

Zero Covid Campaign. 2020. "Zero Covid Campaign: Affiliated organisations". *Zero Covid Campaign*, https://zerocovid.uk/affiliated-organisations/

2

STOPPING THE SPREAD OF HEALTH

Sinéad Murphy

In March 2020, the UK government undertook the extraordinary task of stopping the spread of a respiratory virus in its population of 67 million. In accordance with policies being implemented by governments around the world, restrictions were introduced on the social, personal, political, cultural, and economic lives of people of such severity and on such a scale as had never before been applied – leaving home, staging a protest, attending worship, buying "inessential" items, holding the hand of one's own mother: all outlawed by emergency legislation that neutralised the most fundamental liberties.

Did it work? Evidence suggests otherwise. There is no pattern discernable between the mortality attributed by individual states to infection by the SARS-CoV-2 virus and the extent of non-pharmaceutical intervention by their governments.[1] It may be, as pathologist Dr. Clare Craig has repeatedly stated, that stopping the spread of a respiratory virus is nothing short of an illusion.[2]

But there is a sad irony about governments' great chase after this illusion: notwithstanding the fact that efforts to stop the spread of the SARS-CoV-2 virus were made under the banner of protecting people's health – "Protect the NHS" has was the UK slogan of all slogans during 2020 and 2021 – what these efforts have achieved above all is the devastation of people's health and health prospects.

This is certainly due to what is beginning to be acknowledged by governments and the corporate media: the sudden cessation of diagnostic and treatment programmes for cancer, heart disease, diabetes, and mental illness of all kinds. But it is also due to something that is as yet rarely mentioned: that health as a possibility for individuals in society relies upon precisely the channels of contact and communication that were closed by governments' virus-related interventions; blocking those channels did not stop the spread of the virus, but it did stop the spread of health.

DOI: 10.4324/9781003259336-4

The framework within which governments' efforts against SARS-CoV-2 have been made is that of what is called "public health". "This is public health", tweeted Devi Sridhar, chair of global public health at the University of Edinburgh and COVID-19 advisor to the Scottish government, in January 2021, as if there is little more to be said once public health has been invoked.[3]

But there is much more to be said. Not only because measures taken in the name of public health have, during 2020 and 2021 at least, failed to protect people's health, but because the pursuit of public health is itself a kind of failure. Good health is neither a public matter nor even, perhaps, a health matter, and is therefore profoundly ill-served by a public-health agenda.

In a short essay from the early 1990s, the German philosopher Hans-Georg Gadamer addresses what he identifies as the essentially "enigmatic" or "miraculous" character of health; his insights help to suggest what a category error it may be to assume that the health of people is promoted by public-health policies. More than this, Gadamer's account implies that public-health policies may constitute a direct assault upon people's health.[4]

This assault can be described as operating on two fronts: subjecting to *standard* values and interventions that which is inherently particular; and rendering *explicit* that which is essentially tacit.

On both fronts, the role of contact and communication, of touch and dialogue, is dramatically diminished. Yet, on Gadamer's account, it is precisely contact and communication that are necessary for good health.

First, to the public-health application of standard rules and values to that which is essentially particular:

Public-health policies operate on a very general level and a highly specific level: on the very general level, they establish and appeal to trends in the population at large; on the highly specific level, they isolate and address discrete objects, often discernable only to instruments applied by experts. In being so directed at general trends in the behaviour of specific objects, public health tends to bypass that which ought arguably to be at the centre of healthcare: the individual person, neither inevitably subsumable under general trends in populations nor merely the sum of the specific parts studied and manipulated by experts.

In this context, Gadamer mentions two phrases whose emergence indicates a concerning removal from conventional healthcare of what ought to be essential to it. These relatively recent and, Gadamer observes, "artificial" phrases, "quality of life" and "holistic medicine", suggest that vital consideration of the individual person, taken as a *whole* and in the context of what contributes to making their life *worthwhile*, has been extracted from the normal course of healthcare, consigned to the margins of so-called "alternative" therapies. (Gadamer, 1996: 104–106)

Public-health policies reassemble the human terrain on which care for health operates as a vast conglomeration of biological parts and processes: white cell counts, cholesterol levels, heart rates, fat contents, blood pressure, viral fragments, and so on.

In doing so, public health dissolves the wholeness of individual humans – in whom the discrete parts and processes that are addressed by public health exist and operate in the context of other parts and processes – and of time of life, of hopes and of history and of all the rest, each one of which contextual factors determines the quality of individuals' lives in quite particular ways.

Public health charts the ebb and flow of specific parts and processes as they cluster and spread in and through entire populations. Yet, the individual human is a whole in whom the specific objects of public health do not merely course but are suspended in balance with so many other contingent factors that to isolate them in their specificity and administer to them in their generality is to efface their mode of existence in human beings.

"Holistic medicine" has emerged as a particular offering of marginal medical practices when holism should be a basic principle of any medical practice. This has meant that a person's "quality of life" is only sometimes adjusted for, as an extra consideration of healthcare over and above the continued existence, the mere survival, that is increasingly revealed as the standard of public-health agendas.

With great prescience, Gadamer refers in his essay to the significance of the term "case", which has, during the last two years, been confirmed as the public-health substitute for the individual person – the number of "Covid cases" has been touted endlessly during 2020 and 2021, and these "cases" have been allowed to override the most basic experiences of people living their lives.

The German word for case is "Fall", Gadamer observes, reminding us that illness is that which befalls a person – in English, we say that we "fall ill" (Gadamer, 1996: 107). What does this imply? It implies that illness is that which causes a person to stop in their tracks, to falter, that which interrupts the smooth flow of their daily living. Gadamer informs us that the Greek word "symptom" also refers to that which befalls us (Gadamer, 1996: 107).

Gadamer's analysis suggests that illness is that which primarily affects the whole person, whose life has a particular quality, operating upon their whole so as to impact negatively upon what makes their life worthwhile. One is a case, one has symptoms, when one cannot do what one usually does, when the quality of the daily experiences of an individual is adversely affected, when this person's life is brought low.

As has become painfully evident since the advent of COVID-19, public-health policies establish cases in accordance with the anonymous results of vast measuring procedures aimed at biomedical parts and processes so discrete that they are rarely salient in the experience of individuals and then averaged for the population at large. On Gadamer's account, public-health policies thereby mistake the very nature of illness, which cannot be captured anonymously according to standard rules and values.

This public health mistake about illness participates in the fundamental philosophical problem about the relation between abstract rules and objects and between concrete events and experiences (Gadamer, 1996: 104). This relation must not be one of *mere* application, as Gadamer considers elsewhere, as if all that is to be done is to lay abstract rules and objects over particular events and experiences (Gadamer, 2003: 307–312). There is a qualitative difference between a particular person, taken in the whole and in the context of their lives, and a single element of a population or a conglomeration of specific biomedical entities. This qualitative difference means that what applies to general populations or to specific biomedical entities does not simply apply to particular people; insofar as public-health agendas assume a relation of simple application, those agendas are careless of particular people.

How amplified during the COVID-19 era has been this carelessness with regard to people, inherent in the conception of health as a public phenomenon. The disease COVID-19 – which, according to official government figures, has not resulted in any excess deaths of people in many countries[5] – has been abroad as a "pandemic" primarily by being pegged to the identified spread of the SARS-CoV-2 virus and to the naming as cases not primarily those who fell ill but those who tested positive for a fragment of that virus in accordance with a standardised testing procedure.

Indeed, the figure of the "asymptomatic case" has been the dominant one during COVID-19 times, when the properly intimate connection between cases and symptoms has been dismantled and the determination of cases misconceived as a matter of mere application of standard criteria and a standard measurement protocol. The upshot of this has been that we have spent almost two years now in logging the progress of a biological object so specific that it must often be amplified forty-fold to be salient through a population considered so generally that whether individuals within it were or were not ill was mostly irrelevant.

The COVID-19 era has brought to the fore the general effect of public-health approaches, revealing that when it comes to meaningful healthcare, merely applying standard values is no substitute for the clinical practice in which abstract values and objects are applied with judgement on a case-by-case basis, that is, on the basis of the individual patient taken in the whole and in the context of their life.

This brings us to the fundamental weakness of public health: it prioritises what Gadamer terms "scientific medicine" over what he calls "the art of healing", emphasizing "a knowledge of things in general" at the expense of the "concrete application of this knowledge to particular cases" (Gadamer, 1996: 103–104). This concrete application, which is not mere application, requires all manner of arts currently obviated by the standardised procedures of public healthcare precisely to the extent that it is directed primarily at the particular person and not at specific scientifically isolated objects and general population-level trends.

In a clinical setting, the doctor examines the patient, looks at his pallor, feels his pulse, listens to his heart, presses his flesh. *Behandlung* is the German word for treatment, Gadamer observes, in order to emphasise the importance of touch (Gadamer, 1996: 109). And dialogue is central too. The patient is asked, "How do you feel?" – and his replies, anecdotal and subjective, are accorded at least as much significance as the results of the application of measuring instruments and criteria (Gadamer, 1996: 108). Contact and communication, touch and dialogue, are central to the treatment of illness when illness is understood as that which befalls a particular person.

What, after all, do we mean by "treatment", Gadamer asks.

> Clearly what is demanded is that we treat someone in the "right way". Does this mean that we fulfil a norm or follow a rule? In my opinion it means, rather, that we address the other person in the right way, that we do not force ourselves on them or compel them to accept something against their will, be it an external measure or a regulation…. Treatment always also involves a certain granting of freedom.
>
> *Gadamer, 1996: 109*

Compounding the effect of the COVID-19 advertisement of asymptomatic illness, then, has been the COVID-19-era attack upon the contact and communication that are, on Gadamer's account, essential to the proper treatment of individuals. In the UK during 2020 and 2021, doctors were almost wholly unable to touch their patients. Their surgeries were closed. Their consultations were remote. Clinical examination was more or less abandoned. And what of dialogue? They could ask their patients, "How do you feel?" over the phone or on Zoom. But the distance of the communication and the spectre of asymptomatic illness must surely have diluted the significance of the replies.

Though the disease COVID-19 *befell* relatively few in the UK,[6] the obviation of contact and communication, the abandonment of treatment, that arose from government efforts to stop the spread of the virus identified as causing the disease meant that thousands of "cases" of the illness were found and advertised daily. Indeed, very soon it came to be that everyone was a "case"; the UK government's advice was to "act like you've got it". Fallenness was rolled out as a condition of the population generally; the effacement of the particular person and their proper treatment designated everyone as as-if ill.

Not only that, it caused many people to be actually ill. The sudden cessation of routines, of human relations, the suspension of work, of regular wages, the recalibration of home life: all caused anxiety and distress, at the very least.

The condition of "Long Covid" soon became a talking point after the first COVID-19 patients were identified in early 2020. Certainly, it is not uncommon for respiratory viruses to produce a post-viral effect: loss of appetite, fatigue, aching muscles, shortness of breath. But these were also symptoms of the stress and despair produced by government measures. The across-the-board, grotesquely standardised designation of everyone as a "case" and therefore as subject to quarantine made everyone fall as-if ill, and then made many fall ill.

As a treatment of people, the COVID-19 bypassing of the relevant whole – the individual human being – in favour of general trends and specific bio-entities was utterly disastrous. It could not have been more counterproductive. It did not disrupt the virus, whose unrelenting spread is even still incessantly reported, but it certainly actively made healthy people ill.

But public-health policies do not only standardise that which is essentially particular, thereby causing healthy people to fall ill. They operate also on another front, rendering explicit that which is essentially tacit and thereby dissolving what may be the most vital condition for the possibility of good health.

Consider in this regard that, although our theme in this chapter is that of health, we have so far considered not health but illness. And illness, to state the obvious, is not health. It is, in fact, the opposite of health. This is not only because health involves the absence of illness, but also because health, unlike illness, is not a natural object for discussion or intervention. If we have written half an essay on health and yet still not really focused on health, it is because health is not the kind of experience that lends itself to being focused on.

"Health does not actually present itself to us", Gadamer observes (Gadamer, 1996: 107). Only illness presents itself to us, as that which puts an obstacle in our path, that which causes us to falter. Only illness befalls us. Health is something quite other than illness, and care for health something quite other than treatment of illness.

If this is so, then Gadamer's essay supports the suggestion that care for health has been even more ill served than treatment of illness by the Covid-era advertisement of health as a public phenomenon. If government measures to stop the spread of the virus mistook the very nature of illness, they may even more starkly have mistaken the very nature of health.

Good health, like illness, does inhere in the particular person, that individual whole which public-health measures tend to overlook. But it is present in the particular person so enigmatically that it is essentially hidden in them, not only not inevitably enhanced by the arts of medicine but actually possibly damaged by the practice of those arts as well as by the impersonal policies and pronouncements of the public-health sciences.

"It lies in the nature of health that it sustains its own proper balance and proportion", Gadamer claims. "If health really cannot be measured, it is because it is a condition of inner accord, of harmony with oneself that cannot be overridden by other, external forms of control" (Gadamer, 1996: 107) – not even by the arts of medicine, not even by the clinical examination of a doctor with judgement and feeling.

This hiddenness of health arises from health's essentially background character, its constitutive nature. Health does not befall a person. On the contrary, what it is to be healthy is *not* to have fallen, *not* to have faltered, to have continued with life *un*impeded, to have *not* pursued anything but our usual ways and means.

Health is essentially taken for granted, essentially concealed, that which we do not turn towards or attempt to manage, the underlying condition for our proceeding as we wish to and always do.

Indeed, so hidden is the underlying condition of health that the self-reflection of the person themselves does not reach its shadowy reality – as Gadamer observes, one asks oneself or others, "Do you feel ill?" but not "Do you feel healthy?" (Gadamer, 1996: 113) This is not because health does not manifest in the particular person but because the kind of equilibrium involved in health is buried so deeply that it is almost never brought to the attention even of the person themselves.

"Health is not a condition that one introspectively feels in oneself", Gadamer claims. "Rather, it is a condition of being involved, of being in the world, of being together with one's fellow human beings, of active and rewarding engagement in one's everyday tasks" (Gadamer, 1996: 113). One must be in the world with others to be healthy, and health is being in the world with others.

We may imagine, then, what a tension there exists between the public-health drive to remake health as phenomenon of entire populations, advertised and administered with busy éclat, and the quiet implicitness of good health as a particular personal experience.

Furthermore, we may imagine how greatly this tension was exacerbated by the unprecedented amplification of public-health agendas during 2020 and 2021, which hardly allowed for a moment's quiet on the matter of people's health and captured every medium for the dissemination of health advice of all kinds and for the encouragement of people to attend to their own health and that of others. We became a society whose theme was health, a society in which there was no place left for health to hide.

How counterproductive these government interventions were, if health is, as Gadamer claims, an essentially hidden phenomenon; the very thing that health is, is the very thing that the government suspended. Health's hiding places – being together in the world, living life, getting involved – were disbanded as we were enjoined to *be healthy*. But, on Gadamer's account, one can only be healthy by being together in the world and living life and getting involved…by *not being healthy*, in other words, not explicitly at any rate.

If Gadamer's insights are true, then the measures taken by governments to stop the spread of the SARS-CoV-2 virus were aimed directly against human health. As the misguided notion of the asymptomatic case reframed illness as its polar opposite – that which does not befall a person – so the equally misguided health advice to "stay home" and "keep your distance" reframed health as its polar opposite: that which does befall a person. The upshot, on both counts, was that ill people were poorly treated or not treated at all and healthy people were made ill.

"Health is 'the rhythm of life'", Gadamer observes.

> It shows itself above all where a feeling of well-being means we are open to new things, ready to embark on new enterprises and, forgetful of ourselves, scarcely notice the demands and strains which are put on us. This is what health is.
>
> *Gadamer, 1996: 112*

By closing us off to new (and old) things, by barring us from embarking on new (and old) enterprises, by loudly and unceasingly reminding us not to forget ourselves, and by instructing us to remain constantly vigilant for signs of strain on our body's defenses, government measures to stop the spread of the SARS-CoV-2 virus were nothing short of a decimation of what health is, as public-health policies at last became anathema to people's health.

Yet there is there is more to be said about the enigmatic character of health than is contained in Gadamer's essay, as is suggested in one of the essay's analogies.

Gadamer describes health as being like riding a bike. When one knows how to ride a bike, one rides a bike effortlessly. In fact, any effort to deliberately manage the project can hinder it – one adjusts this way and then that until the equilibrium that had been a background condition of riding the bike is upset and one falls off.

"The attempt to maintain an equilibrium is a highly instructive model for the theme we are concerned with", Gadamer writes, "since it shows the dangers involved in all attempts at intervention" (Gadamer, 1996: 113).

In this regard, our bombardment during 2020 and 2021 by government messaging on the matter of health – the perpetual insistence that we measure our health and determine our health and prove our health and protect our health – might well be described as a direct hit on the equilibrium necessary for health.

But if we consider further what this equilibrium of health is comprised of, we discover an additional aspect of the enigmatic character of health, one that is not dwelt upon by Gadamer but which is as vital to the maintenance of health as is the taking of health for granted that he describes and advocates.

Continuing with Gadamer's health analogy, we might observe that, while there is an essentially tacit quality to riding a bike, the achievement does not sustain itself through *inaction*. The action it requires is smooth and low level and disappears into the easy rhythm of cycling, that is true, but it is not the equivalent of inaction and it is constant and necessary.

If we have been in danger of overlooking this element of action in the maintenance of a background equilibrium, if we might have presumed that what is tacit implies no purposeful activity all, this may be the effect of precisely the scientistic culture in which public-health agendas participate – the culture of making everything explicit and of bringing all action to bear on that project. But, as we have already observed, good health runs against the grain of this scientistic culture; and while there is an essential hiddenness about health, health is also essentially active.

Consider firstly that cycling is both the state of equilibrium that makes cycling possible and the action of cycling that produces and maintains that state of equilibrium. If you do not constantly produce and maintain the equilibrium, then you fall off, as sometimes happens with children who begin to cycle and who, distracted by a sudden sight or sound, forget to pedal and topple to the ground.

Then ask, secondly, what the activity might be that maintains the equilibrium of health and that both contributes to the background life force that is health and is supported by that life force. What is the low hum of health activity that is the equivalent of pedaling a bike? If it is not the explicit questionings and measurings and messagings of the COVID-19 era, and yet it is not nothing, what is it? Here, a short example must suffice.

Two letters were written by Jane Austen to her sister Cassandra during the penultimate week of the year 1798, when the author was 23 and her sister two years older and both were staying with their brother Edward for the holiday season.

The first of these letters includes the following passage:

> My Mother continues hearty, her appetite and nights are very good, but her Bowels are still not entirely settled, and she sometimes complains of an

Asthma, a Dropsy, Water in her Chest and a Liver Disorder. The third Miss Irish Lefroy is going to be married to a Mr. Courtenay, but whether James or Charles I do not know'.

Austen, 2003: 27

The second letter includes this:

Poor Edward! It is very hard that he who has everything else in the World that he can wish for, should not have good health too. – But I hope with the assistance of Bowel complaints, Faintnesses and Sicknesses, he will soon be restored to that Blessing likewise. – If his nervous complaint proceeded from a suppression of something that ought to be thrown out, which does not seem unlikely, the first of those Disorders may really be a remedy, and I sincerely wish it may, for I know no one more deserving of happiness without alloy than Edward is. – My Mother's spirits are *not* affected by her complication of disorders; on the contrary they are altogether as good as ever; nor are you to suppose that these maladies are often thought of. – She has at times a tendency towards another which always relieves her, and that is, a gouty swelling and sensation about the ancles. – I cannot determine what to do about my new Gown; I wish such things were to be bought ready made'.

Austen, 2003: 30

What are we to observe in these light and lively accounts of the health of family members, sent between two young women and nestled among details of the romantic fates of neighbours and the sisters' sartorial woes?

Precisely that: that they are nestled among other of life's details, not brought out solemnly, not dealt with in grave tones, not premised upon the suspension of everything else, not explicit in that sense but woven into the fabric of life. The account of Edward moves seamlessly from the humorous hope that a series of complaints will do him good to the earnest opinion that one of those complaints – of the "Bowel" – really will help to expel that which may be affecting his "nerves". And then it is on to the matter of a new dress with not a pause for breath, the health details of family members mentioned alongside the trivia of everyday life, taken as lightly and as seriously, as casually and as repeatedly, between two women who might by us be judged too young and vibrant themselves to care much for such concerns.

There is no squeamishness about body parts and processes. The Bowel sits comfortably alongside the Gown. The Austen sisters are at home in the digestive system, as they are in the ways and means of muslin.

Gadamer observes that health "is a condition of being involved, of being in the world, of being together with one's fellow human beings, of active and rewarding engagement in one's everyday tasks" (Gadamer, 1996: 113). One must be in the world to be healthy, on his account – health is the condition of being in the world.

But one must also be healthy in the world, we might add. One must be involved with health, be together with one's fellow beings on the matter of health. The bowels and the swellings, the nerves and the faintnessess, must be abroad as easily and as adeptly as gowns and neighbours and whatever else comprises the low hum of activity, the steady rhythm, of our daily lives.

The hiddenness of health, then, is not some mystical condition that is removed from us and in respect of which we are inactive, though Gadamer's designation of health as a "miracle" and a "mystery" might be in danger of making us suppose so (Gadamer, 1996: 103, 115). On the contrary, health circulates openly among us and between us. Only by so circulating is health attended to at the right pitch, with the right balance of humour and sobriety. Health is taken lightly, but it is taken. And when it is taken, when we are involved with health, we bolster the underlying condition of health that makes all involvement possible.

The tacit character of health has, then, a circular structure: in trading on the theme of health as on the many everyday themes that go to make up our being together in the world, we help to maintain ourselves and others in a state of good health, which strengthens health as the underlying condition of our being together in the world, which in turn gives vitality to our circulating between ourselves the many themes of our daily lives.

The overriding public-health tendency to render explicit all matters concerning health dismantles not only the tacit nature of health-as-underlying-condition, but also the tacit nature of health-as-low-hum-of-activity.

If the observations of Jane Austen seem strange to us now and implausible, it is only because we are inured to the effect of public-health agendas, which redirect our concerns for our own and one another's health away from the hue of our skin or the swelling of our ankles and towards the results of measurement procedures that address objects too specific or too general for everyday salience. The framing of health as a public matter has gradually sucked the life from the contact and communication with one another that is not only essential to the proper treatment of illness but vital for the tacit circulation of health.

Public-health measures taken in response to the posited threat of COVID-19 did not invent the decimation of health-as-tacit-circulation any more than they invented the demise of health-as-tacit-condition, though they certainly exacerbated these effects. Indeed, the very first of the major COVID-19 debates revealed how already implausible had become the low hum of active involvement on which good health must rightly rely.

Shortly after the announced arrival of the SARS-CoV-2 virus in the UK came the rapid escalation of discussion about "herd immunity", which continues to this day to be one of the most divisive concepts of the COVID-19 era. Herd immunity is a well-established epidemiological concept and refers to the immunity acquired by a population at large when a sufficient proportion of its people have ceased to be able to be infected by or to transmit a disease for the threat from the disease to be attenuated and an endemic equilibrium to be reached.

From the outset, "pursuing" herd immunity – as it was often put, although herd immunity is typically achieved tacitly – was branded by the UK government and by the corporate media as a policy of "Let it rip". As if, while herd immunity developed, there would be no natural capacities among people to take precautions to protect one another, as if the low hum of health activity was already so anaemic as to offer little by way of grassroots resistance to the spread of a viral disease. How impoverished we were advertised to be; so much so that only the option of massive government intervention was allowed to have a chance of protecting "Granny" from illness and death.

Those of us who resisted this option objected to the defamation of herd immunity as a "Let it rip" approach. But why did our cries in its favour fall so over-whelmingly on deaf ears? Is it because reliance on herd immunity really would have been a case of "Let it rip"? Were we already so out of practice in the tacit circulation of health that we were in fact – or felt we were – without the ways and means for the implicit regulation of the spread of a respiratory virus?

A remarkable aspect of Jane Austen's letters is the range of words that they use to describe states of health: "Dropsy", "a gouty swelling and sensation", "Liver Disorder", "Water in the Chest", and many other descriptors pepper her accounts of herself and those around her. When did we forget how to speak in this way, con-fidently and subtly, of health? And does it indicate that we have we also forgotten how to act, confidently and subtly, for health?

One of Gadamer's seminal claims is that "being that can be understood is lan-guage". (Gadamer, 2003: 474) If this is true, then our having lost the words to talk about health means that we have lost also the ways to understand and to regulate our own health and that of others – and certainly suggests that a highly infectious respiratory virus, left to our devices, really might have "let rip".

This brings us to the most devastating limitation of the concept of public health, which may be at odds with good health not only by misconceiving health as a public matter but by misconceiving health as a health matter. In other words, the ubiquity of the term "health", its dominance over efforts to understand and regu-late so many aspects of our being together in the world, may have so overshadowed other, more varied and nuanced terms that our talent for allowing health to circu-late among ourselves may have grown too blunt for purpose.

In his book *Plastic Words*, Uwe Pörksen describes how certain words – everyday words such as "communication", "information", and "development", and, we might add, "health" – have come to dominate our discourse with their great encompassing effects, displacing all manner of more nuanced designators by having been con-ferred with a scientific aura, an atmosphere of being at the cutting edge (Cayley and Pörksen, 1993: 5).[7]

These words are not technical words, which are often strictly limited to contexts. They are words taken from common parlance, refracted through the scientific realm, and returned to everyday talk with a new, broadened application and a new, somewhat ambiguous authority. Having become thus "plastic", as Pörksen describes them, these words denote nothing at all, but are so comprehensively connotative that they suck the life from the many and varied words that fall beneath their shadow (Cayley and Pörksen, 1993: 3–4).

The result is that our powers of circulating among ourselves the significance of fundamental aspects of our experience are greatly reduced as we are unwittingly rendered the clients of public bodies and their experts even in matters that might be, that ought to be, quite personal and concrete (Cayley and Pörksen, 1993: 4).

To the extent that "health" has become such a plastic word, it operates precisely in the manner that Pörksen describes: in displacing many more particular terms – "Faintnesses", "Sicknesses", "throw[ings] out", "gouty swellings", and the like – it reduces our powers of circulating among ourselves our personal experiences of health. Seen in this light, the concept of 'health' is detrimental to health, sapping health's tacit circulation of its vital subtlety and energy.

In September 2021, chief medical advisor to the UK government Chris Whitty recommended the administering of COVID-19 vaccines to those aged between 12 and 15 years, even though the government's Joint Committee on Vaccination and Immunisation had, only a week before, stated that vaccinating this age group could have no health benefits. What is significant is that Whitty made his recommendation on the basis of the vaccine's alleged benefits to so-called "mental health".

How plastic this word "health" has become when, having refused vaccination on health grounds, it then justifies vaccination on health grounds.

But the most sinister moment in Pörksen's account of the rise of plastic words is his claim that, added to their displacement of the descriptors that oil our low-hum involvement with one another and our world, they also displace silence. There is nowhere, Pörksen argues, that "information" is not important, no corner of the earth in which "development" is not a possibility, no instant when "communication" does not apply (Cayley and Pörksen, 1993: 6).

The growing ubiquity of the word "health" is fulfilling Pörksen's grim prediction, gradually inserting itself as a stake in the most surprising aspects of our lives.

Jane Austen could leave her themes of health as easily as she could take them. She could muse on her new gown or her neighbour's romance. But in the COVID-19 era, there is gradually no theme in which health is not at stake. Even gowns, even romance, fall under its sober shadow as we browse in shops with sanitised hands and masked faces and flick past the vaccination status of love prospects on Tinder. Every nook of our COVID-19 world might now be a hospital ward: our churches and our music festivals and our nightclubs and our shopping malls and our football stadiums and our schools, all repurposed for testing and tracing and vaccinating and screening of all kinds.

If we have chased health to its hiding places by rendering it a "public" phenomenon, now health is chasing us to our hiding places by rendering them "health" centres.

Notes

1 For various studies showing this, see www.pandata.org/infobank-lockdowns/
2 See, for example, TalkTV, 2021, Twitter, May 17, 6:08 p.m., https://twitter.com/talkradio/status/1394339134471385097?lang=en

3 Devi Sridhar, 2021. Twitter, 23 January, 3:30 p.m., https://twitter.com/devisridhar/status/ 1353002258779299845?lang=en

4 Chapter 8 of Gadamer (1996).

5 When adjusted for age and size of population, mortality in the UK in 2020 was only the ninth highest of the previous twenty years, and lower than any year before the new millennium. Despite its misleading headline, this BBC article by Nick Triggle includes this correct information: Nick Triggle, 2021, "Covid: 2020 Saw Worst Excess Deaths Since World War Two", BBC, 12 January, www.bbc.co.uk/news/uk-55631693.

6 When the notorious unreliability of the PCR testing procedure that was used to designate people as "Covid cases" is taken into consideration alongside the relatively normal UK mortality during 2020, the number and age of people who fell ill with COVID-19 is not remarkably different from the number and age of people who fall ill annually of respiratory disease.

7 References are to the transcript of this interview.

References

Austen, Jane. 2003. *Jane Austen's Letters*. Collected and edited by Deirdre Le Faye. London: The Folio Society.

Cayley, David and Uwe Pörksen. 1993. 'Plastic Words.' *Ideas*. The Canadian Broadcasting Corporation. Ontario: CBC, 4 February 1993. Transcript https://static1.squarespace. com/static/542c2af8e4b00b7cfca08972/t/58ffcaf2c149d34329cb4045/1493158644 446/Plastic_Words.pdf.

Gadamer, Hans-Georg. 1996. *The Enigma of Health: The Art of Healing in a Scientific Age*. Translated by Jason Gaiger and Nicholas Walker. Stanford, CA: Stanford University Press.

Gadamer, Hans-Georg. 2003. *Truth and Method* (2nd edn.). Translated by Joel Weinsheimer and Donald G. Marshall. New York: Continuum.

3

PANDEMIC RESPONSE, CULTURAL ANTHROPOLOGY, AND "THE MYTH OF THE CARING SOCIETY"

Peter Sutoris

Pandemic response, sacrifice, and myth

Throughout the COVID-19 pandemic, world leaders have justified prolonged, large-scale lockdowns and other unprecedented control measures by calling the pandemic an extraordinary, once-in-a-century calamity. In light of this crisis, policy elites around the world have asked citizens to empathise with those most at risk and to make sacrifices for the greater good. In the United Kingdom, prime minister Boris Johnson summarised the looming threat in his televised address to the country on 23 March 2020, on the cusp of the country's first lockdown:

> To put it simply, if too many people become seriously unwell at one time, the NHS will be unable to handle it – meaning more people are likely to die, not just from Coronavirus but from other illnesses as well. So, it's vital to slow the spread of the disease. Because that is the way we reduce the number of people needing hospital treatment at any one time, so we can protect the NHS's ability to cope – and save more lives.
>
> *Johnson, 2020b[1]*

The government's stated reason for the drastic measures was that an unchecked spread of the virus would overwhelm the health system. This would mean that many people would not be able to access healthcare and some would die unnecessarily. In other words, the justification for mandating exceptional personal sacrifice was that avoidable deaths needed to be avoided at all costs.

The problem with this reasoning is that avoidable death is very common in non-crisis times. According to the UK's Office for National Statistics data for 2019, 136,146 deaths out of 604,707, or 22.5 percent, were considered "avoidable", and this was in line with the data for the preceding five years. Of the deaths considered

DOI: 10.4324/9781003259336-5

avoidable, 64.2 percent were attributed to "preventable" causes (that is, they could have been avoided if effective public-health services and primary care were available), and the remaining 35.8 percent to "treatable" causes (in other words, they could have been avoided if timely, effective secondary health interventions were available). According to these numbers, avoidable death was very much the norm well before the virus arrived.

What's more, the UK government's criteria for considering a death avoidable exclude any person who dies above age 75, regardless of the cause (Office for National Statistics, 2021b: 2). The median age of COVID-19 victims in England and Wales (up to 2 October 2020) was 83 (Office for National Statistics, 2021a); therefore, a large proportion of those who died from or with COVID-19 would, by the government's own definition, not be included in the category of those who died of avoidable causes.

As SARS-CoV-2 spread, the government took unprecedented action to minimise the spread of the virus – action that would go on to cause much avoidable death and misery. The action was justified by saying it was needed to prevent avoidable death, even as avoidable death was the pre-existing norm. This seems inconsistent: Why did preventing avoidable death trigger a call to action during the COVID-19 pandemic but not when there were hundreds of thousands of preventable deaths in years past?

It could be argued that the government was not responding to avoidable death *per se* but to the prospect of a sudden rise in the number of avoidable deaths – in other words, it was not the *quality* of dying in an avoidable manner but the *quantity* of people who might die unnecessarily that was seen as unacceptable and which needed to be prevented at all costs. Surely a great increase in preventable deaths above a relatively stable level constitutes an abnormal event that demands a strong response, but this would mean there was a threshold, some number of avoidable deaths or rate of their increase within a particular timeframe, which would justify unprecedented interventions and exceptional sacrifices.

However, there is nothing self-evident about such a threshold – how many deaths would mean it has been crossed, and who would decide on that number? Were the 136,146 avoidable deaths of people younger than 75 in 2019 below the threshold? Were those people less worthy of solidarity and sacrifice from the rest of society than those at risk from COVID-19? Shifting the analytical frame to the quantity of people dying from avoidable causes does not explain why, in early 2020, avoidable death due to COVID-19 was framed as a crisis worthy of unprecedented measures.

In this chapter, I point to an alternative explanation of why the spread of SARS-CoV-2 triggered a drastic response which was disproportional to the way society had previously treated avoidable death. The pandemic response became an enactment of the "myth of the caring society" – a story at the core of Western civilisation's self-perceived identity as a uniquely egalitarian society, and an important element of the nationalist imaginary of many modern nation states in the West and elsewhere.

Although I use examples drawn mostly from the UK to advance this argument, many of the ideas that follow also apply to other countries. As Toby Green

(2021) has argued, a "Covid consensus" about how the pandemic should be tackled emerged in early 2020 and soon swept across the world. I refer to Western civilisation in this essay because the myth of the caring society is linked to ancient Greek philosophy, Judeo-Christian ideas, and Enlightenment thought, but this is in fact a myth of global significance and relevance. Other narratives have undoubtedly influenced the pandemic response, some of them originating outside the Western world, such as the narrative of "order" that shaped the initial response in China and set a precedent for the rest of the world. Still, the myth of the caring society can help explain why important elements of China's heavy-handed response to the virus found fertile ground in the West.

Myth, identity, and illumination

In common usage, the word "myth" usually means something untrue, a false belief held by a group of people. But myths are first and foremost stories we tell ourselves which may or may not have elements of truth in them. Examining what myths say about the culture of human societies often produces more salient insights than simply asking how true the myths are. The discipline of anthropology has a long history of studying myth and has produced a good deal of nuanced insight into how people shape myths and how myths in turn shape people.

Bronisław Malinowski, one of the most influential early anthropologists, argued in a 1925 public lecture at the University of Liverpool that "an intimate connection exists between the world, the mythos, the sacred tales of a tribe on the one hand and their ritual acts, their moral deeds, their social organization, and even their practical activities on the other" (Malinowski, 1984: 195). This is arguably as true in today's globalised world as it was in the pre-industrial societies of Melanesia which Malinowski researched a century ago.

Apart from shaping collective and individual identities, myths help people orient themselves within the cultural landscapes they inhabit. According to Clifford Geertz, a key theorist of cultural anthropology, humans are "in need of symbolic 'sources of illumination' to orient themselves with respect to the system of meaning that is any particular culture" (Geertz, 1973: 45). Myths and their symbolic meanings are one such source of illumination that can help members of a society navigate its culture.

This orientating role of myths is perhaps their most salient feature at a time of global upheaval. The global spread of SARS-CoV-2 and the associated pandemic control measures did not just lead to crises of health and the economy, they also unleashed a crisis of culture. In an increasingly globalised world driven by individualism and consumerism, people all over the globe were suddenly asked by their political leaders to make massive sacrifices for the common good. The logic of lockdowns went against much of what the world had come to take for granted in the decades before 2020.

Grand narratives and myths thrive at times of confusion, and this helps explain why the myth of the caring society has been so powerful during the pandemic. In its most generic form, the myth could be summarised in this way:

> Since equality is one of our foundational values, we see all human lives as equally important. We will therefore do whatever it takes to preserve the life of each and every individual, at all costs. Preventable death is unacceptable in our society and it is our duty to do all we can to prevent it from happening.

It is beyond the scope of this essay to analyse the origins of this myth and the many roles it plays in Western culture, but it is important to mention at least a few points. Equality, as a foundational value, runs deep in Western thought, from Plato to the Enlightenment to Thomas Jefferson and contemporary liberal democracy as a pinnacle of the West's political evolution. The value of individual human life is firmly rooted in the Judeo-Christian tradition, going all the way back to the Ten Commandments.

It is impossible to separate this myth from the history of conquest, imperialism, and colonialism. The millennia-old moral fibre that wove the fabric of Western civilisation has been codified, refined, and cemented over centuries, often by contrasting it with other, "inferior" civilisations. Much European colonialism was justified by the moral superiority proclaimed by the West and its "civilising mission" in the rest of the world (Said, 1979) – a thread that continues to run through more recent events, such as the 2003 invasion of Iraq. The myth of the caring society requires other, "uncaring" societies to provide a clear contrast and helps to cement a collective sense of moral superiority within a particular "imagined community" (Anderson, 2006). In other words, the myth goes hand in hand with nationalism.

Myths are crucial to national identities, and collective experiences of hardship and bewilderment provide opportunities for solidifying national unity. "I know how difficult this is, how it seems to go against the freedom-loving instincts of the British people", the prime minister said of the lockdowns in his televised speech on 20 March 2020 (Johnson, 2020a). It is in periods of bewilderment that the powers that be seek to activate, spread, and sometimes weaponise a society's core myths. Meanwhile, people often hunger for stories that help them make sense of the unexpected situation in which they find themselves.

Prior to the current pandemic the myth could be seen at play, for example, in the cases of Westerners imprisoned in foreign countries, as politicians and the media fretted about their fate and emphasised their home country's efforts to free them. This selective attention helped to demonstrate the West's perceived moral superiority, yet it was these same politicians and the same media that often turn a blind eye to human rights abuses at home. In 2020–22, leaders demonstrated their moral superiority by taking measures to avoid one kind of preventable death while ignoring other avoidable causes of death and human suffering.

The story and the ritual

Many anthropologists see myth as "a story connected with a ritual" (Emmet, 1998: 44). If the story at the heart of the myth of the caring society is one of equality, solidarity, and preventing the avoidable deaths of the members of our "tribe" at all costs, through what rituals have we acted out the story since the outbreak of the virus?

The pandemic control measures have been the enactment of our society's ritual of care. The many steps taken by governments and individuals to control the spread of the virus – from lockdowns to politicians' press conferences – carry symbolic meaning. On one level, these actions are motivated by scientific knowledge that has been privileged during the pandemic, such as computer modelling (see Anthony Mckeown's paper in Chapter 1 about performative scientism). On another level, they are the rituals of belonging to a particular culture, signals of being one of "us" rather than one of "them".

If a society stands for virtuous, laudable values – equality, value of life – being a member of that society allows individuals to make a claim to this "goodness". This sense of belonging, of this goodness, can, in the eyes of the individual and their peers alike, compensate for individual moral failings. But to claim these benefits, membership has to be signalled and reaffirmed through symbolic rituals of belonging.

Aside from expressing support for and adhering to pandemic control measures, the world has seen countless such rituals during the pandemic. The applauding of healthcare practitioners and other essential workers became a regular sight in cities around the globe. This gave ordinary people not only an opportunity to express their gratitude to the hard-working and often underpaid workers but also a chance to feel like they were "doing something", participating in a small way in the society's pandemic response by signalling their belonging to the culture of care. It is telling that these public rituals rarely led to increased political support for better funding of public services, as aptly captured in the "Tax, not clap for the NHS" poster I came upon in London in the spring of 2020 (see Figure 3.1).

Hero worship created further opportunities to signal belonging. In India, military planes dropped tonnes of fresh flowers on the roofs of hospitals to recognise the heroic efforts of the country's medical professionals, while in the UK, the figure of elderly Captain Moore became one of the symbols of pandemic-era grassroots care. A retired 99-year-old soldier who raised millions for the country's health service by walking laps in his garden during lockdown, Captain Moore became a hero to many by capturing the spirit of gratitude and of "doing our bit" that characterised the early days of the pandemic. Yet his story, too, raised questions about the extent to which Britain truly embodied a culture of care. Britain's NHS is meant to be funded through taxes and to provide for the needs of all based on the principles of equality and solidarity. If the efforts of private citizens are needed to help fund it, isn't this more of a cause for concern than celebration?

Inequality, consistency, and visibility

Perhaps the narrative of the caring society is simply an aspiration, something to collectively strive for, and perhaps these rituals are simply ways to cultivate a sense of

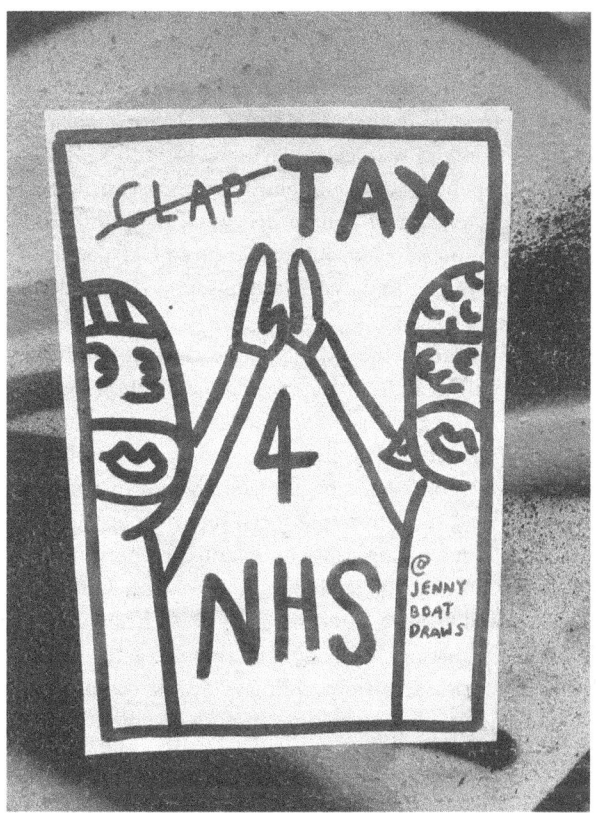

FIGURE 3.1 Tax 4 NHS Poster.

Source: Photo by author.

caring and solidarity. If this is the case, then surely the narrative of the caring society is a force for good?

One way to think about this narrative and the way it has manifested through rituals of care and belonging in response to the spread of SARS-CoV-2 is to ask whether it has brought society closer to or farther away from equality – the value at the very heart of the care narrative. Consider the 23 March 2020 editorial in *The Guardian* which called lockdowns a "necessary hardship" and likened the situation to the introduction of the Emergency Powers (Defence) Act in 1939, a piece of legislation that severely limited individual freedoms. In pondering how the public might respond to such drastic measures, the editorial quoted a 1942 Ministry of Information report: "People are willing to bear any sacrifice if a 100% effort can be reached and the burden fairly shared by all" (The Guardian, 2020). And this, according to *The Guardian*, was what was needed at the time of COVID-19: "During the critical days to come, in the very different Britain of 2020, the present government must trust in exactly the same kind of popular resilience."

This argument assumes that a lockdown could distribute the burden of limiting the spread of the virus fairly among all residents. However, this would only be possible if the myth of the caring society were in fact true, if society had taken care of the vulnerable and marginalised (including those at risk of avoidable death), and if all had entered the lockdown on an even playing field.

This is not what happened. Far from being "the great equaliser", the pandemic and the measures taken to control it have deepened inequality and created additional vulnerabilities among already vulnerable groups of people. This occurred precisely because, in the years and decades leading up to the pandemic, society had in fact not been "caring".

One of the dangers of the myth of the caring society lies in its obscuring many areas in which society fails to address deep-seated inequalities. Even if the narrative is seen as aspirational rather than as a *fait accompli*, it depicts care and equality as core values with a long history; if people in this society have aspired to equality for many generations, surely progress has been made. Even if they are not perfect and there is more work to be done, surely the social support net, the welfare state, and the health system have come a long way. The assumed progress made by those who shared the same aspiration in the past obscures the systemic inequality that renders the idea the burden could ever be fairly shared by all virtually impossible, however much the individuals comprising society might aspire to care.

Equality demands consistency. If preventing avoidable death was the goal – and the reason for the unprecedented restrictions imposed by the authorities – but only visible avoidable deaths received attention, this in itself is an inconsistency incompatible with the goal of equality. Let's return to the 136,146 avoidable deaths in 2019. These deaths were treated very differently from the deaths linked to COVID-19. The government did not limit the personal freedoms of millions of people or run up debts that will take generations to repay to prevent these earlier deaths, as it did in its efforts to slow the spread of SARS-CoV-2.

Such inequality in death shows that the quality that separates the acceptable from the unacceptable, that which is worthy of exceptional measures from business as usual, is not whether a death is avoidable, as the myth of the caring society would have us believe, but whether a death is visible. The tens of thousands of avoidable deaths that occur every year in the UK have become normalised – that is, largely invisible. People who died prematurely because their cancer diagnosis was delayed due to a long wait for a medical appointment or people who were victims of their unhealthy lifestyle usually died quietly, without TV cameras or journalists to report on what happened to them. In contrast, media coverage of COVID-19 deaths was ubiquitous. From the early footage of hospitals in Bergamo, Italy struggling to cope with the surge in COVID-19 patients, to the mounting death figures reported every day for months, COVID-19-related deaths were not just visible but under a constant spotlight. This further overshadowed the many other reasons people die unnecessarily, about which our society seems to be comparatively indifferent.

The visibility of avoidable death contradicts the story about the nature of our society, about what makes it morally superior to other societies past and present, according to which avoidable death is unacceptable. The myth of the caring society can perform its social-cohesion-building function and its orientating role only as long as a critical number of members of the society believe it is true. Avoidable death is not the myth's enemy as long as it is hidden; it is the *visibility* of avoidable death that threatens the myth and therefore the multiple agendas it serves, from nationalism, to helping individuals make sense of a disorienting situation, to making people feel safer in the face of a novel threat.

The problem is not just that the invisible avoidable deaths are neglected but that the pandemic measures added to them. The collateral damage to human life caused by lockdowns, particularly in the low-income countries outside Europe and North America, has been massive. From migrant workers who died of exhaustion on their long journey home on foot when India closed state borders, to countless children who did not receive their vaccinations and may die of preventable diseases, to deaths by starvation because of the economic collapse of fragile low-income economies, lockdowns have cost and will cost many lives. Reports have pointed out that in the UK, too, the healthcare system's narrow focus on COVID-19 will likely lead to tens of thousands of avoidable deaths in coming years due to diagnoses that were missed in their early stage. These potentially avoidable deaths are not receiving nearly the amount of attention or resources that were spent on preventing the deaths predicted to occur if lockdowns were not mandated.

The inconsistencies go even deeper. If unprecedented lockdowns were a just response to the pandemic, why are Western societies reluctant to take much more modest, less intrusive, and less costly measures against other causes of avoidable death? Why are health systems chronically underfunded, and why do epidemics of the "diseases of civilisation", such as obesity and domestic violence, go largely unaddressed? This illustrates that, rather than being a caring society, Western civilisation is structured around countless "us versus them" divisions. It attaches very different value to different lives and often turns a blind eye to preventable tragedies, depending on the who, where, and why of those affected. Indeed, Western civilisation sometimes trades avoidable death for "progress" – for example, in its willingness to normalise traffic casualties as an acceptable price to pay for greater mobility or to justify industrial accidents as part of economic growth.

The myth of the caring society did not just help justify the pandemic control policies of 2020–22; it also provides the cultural grease that helps turn the wheels of the world's globalised economy. While the international community set up a range of international organisations in the wake of the twentieth century's two world wars with the stated aim of promoting prosperity and human rights for all, the same institutions largely fail to challenge, and in some respects help maintain, a global economic system that runs on human sacrifice. By paying sub-subsistence wages to people in low-income countries and letting them work in often highly perilous conditions, the world economy essentially extracts economic value from the workers' shortened lifespans, trading life for wealth. In this system, protecting life is not about care for the individual, or even for entire communities, countries, or regions of the world, but is an imperative for protecting the economic stability of a nation when supranational capitalism is threatened by a mass loss of life – such as during a pandemic.

From myth to reality

In this chapter, I have argued that the pandemic policy of 2020–22 could not be consistently justified by appealing to the myth of the caring society. I have also argued that relying on the myth led to blind spots in policymaking among the elites and a collective sense-making of the pandemic across society, and that these blind spots resulted in deepened inequalities. What does this tell us about the relationship between myth and policy?

We cannot fully separate myth from identity, nor can we formulate policy that does not reflect our collective identity. While we might strive for evidence-based policymaking, the curation of relevant evidence and its interpretation and translation into action are value-laden processes through which society enacts its foundational myths. Put differently, myth-free policy is a myth.

But this does not mean there is nothing we can do to remove some of the collective blind spots resulting from the messiness of our culture. Arguably, preventing all avoidable death at all costs all the time is not realistic. Yet doing so selectively, as has been the case with COVID-19, undermines the very idea of the caring society the myth promotes. Recognising that we are vulnerable to these traps enables us to defetishise the myth and enter into a conversation with it, asking questions like: How do we reconcile care and equality? How can we make avoidable tragedies more consistently visible?

And, ultimately: How do we become a more caring society?

Note

1 According to reports by the investigative journalists Jonathan Calvert and George Arbuthnott (2021), this goal was ultimately not achieved. In their book *Failures of State,* the journalists documented the way British hospitals did get overwhelmed during the pandemic and people were unable to access care. They also pointed out the many years of budget cuts and policy choices that constrained healthcare capacity and had much to do with this outcome, quite apart from the issues of severity and the length of pandemic control measures.

References

Anderson, Benedict. 2006. *Imagined Communities: Reflections on the Origin and Spread of Nationalism.* London: Verso Books.

Calvert, Jonathan, and George Arbuthnott. 2021. *Failures of State: The Inside Story of Britain's Battle with Coronavirus.* London: Harper Collins.

Emmet, Dorothy. 1998. "Anthropologists on Myth". In *Outward Forms, Inner Springs: A Study in Social and Religious Philosophy,* edited by D. Emmet. London: Palgrave Macmillan UK: 44–56.

Geertz, Clifford. 1973. *The Interpretation of Cultures*. New York: Basic Books.

Green, Toby. 2021. *The Covid Consensus: The New Politics of Global Inequality*. London: Hurst & Co.

The Guardian. 2020. "The Guardian View on Lockdown for Britain: Necessary Hardship". *The Guardian*, March 23, www.theguardian.com/commentisfree/2020/mar/23/the-guardian-view-on-lockdown-for-britain-true-leadership-is-required

Johnson, Boris. 2020a. "Prime Minister's Statement on Coronavirus (COVID-19): 20 March 2020". *Gov.uk*, 20 March, www.gov.uk/government/speeches/pm-statement-on-coronavirus-20-march-2020

Johnson, Boris. 2020b. "Prime Minister's Statement on Coronavirus (COVID-19): 23 March 2020". *Gov.uk*, 23 March, www.gov.uk/government/speeches/pm-address-to-the-nation-on-coronavirus-23-march-2020

Malinowski, Bronislaw. 1984. "The Role of Myth in Life". In *Sacred Narrative: Readings in the Theory of Myth*, edited by A. Dundes. Berkeley: University of California Press: 193–206.

Office for National Statistics. 2021a. "Freedom of Information Request: Average Age of Those Who Had Died with COVID-19". *Office for National Statistics*, 11 January, www.ons.gov.uk/aboutus/transparencyandgovernance/freedomofinformationfoi/averageageofthosewhohaddiedwithcovid19

Office for National Statistics. 2021b. "Statistical Bulletin: Avoidable Mortality in the UK: 2019". *Office for National Statistics*, 26 February, www.ons.gov.uk/peoplepopulationandcommunity/healthandsocialcare/causesofdeath/bulletins/avoidablemortalityinenglandandwales/2019

Said, Edward. 1979. *Orientalism*. New York: Vintage Books.

4

DIGITAL SOCIETY, ALGORITHMIC HARM, AND THE PANDEMIC RESPONSE

Mark Wong

This chapter examines how policy responses to the COVID-19 pandemic have deepened the harms and injustice embedded in the exploitative designs of many technological platforms and digital infrastructures. The rapid surge in number of people and frequency of interacting with technologies using data-driven innovations – from big data analytics, automated decision-making, artificial intelligence/machine learning (AI/ML), to deep learning – is not only unprecedented but also deeply problematic. The policy failure to address the impact of this shift, particularly the algorithmic harms caused to people and communities who are most marginalised, has the potential to lead to irrevocable consequences on social justice and equity. The long-term human cost of the pandemic cannot be truly assessed if these harms are not fully accounted for and, more importantly, mitigated through inclusive and equitable innovation and policies.

Drawing on an interdisciplinary approach, this chapter examines the harms caused by the accelerated ubiquity of technologies known as "data-driven innovation" over the course of the COVID-19 pandemic. This chapter will highlight the importance of listening to the social science perspective to prevent exacerbating algorithmic harm in future pandemic and crisis responses and thereby to create a more equitable and inclusive digital society in the long-term.

Introduction

The COVID-19 pandemic had drastic and unequal impacts on people, communities, public health, and the environment, and it demanded urgent policy responses by states and governments across the world. However, these responses have fallen short in protecting the most vulnerable groups, and they have been exacerbating and deepening existing inequalities within and across nations (ILO, 2020). Such lasting impact, which we are only beginning to grasp, is often referred to as the pandemic's

DOI: 10.4324/9781003259336-6

"scarring" effect. The debate to date has largely focused on "economic scarring" – such as further economic precarity, income insecurity, and experiences of unequal opportunities and inequity in the labour market (Cook et al., 2021; Lee et al., 2020).

This chapter offers a new perspective in this debate by addressing how the harms caused by inequitable designs of technology and, specifically, biases embedded in AI and algorithms (that is, algorithmic harm) have been inadvertently exacerbated by the responses to the COVID-19 pandemic. Media and communication scholars, such as Crawford (2021) and Buolamwini et al. (2020), demonstrate that algorithmic harm disproportionately affects people who are most marginalised in society, including women, children and young people, LGBTQ+, disabled people, and Minoritised Ethnic communities. Some of these communities have also been disproportionally affected in regard to their health during the COVID-19 pandemic. The policy failure in many nations to address the negative impact of the surge in usage of technology that adopts data-driven approaches (for example, big data analytics, AI/machine learning, and automated decision-making) will lead to irrevocable consequences if it continues to be neglected. Urgent actions are needed in COVID-19 recovery policies to mitigate the exacerbated effects of algorithmic harm.

This chapter goes beyond merely looking at the issues and policy efforts in addressing the "digital divide" – that is, a narrow focus on the "haves" and "have-nots" in internet connectivity and access to technology (Livingstone and Helsper, 2007). It seeks a deeper and more critical reflection on the harms and injustice embedded, and sometimes *hidden*, in the exploitative designs of many technological platforms. Examples of algorithmic harms can be found in many digital infrastructures intertwined in people's everyday lives during the pandemic – for example, data processes involving algorithmic and automated-decisions in digital services (see Eubanks [2018] on examples in housing and public services), harmful recommendation algorithms with gender and racial biases (for instance in search engines and financial credit checks), and, more generally, the large-scale exploitation of environmental, labour and data resources in the Global North and South (Crawford, 2021).

Issues relating to algorithmic harm and injustice have been made worse by the forced and rapid increase in use of data-driven innovation. For example, access to general practitioners (GPs) and other health services have become "digital-first" in the UK during the COVID-19 pandemic – not only in terms of the shifting of GP appointments from in-person to video calls by default, but also with algorithmic processes being introduced for matching patients to health services and care. This shift is also found in the increased use of automated eligibility checks in financial services and insurance, data-driven approaches in determining allocation of public resources and housing, and automation in customer services, job/CV matching, and other digital services. Many of these services shifted to online and data-driven innovation rapidly, while in-person provisions had to be reduced or removed entirely.

Although some of these shifts were only accelerated in the pandemic, and not necessarily new, many national policies continued to ignore the algorithmic harm caused by digital transformations, which are currently incomplete and inequitable.

This took place in a context that other digital inequalities were also intensifying, for example in online education, digital health and social care, online social networks, and digital public and social services, which disproportionately impacted people who are historically marginalised (Eubanks, 2018; Pink et al., 2021). As will be demonstrated in this chapter, the pandemic response has inadvertently exacerbated algorithmic harm, as more people are being exposed to data-driven innovations that are inequitable in design. This chapter will draw from evidence mainly in Scotland and the UK more broadly to illustrate the extent to which algorithmic harms have been exacerbated by the gaps and inaction in the pandemic response policies. This chapter will discuss evidence that is currently emerging and highlight some early examples of algorithmic harm. While a comprehensive empirical study of the pandemic's impact on exacerbating algorithmic harm has yet to be conducted, it is clear that this concept is relevant to the pandemic as indicated by the emerging evidence available (see the section "Algorithmic harm in automated decision-making" for discussion).

It is worth noting that this chapter aligns with the position of many activists, community organisations, and media and communication scholars that benefits and opportunities afforded by technologies are not yet, but can be, equally shared. However, wealthy individuals and nations are currently most likely to benefit from technological innovation (Homes and Burgess, 2020; Kinyondo and Pelizzo, 2021; Matthewman and Huppatz, 2020). These innovations include applications of data science and big data analytics, artificial intelligence/machine learning, automated decision-making, and the Internet of Things – broadly defined as "data-driven innovations" in the social science literature and policy documents (Usher et al., 2020).

This chapter will argue that the long-term human cost of the pandemic cannot be truly assessed if the harms caused by data-driven innovations to equality, social justice, and well-being are not fully accounted for and, more importantly, mitigated through inclusive and equitable design of innovation and policies. Drawing on an interdisciplinary approach, this chapter brings together theories and concepts in digital sociology, science and technology studies (STS), media and communication studies, and social policy to present a new understanding and perspective on this debate. This chapter will highlight how these perspectives can improve policy responses and inform required actions, particularly in Scotland and the UK; as such, these perspectives may inform policy in other countries but need to be more specifically tailored to other cultural, geographical, and social contexts.

Listening to the perspectives of social sciences and humanities from the beginning in the policymaking and innovation process would help prevent exacerbation of algorithmic harm in future responses to pandemics and global crises, and would create a more equitable and inclusive digital society in the long term.

What are digital society and data-driven innovation?

The concept of digital society describes a new era in which we have witnessed a rapid global transformation of technology and society at the beginning of the twenty-first century (Redshaw, 2020). The nature, extent, and inequalities of the socio-digital transformation have attracted extensive public and academic debates across disciplines, from digital sociology, media and communication studies, STS, politics, and philosophy, to computer sciences, studies of human-computer interactions (HCI), and ethics (boyd and Crawford, 2012; Duncan, 2015; Nelson, 2002; Noble, 2018; Vallor, 2016). What is distinct about this era is the increased use and pervasiveness of technology in everyday life – from digital devices and social media to large-scale digital infrastructure based on a myriad of data, algorithms, and advanced computational tools such as artificial intelligence and automated systems (Campolo and Crawford, 2020). There is also an increased prevalence of smart technologies in our physical and social environments, such as the Internet of Things, environmental sensors, and facial recognition. This creates new realities and experiences in the age of digital society, as the "digital" becomes an integral part of what we do every day, how we communicate, and interweaving with the fabric of our societies and how we connect with one another as human beings (Wong, 2020; Couldry and Hepp, 2017).

During the COVID-19 pandemic, we witnessed a rapid and accelerated transformation of the frequency with which technology is used in our daily lives. Smartphones, virtual AI assistants, smart home devices, wearable technologies, and virtual and augmented reality and gaming, created by "big tech" companies and start-ups, were introduced into households and personal lives at a rapid and unprecedented speed while disguised in a grand vision of creating more and better social connections. However, this also means more data is being extracted from people during the pandemic, with little understanding of the ramification by those who are extracting or interpreting it, in order to seek understanding of a wide range of social, political, cultural, and economic activities and to predict human behaviours across the globe (Mejias and Couldry, 2019). This has created new opportunities to utilise data and data-centric approaches to interpret human life and potentially assist services in public, private, and third sectors such as health and education (Usher et al., 2020). In Scotland, for example, the COVID-19 vaccination programme has presented unprecedented opportunities for the Scottish Government and Public Health Scotland to collect a vast amount of new data on the population, with an aim of addressing health inequalities and the disproportionate impact of COVID-19 on certain groups, such as Minoritised Ethnic communities (Scottish Government, 2020).

The debate on the opportunities versus the risks of data-driven innovation is linked to the concept of *datafication* in media and communication studies. Mejias and Couldry (2019) highlight that data-driven innovation is underlined by the "processes of datafication that create digital data out of human life", and the authors go on to argue that as these processes and online platforms keep expanding, they perpetuate "the wider transformation of human life so that its elements can be a continual source of data" (Mejias and Couldry, 2019: 2).

The concept of human life becoming a continual source of data highlights one of the key causes for concern regarding data-driven innovation during the COVID-19 pandemic. More people, and hence more data, are becoming the targets of large-scale data extraction by not only the private sector and big-tech companies but also increasingly public and third sectors. For example, when citizens access digital services embedded in data-driven innovation and automated decision-making, their interactions with public or private services become subjected to datafication, often unknowingly or in a manner that is opaque to the users. This unprecedented surge in collection of data increases people's exposure to algorithmic harm embedded in the current designs of many data processes, AI, and digital infrastructure (Zuboff, 2019).

There are, therefore, two key concerns associated with the increased ubiquity of data-driven innovation during the COVID-19 pandemic. Firstly, the hasty and unquestioned pursuit of the transformation of human life into data, sped up manyfold compared to before, as will be further illustrated in the rest of this chapter. Secondly, the generation of various kinds of value, especially economic profits, in the ludicrous operations of collecting, mining, harvesting, storing, analysing, and selling data. Many online platforms and "big tech" companies (for example, Google, Facebook, Amazon, Apple, Tencent, and Alibaba) have been cunningly embedding these processes in the designs of their platforms and services. But due to the circumstances of the pandemic, these platforms have had a significant *boost* to how much data they are able to extract, and thereby exploit, from people across the world. The concept of datafication is, therefore, necessary to signal a historically "new method of quantifying elements of life that until now were not quantified to this extent", which is distinctly celebrated in the era of digital society and exacerbated, in terms of reach and speed, by the COVID-19 pandemic (Mejias and Couldry, 2019: 3).

How did the pandemic exacerbate algorithmic harm?

The pandemic led to a forced and accelerated reliance on technology in many aspects of people's everyday lives. This includes, for example, digitisation of work and hybrid working, communication and social interactions, online/blended learning, streaming entertainment, purchasing of goods, and access to health, financial, and public services (Bengtsson et al., 2021; Nguyen et al., 2021). Emerging evidence points to a conclusion that echoes many people's experiences of the COVID-19 pandemic, albeit in different ways, indicating a "surge in the use of digital technologies due to the social distancing norms and nationwide lockdowns" (De et al., 2020: 102171).

To highlight the scale of the increased levels of digitisation and datafication in the UK, for example, Ofcom's *Online Nation 2021* report estimated that "UK adults on average spent 4 hours 2 minutes online per day in April 2020" (Ofcom, 2021: 12). This was the greatest amount of time spent online in the UK ever recorded by its communication regulator, Ofcom. The pandemic has increased the population's reliance on digital platforms and hence their exposure to datafication and potential algorithmic harm. The *Online Nation 2021* report, using Comscore MMX Multi-Platform data, highlights a similar trend in other countries, including the United States, Canada, Brazil, Spain, France, and India, where the average time spent online per day has increased drastically since the start of COVID-19 pandemic (further illustrated in Figure 4.1). Some cities in the Global South, such as

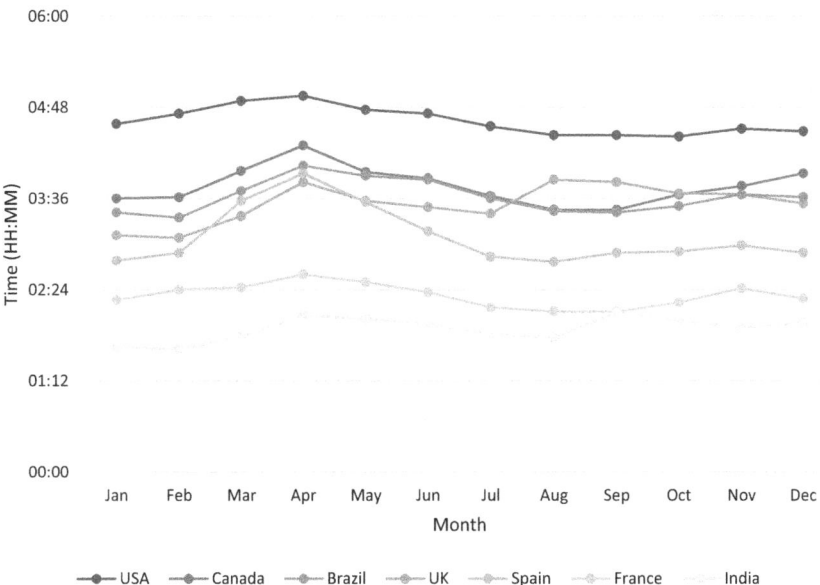

FIGURE 4.1 Average time spent online per day, by country, in 2020.

Source: Adapted from: Ofcom 2021, 16.

Bangalore, have seen an increase of up to 100 percent in online and internet traffic (De et al., 2020).

This evidence highlights an increased number of people across the world using technology and being more frequently subjected to datafication in their daily lives. This took place in a context where some people had been *forced* to access public, health, and financial services solely through online platforms while in-person services were shut-down, and some may never return to in-person provision. Similarly, the shift towards hybrid working, and increased reliance on remote-working technology that arguably increases workplace surveillance, is another alarming pattern that is affecting many people and can have a significant impact on the global geopolitics of work and datafication (Woodcock and Graham, 2019).

Regarding different types of technology, the surge in the use of digital platforms with video-calling functions has been one of the most drastic during the pandemic. Although they serve as an important means for communication and interpersonal interaction for people in countries where in-person gatherings have been restricted, their use significantly increased the data flow *relentlessly* extracted by these platforms for monetary value or training of AI and machine learning algorithms. In the UK, the proportion of people making video calls using online platforms (for example, Zoom and Microsoft Teams) was doubled (Ofcom, 2021). Zoom's total users increased to 13 million adults, representing a growth of nearly 2,000 percent in the UK alone in the period of the UK's spring 2020 lockdown (note that lockdown measures were a devolved matter in the UK, meaning England, Wales, Scotland,

and Northern Ireland had different lockdown measures but at times coordinated across the four nations). Microsoft Teams reached 13.7 million UK adult users in March 2021, with a drastic increase in usage in workplaces as well as in personal communications. Similarly, in the United States, Nguyen et al. (2021) found surges of a similar scale in uses of digital and online platforms, especially for personal communications.

What is the problem of accelerating digitisation and datafication?

What is left unchallenged in this surge are the harms and injustice that are *embedded* in these digital services and platforms, which people have been forced to use more frequently over the course of the COVID-19 pandemic. As the reliance on these platforms have grown, the datafication processes embedded in these platforms are subjecting more people to more harms, and thereby *amplifying* hidden structures of injustice. Inequitable and inherently exploitative power relations (such as the lack of transparency and access to data for users) are built into many of the current designs of data-driven innovations – whether intentionally or unintentionally. However, these platforms and data infrastructures have been left unchallenged to grow in both numbers of users and hours of usage during the pandemic. The process of replicating inequalities and power asymmetry in the design and use of data-driven innovation is what Virginia Eubanks (2018) calls "automating inequality".

When data and AI are used ethically, there are opportunities to design data-driven innovation for social good and for the benefit of people and our society (Usher et al., 2020). This has, however, not been considered or accounted for when the adoption of data-driven innovation sped up rapidly during the pandemic. The problems emerged and intensified when our everyday encounters became increasingly decided by machines and not by humans, and when digital services and data-driven innovation permeated more frequently and deeply into people's everyday lives during the pandemic. The automation of decision-making makes *complex* issues of social injustice into technological and system-engineering problems. The result is that it can harm people who are the most marginalised and deepen existing inequalities (Williamson, 2021).

The inaction of many national pandemic responses in addressing how technologies amplify and automate inequalities has enabled exploitative practices embedded in data-driven infrastructure to perpetuate. The pandemic response continued a long-standing pattern of turning a blind eye to the problems and harms associated with technological platforms, data processes, and algorithmic and AI biases, even when ample evidence demonstrates that they deepen systemic inequalities. The forced increase in the reliance on and use of data-driven innovation during the COVID-19 pandemic has led to an increased use of databases that can target, track, and punish people who are most vulnerable and in need of support and services. More importantly, the mining, storage, and linkage of data about people's behaviours and choices – on a second-by-second basis – have been magnified, with minimal scrutiny and policy regulation, as the time people spend on online platforms has surged. These data-driven innovations inevitably perpetuate and reproduce a system of power and control which compromises people's sense of self-determination (Eubanks, 2018).

Exploitative relations in data and algorithmic harms in a pandemic

It is important to recognise that the problem of neglecting the harms of technologies and data-driven infrastructure in policy is not new. However, it has become an "unintended consequence" to speed up the spread and reach of algorithmic harm during the COVID-19 pandemic, without the critical voices to question this shift. Such harms and injustice embedded in the design of many data-driven innovations have affected the everyday lives of billions of people across the world more intensively and deeply as people use technology more frequently (De et al., 2020; Ofcom, 2021). In some cases, the rapid surge of new users, such as for online learning platforms (for example, Google Classroom), is exposing more people to algorithmic harm for the first time (Williamson, 2021). Williamson also questions the "viral surge" in the use of – and misplaced trust in – algorithmic processes in education technology during the pandemic, and he highlights that

> the turn to algorithms as seemingly efficient and effective responses to public policy questions is a form of technological solutionism. This algorithmic worldview assumes that quantitative data analysis can provide accurate, objective, precise solutions to highly complex societal problems. But this assumption…obscures the fact that algorithms reflect the social contexts in which they are produced.
>
> *Williamson, 2021: 16*

The harms and injustice embedded in data-driven innovation, despite being neglected by policies, are in fact multifold (O'Neil, 2016; Crawford, 2021). This is a deeply problematic trend, as more people are becoming not only targets of exploitative datafication but also subjects of potential algorithmic harm. Exploitative relations of data embedded in people's use of technology have been allowed to grow – while policies have continued to sidestep them – and have been worsened by the increased reliance on data-driven innovation in the pandemic. Eubanks (2018) argues such inaction can be classified as form of "rational discrimination", as she highlights that

> rational discrimination does not require class or racial hatred, or even unconscious bias, to operate. It only requires ignoring bias that already exists. When automated decision-making tools are not built to explicitly dismantle structural inequities, their speed and scale intensify them, as discrimination and bias continue to be ignored.
>
> *Eubanks, 2018: 190*

This means that inaction in the pandemic response towards the exploitative and extractivist practices of data-driven infrastructure can, in fact, been seen as a form of rational discrimination. What could have been addressed in policies was the prevention and regulation of the escalating exploitation of data from people during the pandemic, especially of what is called behavioural data by Zuboff (2019) – for instance, clicks, app tracking, eye movement, finger gestures, and scrolling patterns. The vast amount of new data being collected by online platforms, data processes, and AI that we encounter as part of our everyday interactions in the pandemic is unfair and unjust.

By using these platforms and services more intensively during the pandemic, people are handling over their data, or more accurately, the *datafication* of their habits and behaviours, to these platforms – free of charge or at a cost to themselves. More users, across the world, are essentially turning into free labourers to generate the data that data-driven innovation mines, sells, trains AI with, and generates huge profits from. This is a form of exploitative global operation termed *data extractivism*. What is worse, many users have been scarcely aware that they are working for someone else's gain with every click they have been making throughout the course of a global pandemic.

Issues of data extractivism and algorithmic harm

Issues of data extractivism and algorithmic harm are most apparent in how data is being mined and harvested by commercial and "big tech" companies to create predictive insights and classifications of people (Crawford, 2021). Over the course of the COVID-19 pandemic, while more people use online platforms for longer period of time, more people are in fact being subjected to exploitative practices of data extraction and, worse, being exposed to harms embedded in the classifications of people by algorithmic and data processes. Such harms, often based on prejudiced and biased classifications of people into clusters of data points, are embedded in many of the designs of data-driven innovation being used more frequently and by more people during the pandemic. This has increased exposure of disproportionate harm to people and communities who are historically marginalised, especially Minoritised Ethnic communities, women, children and young people, LGBTQ+, and disabled people (see Noble [2018] for a detailed account of how algorithmic processes reinforce bias and prejudice against women and Minoritised Ethnic communities, for example).

In highlighting the risks of this shift, Zuboff's influential monograph *Surveillance Capitalism* underlines that "rights to privacy, knowledge, and application have been usurped by a bold market venture powered by unilateral claims to others' experience and the knowledge that flows from it" (Zuboff, 2019: 20). This evasion of people's rights is being strengthened and is permeating into more people's lives during the COVID-19 pandemic, and has hardly faced any resistance in pandemic policy responses. In this emerging economic order, private corporations claim even more human experiences as raw materials for endless extraction, prediction, and marketing and sales. This reinforces a power asymmetry between the companies and organisations that have the ability to extract and exploit people's data and the people who generate this data in the first place. The COVID-19 pandemic has meant more people are being forced into this inequitable transaction, and many people are becoming new data points in the planetary-scale datasets that private companies are creating, profiting from, and ultimately gaining more power based on.

Data-driven innovation is, therefore, not only transforming how we connect with one another; the algorithms and data architecture underpinning these connections are utilising surveillance of human and social interactions to generate several private corporations' own gains. What is worse, the expansion of datafication in social life during the COVID-19 pandemic has been reinforced and celebrated as the new logic of profiteering. Many companies collecting, storing, and selling data are benefiting from and growing rapidly over the course of this global crisis (Zoom and Microsoft being prime examples). However, the basis for monetisation is fixated on extracting as much data as possible from the human experience. The increased uses of online platforms and services during the pandemic has only perpetuated this hegemonic economic enterprise and sped up the adoption of these technologies.

This accelerated shift during the pandemic is best described by what Couldry and Mejias (2020) call *data colonialism*. They theorise the continuous appropriation of human life for the benefit of the few as a new mode of colonialism, and they argue that

> instead of territories, natural resources, and enslaved labour, data colonialism appropriates social resources. While the modes, intensities, scales and contexts of data colonialism are different from those of historic colonialism, the function remains the same: to dispossess.
>
> *Mejias and Couldry, 2019: 6*

As witnessed during the COVID-19 pandemic, governments and companies alike are increasingly seeking to use data-driven innovation tools, such as AI and facial recognition, to extract as much data as fast as possible, as this is one of the fundamental tenets of data-driven innovation. Couldry and Mejias (2020) compare such large-scale data-extractivist operations to "land grabbing", but what is being appropriated is human life through its conversion into data by many different sectors.

The COVID-19 pandemic, and more importantly the failure of pandemic response policies to address algorithmic harm, have created unprecedented conditions for data colonialism to *thrive* and to extend its reach and speed. More people are being exposed to the harms associated with data colonialism encoded into the logic of data-driven innovation, not only in the private sector and "big tech" companies but also increasingly in digital services in the public and third sectors. The extent to which these harms are being reinforced and replicated by the adoption of these technologies in the COVID-19 is yet to be fully determined. However, the lack of recognition of these harms in the pandemic response has only allowed them to perpetuate and grow.

The second, but arguably greater, issue at stake is the direct negative impact of algorithmic harm on people's livelihood and well-being. The exposure of more people to algorithmic harm, and more frequently, is increasing the risk that people will be denied access to much-needed health services, housing, financial products, insurance, and job opportunities, especially as people's need for these services has grown and changed with the economic impact of the COVID-19 pandemic (Cook et al., 2021).

Prejudice and unconscious bias can be encoded in data-driven innovation and data processes, which can reinforce sexism, racism, ableism, ageism, and other forms of injustice. When more people are being required to use (and are subjected to) automated decision-making to access services (for instance, automated eligibility checks and decisions on resource allocation) during the pandemic, the harm they can cause to people can be more direct and impactful. Evidence of the devastating impact of algorithmic harm on people who are historically marginalised is overwhelming (Noble, 2018). Unconscious bias is shown to be replicated in the algorithmic and data processes built into many digital services and platforms. These data infrastructures, which are being increasingly used during the pandemic, can be inequitable and socially unjust by design, especially as biases and prejudices are often not mitigated before the platforms and services are in use.

The failure of pandemic responses to protect citizens from deeper and more widespread algorithmic harm is, therefore, urgent. There is a need to strengthen regulations of large-scale data extractivism and surveillance capitalism, and to ultimately promote *inclusive* and *equitable* designs of AI and data-driven innovation, which have inevitable caused more harm to people during the COVID-19 pandemic than before. Pandemic policies have fallen short in safeguarding citizens from issues of bias, harm, and unjust social outcomes embedded in many automated decision-making systems and other forms of data-driven innovation. Citizens continue to have little or no access to or ownership of the data that is being extracted from them. The issues of inequity encoded in the design of many digital platforms, which have grown and expanded during the pandemic, can no longer be ignored.

Algorithmic harm in automated decision-making

It should be cautioned that algorithmic harm is particularly prevalent in automated decision-making systems, and this is where harm is mostly likely to occur and be detrimental to people's lives during the COVID-19 pandemic. One of the key reasons that data-driven innovation has gained momentum across the sector is its promise to make decisions, arguably more precisely, based on insights from real-time data. This is underpinned by the principle of enabling organisations and companies to automate decisions in their services based on probabilistic predictions about people generated from a large amount and various sources of data. For example, algorithms can be used to compute an individual's probability of repaying a loan or of having a certain health condition. This is seen as having the potential to remove the need for humans to make decisions and judgements, and it has become more commonly used and somewhat more attractive to different sectors during the COVID-19 pandemic, including governments and public organisations, health and social care services, energy companies, and the third sector. Increasing numbers of organisations in the UK are deploying and integrating data-driven approaches and automated decision-making. This approach claims to remove the need for interactions between humans in each transaction, and provides an arguably timely alternative that reduces workforce demand, which had become increasingly strained during the pandemic (e.g., technologies that check eligibility for insurance, process loan applications, and recommend decisions for referral to health services).

However, the use of data-driven approaches to automate decisions and services – despite becoming more widely adopted and accepted because of the pandemic – relies on algorithmic predictions. Algorithmic prediction produces hierarchies of "worth" and "deservingness" using statistical techniques, AI/machine learning, and data to make decisions or recommendations. These algorithms and data-driven infrastructures are found in social media, streaming platforms, and, increasingly since the pandemic, in public, housing, and financial services. They make decisions by creating profiles and classifications of people that not only measure the behaviour of individuals but also group "like with like". This approach creates an inherent power imbalance; evidence shows that it disproportionately harms the most vulnerable and historically marginalised communities, who are also most likely to be in need during the pandemic because of systemic injustice (Cook et al., 2021).

Crawford (2021) highlights that classicisation in AI and data-driven innovation is a problematic form of power, as it produces and limits ways of *knowing* and *constructing* identities, such as ethnicity and gender identities. Data about people, such as their ethnicity, genders, sexuality, and other characteristics, are *not* objective or neutral, however tempting it may be to assume otherwise. These are complex, political, cultural, relational, and dynamic identities. Algorithmic harms can intensify when these classifications of people are built into the designs and processes of data-driven innovation to make decisions during the pandemic (Commission on Race and Ethnic Disparities, 2021). They can replicate systemic racism, sexism, and other oppressive forms of injustice through classifications of people, and such unjust power structures are being intensified during the COVID-19 pandemic by the increased use of automated decision-making.

The existing evidence points to the prevalence of gender and racial biases in particular in decisions made by algorithms and AI, which can miscategorise people and reinforce sexist and racist assumptions. They reproduce systemic forms of oppression, such as those found in algorithms used in policing, criminal justice systems, and facial recognition technology (Crawford, 2019). Gaps in the pandemic response are particularly apparent in this case, as algorithmic injustices are neglected while harms are amplified by these systems being increasingly used and developed. Emerging evidence of algorithmic harm has been highlighted in facial recognition and automated decision-making introduced in the pandemic in education technology (Williamson, 2021). The Commission on Race and Ethnic Disparities' (2021) report also cautions against algorithmic harm caused to Minoritised Ethnic communities by the increased use of automated decision-making in the UK's public sector, calling for more transparent and fair algorithms and AI.

The fundamental problem, therefore, lies in the approach of automating decisions based on data and algorithms, especially when the users and people who these decisions are being made about have not been involved in their design. The inequitable design process of data-driven innovation ignores the unequal outcomes and harms caused to people in the data process and classification parameters. Algorithmic harms embedded in data-driven innovations need to be addressed and accounted for in any formulation and evaluation of pandemic responses, in order to fully mitigate the "scarring" effects of the pandemic.

Conclusion

This chapter concludes that the policy community needs to urgently address the issue of algorithmic harm due to the increased and intensified use of data-driven innovation technologies and automated decision-making during the COVID-19 pandemic. As the world continues to discuss "Covid recovery", we must acknowledge and rebalance the power and harms caused to individuals and communities, especially those who are historically marginalised.

We need to rebuild an inclusive digital society after the pandemic that does not cause more algorithmic harm, and to support people to mitigate such harm. This has to be one of the priorities in every nation and multinational organisations' plans for recovery from the COVID-19 pandemic (and from any future pandemics and global crises) in order to promote equity and social justice.

There are five value-led principles that are urgently needed, and which are the key policy recommendations of this chapter:

- Our innovation process needs to change by making sure the use of data and data-driven innovation is inclusive, fair, and equitable, and that data-driven innovation is used to benefit and meet the needs of people and communities, not just the few.
- Policymakers, industry, and the third sector need to work together to put policy, regulation mechanisms, and ethical standards and codes of practice in place to make sure data-driven innovation and digital services are *ethical by design*. The designs of all online platforms and digital services should be – by default – inclusive and non-harmful, and should meaningfully engage with citizens and marginalised communities in their design and development, rather than retrospectively working to reduce harm once the platforms are in use.
- We need to design platforms, services, and data processes that will not replicate or create new patterns of discrimination based on ethnicity/race, gender, age, and other intersectional factors.
- Bias need to be understood not just in terms of the accuracy of the data but also in terms of its outcomes for different groups of people. Data-driven innovation and AI need to be inclusive, accountable, and fair for all in both their design and the implications of their application.
- We need to recognise that data and classification (such as of ethnicity and genders) are *not* objective, neutral, or biologically detectable measurement and categories. Citizens should be included and heard in the development of any

classifications of people, and self-identification (and people's own perceptions of their identities) should be prioritised in data collection, analysis, and development of any predictive models.

One of the best ways to achieve the principle of "ethical by design" is to include the voices and input of people and diverse communities right at the start of the design and innovation process, rather than at the end (see Berditchevskaia et al. [2021] as an exemplary framework of a participatory approach to the design of AI for humanitarian crises). Policies should encourage, if not mandate, that citizens be engaged throughout the development pipeline of all AI and data systems. One example of this is the establishment of citizen panels (sometimes called citizen juries) and social living labs. Social living labs can be used as a participatory methodology in the research and development process. They encourage dialogues and deliberations among citizens, researchers, professionals and practitioners, policymakers, service and practice leaders, computer/data scientists, developers, and the industry to co-create practical solutions for social problems. *Social* living labs intentionally extend beyond the commercial and product-centred goals of more traditional living labs, and they seek to co-create *citizen-led* solutions and innovations to address issues identified by citizens; they help create solutions that prioritise the needs of communities and people (Hughes et al., 2018). Key to this is strengthening the capacity of historically marginalised groups to understand, articulate, and be supported and trained to help identify and reduce the biases and harms in data-driven innovation. Historically marginalised groups, with expertise in their lived experiences and other skills, should be considered *key* actors in an inclusive innovation and policy ecosystem.

There also needs to be a clear commitment to non-harm principles in digital policies – that is, platforms, companies, and organisations should have to show evidence that their use of data-driven intention is not and will not be harmful. If they cannot be sure, then they should not be allowed to do so. Regulatory bodies, such as Ofcom in the UK, should be given statutory responsibilities to regulate and approve ethical and fair use of data-driven innovations.

There needs to be more concrete and specific protection of people from algorithmic harm and injustice in policies, particularly in "covid recovery" policies. Such policies should regulate and monitor the exploitative practices of data-driven infrastructure and AI, not only from the "top down", from a policymaking or regulatory point of view, but they should also create ground-up solutions that involve the active participation of citizens and marginalised communities to uphold accountability and fairness. Fairness and equity should be prioritised over design convenience when designing and delivering digital services (Eubanks, 2018). The issues of justice, ownership, privacy, and digital rights of people should be more fully addressed as a priority in the pandemic response to reduce the effects and exacerbation of algorithmic harm.

To conclude, the urgent priority is to enable different sectors and communities to understand the lived experiences of people and the concerns, frustrations, and lived realities of digital technologies in people's lives during and after the pandemic. This understanding is crucial to help societies to truly realise the aspirations and opportunities that data-driven innovation can provide and to make sure these benefits of data are shared and inclusive for everyone. Inclusive innovation is key to mitigating the algorithmic harms that have been exacerbated by the pandemic response.

References

Bengtsson, T.T., L.H. Bom, and L. Fynbo. 2021. "Playing Apart Together: Young People's Online Gaming During the COVID-19 Lockdown". *YOUNG* 29 (s4): S65–S80.

Berditchevskaia, A., E. Malliaraki, and K. Peach. 2021. Participatory AI for Humanitarian Innovation. London: Nesta: https://media.nesta.org.uk/documents/Nesta_Participatory_AI_for_humanitarian_innovation_Final.pdf

boyd, d., and K. Crawford. (2012) "Critical Questions for Big Data". *Information, Communication & Society* 15 (5): 662–679.

Buolamwini, J., V. Ordonez, J. Morgenstern, and E. Learned-Miller. 2020. Facial Recognition Technologies: A Primer. https://global-uploads.webflow.com/5e027ca188c99e3515b40 4b7/5ed1002058516c11edc66a14_FRTsPrimerMay2020.pdf

Campolo, A., and K. Crawford. 2020. "'Enchanted Determinism: Power without Responsibility in Artificial Intelligence". *Engaging Science, Technology and Society* 6: 1–19.

Commission on Race and Ethnic Disparities. 2021. *The Report of The Commission on Race And Ethnic Disparities*. London: Commission on Race and Ethnic Disparities: www.gov.uk/government/publications/the-report-of-the-commission-on-race-and-ethnic-disp arities

Cook, J., S. Threadgold, D. Farrugia, and J. Coffey. 2021. "Youth, Precarious Work and the Pandemic". *YOUNG* 29 (4). Advance online publication. doi: 10.1177/11033088211018964.

Couldry, N., and A. Hepp. 2017. *The Mediated Construction of Reality*. Cambridge: Polity Press

Couldry, N. and U.A. Mejias. 2020. *The Costs of Connection: How Data is Colonising Human Life and Appropriating It for Capitalism*. Stanford: Stanford University Press.

Crawford, K. 2019. "Halt The Use of Facial-Recognition Technology until It Is Regulated". *Nature* 572 (565).

Crawford, K. 2021. *The Atlas of AI: Power, Politics, and Plenetary Costs of Artificial Intelligence*. New Haven: Yale University Press.

De, R., N. Pandey, and A. Pal. 2020. "Impact of Digital Surge during COVID-19 Pandemic: A Viewpoint on Research and Practice". *International Journal of Information Management*. Advance online publication.

Duncan, J. 2015. "Debating ICT Policy First Principles for The Global South: The Case Of South Africa". *Communication* 41 (1): 1–21.

Eubanks, V. 2018. *Automating Inequality: How High-Tech Tools Profile, Police, and Punish the Poor*. New York: St Martin's Press.

Homes, H., and G. Burgess. 2020. Coronavirus Has Highlighted The UK's Digital Divide. Cambridge: Cambridge University Press: www.cchpr.landecon.cam.ac.uk/Research/Start-Year/2017/building_better_opportunities_new_horizons/digital_divide

Hughes, H., M. Foth, M. Dezuanni, K. Mallan, and C. Allan. 2018. "Fostering Digital Participation And Communication Through Social Living Labs: A Qualitative Case Study from Regional Australia". *Communication research and Practice* 4 (2): 183–206.

ILO. 2020. ILO Monitor: COVID-19 and The World Of Work. Geneva: ILO: www.ilo. org/wcmsp5/groups/public/@dgreports/@dcomm/documents/briefingnote/wcms_ 740877.pdf

Kinyodo, A., and R. Pelizzo. 2021. "How COVID-19 Has Affected Africa's Development". *World Affairs* 184 (1): 57-76.

Lee, S., D. Schmidt-Klau, and S. Verick. 2020. "The Labour Market Impacts of the COVID-19: A Global Perspective". *Indian Journal of Labour Economics* 63 (s1): 11–15.

Livingstone, S., and E. Helsper. 2007. "Gradations in Digital Inclusion: Children, Young People and the Digital Divide". *New Media & Society* 9: 671–96.

Matthewman, S., and K. Huppatz. 2020. "A Sociology of COVID-19". *Journal of Sociology* 56 (4): 675–683.

Mejias, U.A., and N. Couldry. 2019. "Datafication". *Internet Policy Review* 8 (4): 1–10.

Nelson, A. 2002 "Introduction: Future Texts". *Social Texts* 20 (20): 1–15.

Nguyen, M.H., J. Gruber, W. Marler, A. Hunsaker, J. Fuchs, and E. Hargittai. 2021. "Staying Connected while Physically Apart: Digital Communication when Face-to-Face Interactions Are Limited". *New Media and Society*. Advance online publication.

Noble, S. 2018. *Algorithms of Oppression: How Search Engines Reinforce Racism*. New York: New York University Press.

O'Neil, C. 2016. *Weapons of Maths Destruction*. New York: Crown Publish Group.

Ofcom. 2021. Online Nation 2021. London: Ofcom. www.ofcom.org.uk/__data/assets/ pdf_file/0013/220414/online-nation-2021-report.pdf

Pink, S., H. Ferguson, and L. Kelly. "Digital Social Work: Conceptualising A Hybrid Anticipatory Practice". *Qualitative Social Work*. Advance online publication.

Redshaw, T. 2020. "What Is Digital Society? Reflections on The Aims And Purpose Of Digital Sociology". *Sociology* 54 (2): 425–431.

Scottish Government. 2020. *Expert Reference Group on COVID-19 and Ethnicity: Recommendations to Scottish Government*. Edinburgh: Scottish Government: www.gov.scot/publications/ expert-reference-group-on-covid-19-and-ethnicity-recommendations-to-scottish-gov ernment/

Usher, K., J. Clark, G. Collinson, and A. Lang. 2020. Powering Good: Insights from Nesta's AI for Good programme. London: Nesta: https://media.nesta.org.uk/documents/Poweri ng_Good_h7LLOiP.pdf

Vallor, S. 2016. *Technology And The Virtues: A Philosophical Guide to A Future Worth Wanting*. New York: Oxford University Press.

Williamson, B. 2021. "Education Technology Seizes a Pandemic Opening". *Current History* 120 (822): 15–20.

Wong, M. 2020. "Hidden Youth?: A New Perspective on The Sociality Of Young People 'Withdrawn' In The Bedroom In A Digital Age". *New Media and Society* 22 (7): 1227–1244.

Woodcock, J., and M. Graham. 2019. *The Gig Economy: A Critical Introduction*. Cambridge: Polity.

Zuboff, S. 2019. *The Age of Surveillance Capitalism: The Fight for a Human Future at the New Frontier of Power*. London: Profile Books.

5

AGAINST THE LOGIC OF IMMUNITY

Philosophy and the Epidemic

Michael Lewis

Introduction: *Quod* and *quid*

What can philosophy teach us about the events of the past two years?

Over the space of a very few months at the beginning of 2020, a consensus was formed regarding both a "novel coronavirus" and the response that was to be made to it. With the passing of time, along with the retention and recurrence of the measures taken, this consensus has hardened into a twofold dogma, affirming that one and only one conception of the pandemic and of the response to it is viable.

Both aspects of the COVID-19 dogma involve positing a certain differentiated multiplicity as if it were an undifferentiated unity or totality. The first aspect affirms that the dissemination and peril of the virus are total and it expresses this by employing the word "pandemic". This term connotes that disease is everywhere and a risk to everyone equally. The second aspect of the COVID-19 dogma affirms the same totality with respect to the predominant response to the virus: the police strategy of "lockdown" – legal confinement, isolation, and separation.[1] This was presented overwhelmingly as the only adequate response, and as applying everywhere to everyone.

But for philosophy, no dogma, nor indeed any statement, should in principle remain unquestionable. The very first questions that philosophy asks of any phenomenon fall under two headings: the "that" (in Latin, *quod*) and the "what" (*quid*): does it exist, and if so, what is its nature or essence? This makes it all the more surprising that most philosophers speak without blinking of a "pandemic" or in an even tone of "lockdown", as though these were affairs that went without question, to be doubted only by the illogical and the immoral – in a deranged howling that emanates from the margins of respectable discourse.

DOI: 10.4324/9781003259336-7

We might then summarise the thrust of the present work with the following questions: What is a pandemic (*quid*), and are we living through one (*quod*)? What is a lockdown (*quid*), and has there truly been one (*quod*)?

Quid: What is a "pandemic"?

Things are by no means straightforward here: the definition of "pandemic" has a history and is thus demonstrably mutable. The official definition was changed quite recently for the sake of a virus similar to the one that has come to monopolise our attention.[2] This alteration allowed a certain body (the World Health Organisation) to authorise itself in pronouncing the spread of that virus to constitute a pandemic.

The art of rhetoric demonstrates that the way in which one speaks about an event can have material effects. A pandemic encompasses all (*pan*) of the people (*demos*), everywhere. It is a powerful term, capable of justifying mitigation measures with an equally global, undifferentiated reach. The very utterance of "pandemic" was a crucial component in allowing unprecedented government measures to appear acceptable, even in liberal democratic regimes. As David Cayley has it,

> The declaration by the World Health Organisation that a pandemic was now officially in progress didn't change anyone's health status but it dramatically changed the public atmosphere. It was the signal the media had been waiting for to introduce a regime in which nothing else but the virus could be discussed.
>
> *Cayley, 2020a; compare Lévy, 2020: 79ff*

The use of the word "pandemic" has rendered the novel coronavirus especially visible, in such a way as to cloak in shadow every serious disease other than COVID-19. The virus was constituted as *the* pathogen of overriding importance, to the government, the media, and even the health services themselves.

Quod. Have we lived through a pandemic?

It is true enough to say that there is such a thing as a virus which received the abbreviated name SARS-CoV-2, although a virus is a particularly difficult entity to classify and even to isolate: it is neither living nor dead, and is in some respects a literal "non-entity". But is there a viral pandemic?

Seeing the future

The existence of such an event as a pandemic, the apparent effects of which we are continuing to live through, should be uncontroversially questionable. This is at least due to the fact that measures implemented in response to it are taken precisely in order to *pre-empt* the event's complete occurrence. Thus, no advocate of the *efficacy* of lockdown can straightforwardly assert that the pandemic is happening.

The actions that were taken to prevent the pandemic were, then, grounded not on something actual but on something possible, which was laid out in the form of a prediction that was based on a very particular model. In turn, these actions have been so extreme, and so prolonged, that they cannot but have retroactive effects on our perception of the magnitude of the event (the pandemic) that might have been but presumably was not (compare Cayley, 2020a).[3]

The model used for predicting the future is crucial here: the model chosen as the basis for government action against the spread of the virus predicted a future that was far enough beyond the scope of what could be addressed by conventional means that it was taken to justify the cruel and unusual actions that followed. It is one thing to attempt to present a reported state of the present as a pretext for action, but here action has been taken on the basis of a prediction with regard to the future which can never be verified, by definition, and which indeed was vigorously disputed.

Yet far from this ambiguous, forestalled status of the event leading to questions regarding the justice and proportionality of lockdown, it led, after a moment's uncertainty, to an exacerbated *faith* in lockdown's efficacy: it seemed to be implicitly believed that, in the absence of certain knowledge, what was needed was not critical appraisal but a simple and obedient belief in the rectitude of one particular set of predictions. Despite their very repetition and ongoing existence demonstrating them to be ineffective in terms of what they were said to be able to achieve, that these measures were the only ones taken (at least according to the mainstream media) and, at the same time, that the modelled predictions did not come to pass were accepted, implicitly or explicitly, as testimony to the correctness of those predictions and the actions which they urged.

Science and religion

Faith stands at the limits of reason, where predictions come to play the role of prophecy and scientists that of prophets. Accompanying faith are endless commandments simply to obey, promised messiahs, and the ostracising of heretics. This, together with the role given to "the Science" in political decisions, at least partly explains why the Italian philosopher Giorgio Agamben speaks of "Science as religion" in this context.[4]

The virus and the modelling of its predicted course were presented by those in power on the basis of what they described, in their infantilised and infantilising jargon, as "the Science" (often capitalised so as to stress its supposed univocity and authority). Here we find yet another one of the consensuses whose apparent totality philosophy is obliged to put in question. Science does not speak with one single voice; but it has been made to seem as if it does, with all dissenting voices drowned out by the combined forces of government pronouncements and an overwhelmingly subservient media.

Cayley, following Ivan Illich, has devoted himself to determining how the natural sciences in particular could have achieved such a hold over our political life.[5]

He demonstrates that in order to achieve sovereignty, one must first be seen to acquire *unity*, indivisibility. Political leaders can then allow themselves to say that in their actions they are simply "following" something unambiguous and unambiguously correct – "the Science". "Contemporary society is 'stunned by a delusion about science' [Illich]; this delusion takes many forms, but its essence is to construct out of the messy, contingent practices of a myriad of sciences a single golden calf before which all must bow" (Cayley, 2020a 2020b; compare Green, 2021: 15).

In the case presently under consideration, two moments in this construction of "the Science" may be identified as "political". Firstly, consider a panel such as the United Kingdom's SAGE committee (Scientific Advisory Group for Emergencies). A panel implies a multitude of voices; those in power must decide which views to give prominence to, which to represent, and which to act upon. Even if the decision simply amounts to a choice to go with the "majority", this very choice is itself political, or meta-political in the sense that it involves a decision regarding how politics should be conducted.

Secondly, consider an even earlier political decision, and one more likely to recede into a still deeper obscurity as a result: choices had to be made as to the very constitution of the panel itself, which determined the breadth of options from which the first decision selects, as well as the range of voices to be heard.

In both of these moments, some are heard while some are denied a hearing; in the first case, they speak and then are silenced, while in the second they are never allowed to speak at all.

Once this vision of "the Science" is presented by those who authorise themselves to enunciate it as such, the government and media can present a very particular "scientific consensus". This thrusts the voiceless alternative accounts into obscurity or, in order to avert this absolute violence, the fringes of "respectability" – the internet and its like – an advantageous gesture in that it allows them easily to be ruled out as merely crankish and the hegemonic position to be bolstered.

Statistics

Against this vision, Agamben has insisted on the concealed disunity of science: "There is no consensus among scientists – even if the media are keeping quiet about this" (Agamben, 2021a: 45; compare p. 10). It is this conflict and dissensus among scientists which allows the philosopher to open a question as to the nature and existence of the pandemic.

Agamben himself supplements the media's silence on dissenting scientific accounts of the virus by providing what he suggests should have been presented all along, and that is the overall daily mortality rates (1772 in Italy) (Agamben, 2021a: 43). He thus makes a point about the most basic intellectual "hygiene": figures presented in isolation, in sloganistic or imagistic form, are drained of significance. "The real texture of the epidemic can only be ascertained by comparing, in each instance, the communicated data with statistics (categorised by disease) concerning the annual mortality rate" (Agamben, 2021a: 44; compare pp. 47, 18;

compare Benvenuto, 2020). As an example, Agamben places the data relating to the recent coronavirus alongside those from previous years for cardiovascular disease, cancer, and respiratory diseases in general.

In addition to this, one has every right to question the reliability of whatever tests generate the ultimate number of cases, or more precisely infections, which do not necessarily lead to actual disease – another elided distinction, perhaps due to the obscure and motivated notion of the "asymptomatic", or a studied exaggeration designed to instil fear. These "cases" inevitably include false positives as a result of remnant RNA from earlier encounters with the same and related viruses. And we should not forget the well-known affair of the real causes of "Covid deaths" – with post-mortems barely carried out, if at all, comorbidities dismissed as irrelevant, deaths often simply presumed to be "*of* Covid" and sometimes urged to be or even rewarded for being so, the figures then presented in isolation from all other deaths, in a short-term manner, indeed daily, with all the distorting vulgarity of the running tallies presented in the morning papers.

Only answering such questions, which arise from the rejection of the very possibility of "the Science", would allow one truly to say that a pandemic is taking place.

Quod and *quid*: Lockdowns

The two philosophical questions that we have asked of the pandemic must also be asked of the response to it, and here they are still more tightly intertwined. This is because the relation between reality and (mere) appearance is rather intricate in the case of a lockdown. A lockdown cannot but present itself as total, and yet it can never be total. Thus, while it cannot strictly come to pass, it *can* come to pass in the sense that the very appearance of the existence of the totality that is a lockdown has serious material effects.

Any philosophical response to the mass enclosure of human beings has to begin from the fact that it is *not* universal – and from the fact that it was presented precisely as if it were, as if the command to "stay at home" could possibly be heeded by everyone. A lockdown is possible only if it excludes some people, and perhaps more than half the population: those who maintain "our" "essential services" – which is to say, those who allow us merely to survive. This is in large part the working class, to whom the message was never addressed and upon whom the potential for virtue and its all too public performance ("virtue signaling") were never bestowed.[6]

But the lockdown was applied beyond the boundaries of an individual culture. As the one single strategy of non-pharmaceutical intervention, it was applied globally. Everywhere it has produced desperately deleterious effects, even for the very physical health that it was supposed to be protecting, but in each case to different degrees depending on the character of the culture in question and on the consequent nature of the partiality of the lockdown. These effects and these differences, which testify to the partial character of a measure that must always appear to be total, have, like so much else, been thrust into obscurity.[7]

The essence of a lockdown is that of something which *cannot* be total: it destroys itself if it is; and yet it is something which must *present* itself as total, for any acknowledgement of an alternative strategy risks undermining its observance. In this sense, we can say that the lockdown both did exist and yet never could.

The time of lockdown

The strange totality of the lockdown also has a temporal aspect. These restrictions could be embarked upon only if a promise was made that they would eventually come to an end. This was presented as the moment at which non-pharmaceutical interventions could restore to the pharmaceutical its rightful place: the arrival of the vaccines. As must happen when such a role is assigned to an advent, the apparent arrival of the messiah in actuality introduces problems of its own, since the question must arise as to whether *this* messiah is true or false.

But irrespective of their quality and effects, given the function that they serve in bringing with them the promised end, the vaccines are urged – and even forced – upon adult and child, with a tireless manipulative aggression perhaps even more total than that with which the lockdown was urged. The vaccines are in no sense purely a medical matter: they are political in embodying the price for re-entering human community following its closure. Their function is not simply – perhaps not even primarily – to eradicate the disease but to restore normality, or at least to reiterate the promise of normality, or to render that promise more concrete.

The rhetoric of civil war

Given its untested nature and the immense damage that it was always certain to cause, and given that it cannot even exist in its supposed totality, how could lockdown have been presented and accepted in such a unanimous way? We have no space to deal with all of the strategies employed, in a way and through channels so numerous that they truly warrant the title "totalitarian" (compare Caduff, 2020, 467–487; Han, 2021a: ch.15), but we might profitably investigate a certain pervasive rhetoric that has been used effectively to quell dissent and to marginalise opponents, as well as to conceal the partiality of what is rightfully total: the language of war. The particular character of this discourse may supply the clue that leads to the heart of the epidemic itself.

The language of war has in general proliferated after the dissipation of the Cold War, which spelled the end of international war and marked the beginning of an era of "civil wars". In this context, the language of war has been generalised and turned on the unity of the social body itself, so as to instigate a battle designed to exclude certain parts of it as (internal) "enemies". We can wage war on crime, on drugs, on terror, on certain social attitudes, and finally on the virus – and by extension on those who appear to us as its advocates, who would let it roam free rather than keeping it locked up and controlled, along with its potential bearers. Thus, the body politic is purified of immanent disorder.

As Cayley points out, the rhetoric of war immediately affirms that the situation is one of crisis, and that there are only two sides, friend and enemy, *pro* and *contra*, diametrically opposed, without any third position available. This patriotic language stirs and sways us by means of its emotional character, and it "moralises" the entire situation: to be on the "other side" is not simply to adopt a position which is false, it is to be guilty of disloyalty and immorality (Cayley, 2020a).[8] Even if dissent were grounded in something true, to give voice to it would be wrong.

The logic of immunity

A body can be at war with itself such that a certain part of it must be sacrificed in order for it to survive. This would be to restore the body to full health by "immunising" it. The efficacy of the language of war in the context of the police strategy, together with its pervasive character, may be explained by the fact that it reflects something of the logic of the lockdown itself.

What was the general structure of the argument for the restrictions placed on human life over the last two years? It was that certain aspects of human life had to be sacrificed if they were ever to be enjoyed again. Crucially, even if the promise of this future was indefinite, the promise had to be at least implicitly made in order to ensure that the measures would appear temporary.[9]

That a certain portion of ourselves should be sacrificed, temporarily or in part, in order that our identity might be protected is a logic that Jacques Derrida was among the first to speak of by analogy with *immunisation*.[10] If one is fighting against an enemy – a disease, for example – one does not reject it altogether, but rather one takes within oneself a milder form of that disease. One does this in order to build up a certain protection against any more extreme version of the same that one might encounter in the future.

Generalising this logic, any notion which attempts radically to exclude its opposite from its own identity from the very outset can only fail to be what it is.

To render this more concrete, let us return some flesh to the bare bones: democracy can never be *purely* democratic *if it is to be democratic*; the cases which demonstrate this most clearly are those in which a non-democratic party seems likely to be democratically elected, having promised, if elected, to abolish the democratic process. In order to avert this greater evil, democracies have to be prepared to *suspend* democracy, temporarily, in order to save themselves, and thus they are required by democracy itself to act undemocratically.

Analogously, contemporary advocates of lockdown assume that to reduce human life temporarily to a subhuman life of isolation, distance, and invisibility is an acceptable price to pay for the survival of humanity. Indeed, this is the only way to achieve an immunity that "we" apparently do not yet possess. We simply have to survive in order later on, perhaps, to live more fully.[11]

But such an immunising, sacrificial procedure is not without its risks, for even though it may be intended to save the very thing that it sacrifices, it is always possible that one becomes so rigid as to permanently assume the guise of one's opposite: the logic of immunity always risks slipping into an excessive version of itself that would amount to *auto*-immunity. In this state, the imbibing of the poison fails to function as it ought, perhaps due to excessive incursion or an adverse reaction *to* that ingress on the part of the organism's immune system. Thus, the measures taken to protect one's identity end up destroying it: democracy tips over into tyranny; the temporary suspension of human life becomes permanent; the exception becomes the rule or the "new normal".

Against the logic of immunity

Agamben has identified something like this auto-immune and self-sacrificing loss of identity in the recent epidemic: the scandal of churches closing their door to the new lepers or Jews – those actually ill and those only potentially ill; the cancellation of funerals and marriage; the closure of education and most aspects of human culture; the prohibition of love and friendship. All of which has legally or normatively *demanded* that human beings sacrifice crucial parts of their very humanity. Agamben tends to accept, in his own way, Aristotle's enduring definitions of the human being as the linguistic and rational animal (*zōon logon echon*) and as the political animal (*zōon politikon*); the lockdown, which separates human beings from one another, has undoubtedly stifled the very conditions for linguistic and political life.[12]

Although Agamben himself does not put it in quite these terms, we might elucidate his opposition to the lockdown by demonstrating how his own logic differs strikingly from the logic of immunity.[13] This will help us to elucidate such statements as the following, which in his writings on the epidemic themselves Agamben tends to leave unexplained: "The false logic is always the same: just as it was asserted in the face of terrorism that freedom should be abolished in order to defend freedom, now we are told that life has to be suspended in order to protect life" (Agamben, 2021a: 28); "A norm which affirms that we must renounce the good to save the good is as false and contradictory as that which, in order to protect freedom, imposes the renunciation of freedom" (Agamben, 2021a: 37).

Bare life

To establish the falsity of this logic of immunity, Agamben identifies a presupposition tacitly made by the advocates of lockdown: that a particular form of life, like the human being's, can be distinguished from the *un*qualified, *un*formed life upon which it would be founded. This presupposition must be made by any argument which advocates the temporary reduction of a full human life to sheer naked survival, in accordance with the logic of immunity, which demands that we constrain the same for the sake of the same.

This diminished life of sheer survival is in some contexts described by Agamben as "bare life" (*nuda vita*), a life denuded of any potential beyond that of simply dying, with even that terminal decision lying in the hands of whoever it is that wields power in that particular community or setting: the "sovereign", whether it be a single figure, as in monarchy, autocracy, or tyranny, a group of people, as in oligarchy and aristocracy, or the whole civilian body, as in a certain kind of democracy; it can even be a doctor or a scientist.

Biopolitics

The manner in which the administration of life and health is not just a "good" or a right but also a political and legal *obligation* is investigated by the theory of "biopolitics".[14] This is the doctrine according to which matters of life and death have become – or have always been – the concern of (political) power.

As Michel Foucault puts it, in the Modern Age, beginning, in his categorisation, around the end of the eighteenth century, power is applied in the name of *life*, in all its variegations, and of the vitality of this life – its health: "Power is situated and exercised at the level of life, the species, the race, and the large-scale phenomena of population. [...] One might say that the ancient right to *take* life or *let* live was replaced by a power to *foster* life or *disallow* it to the point of death" (Foucault, 1998: 137–138).

For Agamben, biopolitics is much older: a certain sovereign power over life and death may be found from the very beginning of the history of the West.

In the Ancient Greek world, according to Agamben, life, along with its various capacities, from nutrition to reproduction, was not regulated by the laws instituted by the sovereign to govern the life of the city (*polis*); life was instead fostered in the home (*oikos*). And yet, this very distribution was effectively carried out *by* the sovereign himself.

We can understand the significance of this in the following way: the private biological life of the home and the political and linguistic life of the city might – at least in hindsight – be identified with the Greek terms *zōē* and *bios* respectively. If so, then the act of distinguishing between these two notions, the act of separating bare life from a fuller kind of life, presupposes that the one who makes the distinction wields a certain amount of power over *both* forms. This includes the life of the home and those associated with its upkeep – in the Greek world, women and slaves – for those confined to the home were thereby forcibly excluded from civic life, which alone counted as properly human. What these domestic animals were was effectively decided upon by the sovereign, even if the laws he made were null and void once the threshold had been crossed.

For Agamben, what has changed in the Modern Age and even more so in the twentieth century is that this exclusion is carried out by different and more paradoxical means: the bare life that was included within the purview of the sovereign's power purely by means of exclusion is now quite explicitly included within it. Indeed, the sphere in which political power operates most fulsomely is that of "mere life" – the health, life, and death of human beings understood in the statistical form of populations or demographics. What was once considered to be an external separation between two spheres and two distinct groups of human beings, the *polis* and the *oikos*, has now become a division *internal* to each human being: one has one's properly human life, and, distinct from that and absolutely subjected to political power, one's anonymous bare life. It is by virtue of this bare life, remarkably, that one participates in civil life, since it comprises the primary mode whereby one falls within the dominion of the sovereign.

All of this is to say that the very separation between qualified human life and subhuman bare life is itself effectively the deed of the sovereign, or at least the result of a certain history of this power's transfigurations, and an incontrovertible sign that sovereign power is in play.

Speaking of the separation of life "into a purely biological entity on the one hand, and a social, cultural, and political existence on the other", Agamben suggests that, "what the virus has shown clearly is that people believe in this abstraction".[15] And for good reason: (medical) technology has made such a separation effectively possible, with artificial respiration and other technologies which suspend the half-dead in a kind of undead life, a zone halfway between life and death or at the point of their overlapping. Such is the power of modern medicine.

But what is crucial for Agamben is that this separation of bare life and qualified human life – and the power of the doctors and scientists who were able to install it – be rigorously confined within the walls of the hospital and *not* allowed to operate within the city beyond. And yet this is exactly what has happened over the last two years, with the result that bare life, held within the grip of the sovereign medico-scientific power, has become the model, legally mandated in many cases, for all social life: "This body, artificially suspended between life and death, has become the new political paradigm by which citizens must regulate their behaviours" (Agamben, 2021a: 64).

On Agamben's account, any argument which appeals to this separation is effectively relying upon – and by extension accepting – both sovereign power and its attribution to medicine and science. Agamben's entire political philosophy has devoted itself to finding a way, once and for all, to *disable* this type of power structure and to seek out new ways in which communities may be bound together – beyond sovereign power, its law, and the separation of public and private life, and thus beyond the production of any such thing as bare life.

Thus, Agamben's critics misunderstand his reproach to *them* when they protest that they are not solely valorising the survival of bare life over human life but are merely protecting that bare life in order later to restore a properly human life (compare Berg, 2020). Agamben's reproach is most fundamentally that this temporary suspension of human life amounts to an endorsement of the existence of a transcendent sovereign power.[16]

This may be presumed to be one of the principal roots of Agamben's repeated assertions that the conditions imposed by lockdown and its logic of immunity cannot provide the foundation for a *new* community, as many of his fellow philosophers at least temporarily allowed themselves to believe: "I do not believe that a community based on 'social distancing' is humanly and politically liveable" (Agamben, 2021a: 31). Elsewhere, he speaks of the community that follows when one is subjected to that most renowned image of sovereign power, the Leviathan: "Only tyranny, only the monstrous Leviathan with his drawn sword, can be built upon the fear of losing one's life" (Agamben, 2021a: 24–25).[17]

Visions of an immune community are ultimately visions of a society under the sway of sovereign power and so hinder us in thinking a new form of communal relation. They prolong the old in a distorted form that emphasises its most malign aspects, while stifling the new.

Notes

1 The official jargon makes no secret of the fact that this is a police response: "lockdown" was a term blessedly unfamiliar to English audiences before March 2020, and it comes to us on loan from the lexicon of American law enforcement. To underline this point, Donatella Di Cesare speaks of "house arrests" (*arresti domiciliari*) (Di Cesare, 2021: 84; compare 89, 90), as does Peter Sloterdijk, speaking of France's "*Hausarrestregeln*" (Sloterdijk, 2021: 20).
2 For a summary of this history, compare Green (2021) pp. 163–166.
3 Much ink has been spilt over the question of whether the epidemic constitutes an "event". Those who affirm that it does seem largely to do so in order to accuse those who attempt to understand it (in terms of their own established position) of a "philosophical narcissism" which refuses to accept that (their) thought and philosophy cannot truly conceive it (Penzin, 2020; compare inter alia, Ronchi, 2020; Smith, 2020). Without prejudging the matter, this approach runs the risk of a certain piety regarding the event which in other forms may bolster the religious aspects of the police response that we identify elsewhere.
4 Agamben speaks of the religions of both science and medicine (Agamben, 2021a: 45, ch. 12 passim, inter alia), and even "health-religion" (ibid., 97), even though he does not explicitly draw the analogy between prediction and prophecy.

Agamben's writings are among our principal inspirations in the present work. Those of his texts on the epidemic not collected in *Where are we now?* may for the most part be found on the website of his publishers, Quodlibet: www.quodlibet.it/una-voce-giorgio-agamben, while his most recent interventions with Massimo Cacciari on vaccination and its certification may be found here: www.iisf.it/index.php/progetti/diario-della-crisi/date/2021/8.html?catid=35

Of all the philosophers who have written about the events here under discussion, Agamben has been the most unwavering opponent of the measures taken. A greatly expanded version of the present article, under the title 'Review-Essay: Giorgio Agamben, *Where are we now?* & Other Writings (Journal of Italian Philosophy 5 (2022), may be consulted by the reader interested in gaining a more acute sense of the scope of Agamben's interventions, and of their consequences, which have involved him effectively being ostracised from international academia and respectable society more generally.

That said, the experience of expulsion has allowed him to formulate a new and critical relation to the institution as such, as he has found refuge in other, para-institutional groups. These associations have proliferated within the largely stifled resistance to the extreme measures that continue to be inflicted upon Italian social life: "In these conditions, without laying down every possible instrument of immediate resistance, the dissidents need to think about creating something like a society within society, a community of friends and neighbours within the society of enmity and distance. The forms of this new clandestinity, which will have to become as autonomous as possible from institutions, will have to be meditated upon and experimented with in each case, but only they can guarantee human survival in a world that has devoted itself to a more or less conscious self-destruction"

(Giorgio Agamben, 'Una comunità nella società' [A Community Within Society], www.
quodlibet.it/giorgio-agamben-una-comunit-14-ella-societa?fbclid=IwAR3YdHDt
3XO2q8AQTXsc_kPG3StvVndUV5NUP39-MJPxPd2Ef2jOFduDUyk, 17th
September 2021).

The text by the present author referred to above broaches the larger question of
an innovation in the realm of *logos* (thought and language) – although its real age is
uncertain – which has adopted as its strategy a relegation of a perceived enemy to the very
margins of *logos* itself, such that rational discussion between opponents is no longer even
countenanced. Thus we witness the most extreme form of *negation* imaginable (which has
taken the name, once raised by Hegel to the most elevated level of philosophical terminology, "cancellation" [*Aufhebung*]) in which a proposition or set of statements is simply
expelled from the realm of what can be entertained rationally, and banished to the realm
of the illogical and the immoral – effectively the mad, bad, and dangerous to know. We
have seen nothing but this logic from the very start of the recent dalliance with totalitarianism as a remedy for illness. Perhaps this exacerbation of a failure within reason itself
(or its widespread acceptance) will in the long run prove to have been the most serious
aspect of the whole affair.

We have yet to discover the proper way in which to speak of this frightening turn of
events, or to unearth its genealogy, which might be traced back as far as the notion of
"excommunication" or even "exile" more generally (this is why we evoke the uncertain
vintage of this phenomenon). Agamben's case stands as a troubling metonym for this
experience, which has been much more broadly felt by anyone who has been moved to
adopt an attitude that is in any way critical of a hegemonic position with regard to the epidemic and much else besides, particularly in the contemporary academy. For *philosophers*,
obliged to ask for reasons and thus to engage critically with any statement, even one
that presents itself or is presented with an air of unimpeachable obviousness, the risk of
ostracisation is particularly acute.

5 Donatella Di Cesare has devoted an important chapter to the topic of "Government by
Experts: Science and Politics" (Di Cesare, 2021: 50ff), which is more than can be said for
anglophone philosophers of science, who should at precisely this moment have come into
their own.

6 Slavoj Žižek, in his generally confused contributions, has at least insisted upon this point
from very early on (Žižek, 2020: 26; compare 122). Working at home was always a middle-
class prerogative, and this allowed a group whose voice was more readily heard in the
media to embrace the transvaluation of values that occurred in almost every aspect of our
relations to our fellow man in a way that the working class could not.

7 On the impact of the police response on the third world, compare Green (2020), especially Chapter 3. Compare Broadbent (2020). And in relation to the differential effects of
a single action when it comes to sex, race, and immigration, compare the Introduction to
Mitropoulos (2020).

8 Along with Agamben, Byung-Chul Han has written on the analogies between the war on
terror and the supposed war on the virus: "At airports everyone is treated like a potential
terrorist. […] The virus is a terror in the air. Everyone is suspected of being a potential
carrier of the virus, and this leads to a quarantine society, which, in turn, will lead to a
biopolitical surveillance regime" (Han, 2021b: 18). Here we are a step beyond even the
war on terror, for here we must treat even *ourselves* with suspicion.

9 Toby Green, having shown that the damage to bare life caused by lockdowns outweighs
the most extreme predictions of what might have been inflicted by the disease itself,
understands this not as the sacrifice of the present to the future, but of the future to the
present (Green, 2020: 28, 80).

10 To spare the reader a long series of references and citations, let us refer here to the present author's "Of (Auto-)Immune Life: Derrida, Esposito, Agamben" (Lewis, 2015).

11 "Today – waiting for a vaccine, that is, induced immunity – immunisation by distancing is the only line of resistance behind which we can, and must, barricade ourselves. At least until the threat subsides" (Esposito, 2020b: 77). Esposito pits his own position directly against Agamben in these terms: "I personally believe that the defence of life is a value superior to any other – if only because it is presupposed by them [these other values]: in order to be free or to communicate with others, one must first be alive" (Esposito, 2020b: 78). Though, for a nuance of this position, compare Esposito (2020a) and (2021). For a representative but less philosophically interesting example of the same kind of critique of Agamben, compare Berg (2020).

12 Agamben (2021a), Chapter 19; compare Agamben (2021c).

13 This perhaps casts a new light on Agamben's response to the vaccine as it developed from Agamben (2021b) onwards, which treats it solely in the context of the human being's reduction to bare life, before gradually developing an increasing concern regarding its safety (Agamben, 2021f) and the way in which a certain coercion replaced actual legislation that could simply render vaccinations compulsory but at the cost of rendering the state liable for the consequences (Agamben, 2021d, 2021e, 2021g, culminating in two texts written with Massimo Cacciari, op. cit., inter alia).

14 "The citizen no longer has a right to health[…]but is instead forced by law to be healthy ("biosecurity")", to secure and protect health and the services which maintain it (Agamben, 2021a: 56). Even the *potential* for unhealthiness is enough to warrant legally mandated confinement or curfew. For similar worries concerning a legally obligatory, fully immune community, compare Di Cesare (2021), 63, 76–77.

15 Compare: "We have divided the unity of our vital experience – which is always and inseparably corporeal and spiritual – into a purely biological entity, on the one hand, and a social [*affettiva*] and cultural life, on the other" (Agamben, 2021a: 35), "If this condition is extended beyond the spatial and temporal boundaries that pertain to it – as is presently being attempted – so that it becomes a sort of social behaviour principle, we may fall into contradictions from which there is no way out" (Agamben, 2021a: 35, translation modified).

16 This is why we should not presume that Agamben himself is making the same separation that he accuses the current regime of making and simply valorising the other (separated) half. To demonstrate this and explicate its meaning would take a much more extended reading of Agamben (one which has only just begun to take place), but it rules out the reciprocal accusation according to which sacrifices are taking place on both sides.

Here one would have to raise the whole question of what alternative "solution" to the problem of the epidemic we might be offering, and this would be the place for a proper consideration of "herd immunity", even at the risk of establishing the simple opposition that proponents of lockdown have created precisely by rubbishing this alternative to the police strategy, one in which effectively one either controls or loses control (a telling way of putting the matter). The reasoning behind this points towards yet another false totality in which the differentiated susceptibility of the civilian body was elided so as to depict an almost entirely fabulous situation in which "we" were "all in it together", and in which everyone had to keep the other safe and be kept safe in turn: to acknowledge this differentiation is to allow the strategy effectively to draw nearer to that of "*focussed* protection", and to elide its supposedly "sacrificial" character.

It is not clear that dying as such was not simply understood as something that could or should ideally not happen at all. This positing is at least something that is risked by the extreme character of the taboo on death in our culture. The absolute aversion to death's public visibility is a significant factor in at least the efficacy of the media strategy in bolstering the repressive "solution" to the epidemic.

17 On the connection between tyranny and fear, compare Dodsworth (2021), p. 94. Agamben has been accused of exaggerating the connection between the now proven manufacturing of fear and true "totalitarianism", but this book, for all its journalistic limits, demonstrates that those charged with "behavioural control" found themselves compelled to employ a similar vocabulary (compare Rayner, 2021).

References

Agamben, Giorgio. 2021a. *Where are we now? The Epidemic as Politics.* Translated by Valeria Dani. London: Eris.

Agamben, Giorgio. 2021b. "La nuda vita e il vaccine". Quodlibet, 16 April, www.quodlibet. it/giorgio-agamben-la-nuda-vita-e-il-vaccino.

Agamben, Giorgio. 2021c "Il volto e la morte". *Quodlibet*, 30 April, www.quodlibet.it/giorgio-agamben-il-volto-e-la-morte?fbclid=IwAR2jSwf_yQnm2CwDascKhLMQjds0dsZO bO70ClEuIPfRmv0RUv8j3Dxoj7A, 3rd May 2021

Agamben, Giorgio. 2021d. "Cittadini di seconda classe". *Quodlibet*, 16 July www.quodlibet. it/giorgio-agamben-cittadini-di-seconda-classe?fbclid=IwAR3EyZ1PBQFb3qjdbeXIu zKxvhPPQhfSiNBaT0YHvyZ4i_WrKzy8i27_ApA

Agamben, Giorgio. 2021e. "Tessera verde". *Quodlibet*, 19 July, www.quodlibet.it/giorgio-agamben-tessera-verde?fbclid=IwAR0Aiue5ZXKeT3jEzqp9c0Lrvets2klmmofG-oLZ oFhCom5rzTwYbDfImdY

Agamben, Giorgio. 2021f. "Uomini e lemmings". *Quodlibet*, 28 July, www.quodlibet.it/giorgio-agamben-uomini-e-lemmings?fbclid=IwAR2yon-vSihGKn0tE0LUENgMmojSIMZ9 oEml2Q8T5jpioHTRmx0FNkmxThw

Agamben, Giorgio. 2021g. "Non discutiamo le vaccinazioni ma l'uso politico del Green Pass". *La Stampa*, 30 July.

Agamben, Giorgio. 2021h. "Una comunità nella società". *Quodlibet*, 17 September, www.quodli bet.it/giorgio-agamben-una-comunit-14-ella-societa?fbclid=IwAR3YdHDt3XO2 q8AQTXsc_kPG3StvVndUV5NUP39-MJPxPd2Ef2jOFduDUyk

'Benvenuto in clausura', Antinomie, https://antinomie.it/index.php/2020/03/05/benvenuto-in-clausura/, 5 March 2020. 'Welcome to Seclusion', European Journal of Psychoanalysis, https://www.journal-psychoanalysis.eu/articles/coronavirus-and-philosophers/, 3 March 2020.

Berg, Anastasia. 2020. "Giorgio Agamben's Coronavirus Cluelessness". *The Chronicle of Higher Education*, 23 March, www.chronicle.com/article/giorgio-agambens-coronavirus-cluel essness/?bc_nonce=pb1u7aangzpjor9revr5wp&cid=reg_wall_signup

Broadbent, Alex. 2020. "Lockdown is wrong for Africa". *Mail and Guardian*, 8 April, https:// mg.co.za/article/2020-04-08-is-lockdown-wrong-for-africa/

Caduff, Carlo. 2020. "What Went Wrong: Corona and the World after the Full Stop". *Medical Anthropology Quarterly* 34 (4), 467–87.

Cayley, David. 2020a. "Questions about the current pandemic from the point of view of Ivan Illich". *Quodlibet*, 8 April, www.quodlibet.it/david-cayley-questions-about-the-curr ent-pandemic-from-the-point

Cayley, David. 2020b. "Pandemic Revelations". *David Cayley*, 4 December, www.davi dcayley.com/blog/category/Pandemic+2?fbclid=IwAR2fID6gWCw4AjCSIl-_ QYlfQgtUv04PsmtsAaoFDZvdnhpY9HqFUE1QZT4

Di Cesare, Donatella. 2021. *Immunodemocracy: Capitalist Asphyxia*. Translated by David Broder. Pasadena: Semiotext(e).

Dodsworth, Laura. 2021. *A State of Fear: How the UK Government Weaponised Fear during the COVID-19 Pandemic*. London: Pinter & Martin.

Esposito, Roberto. 2020a. "Vitam instituere". Translated by Emma Catherine Gainsforth, *European Journal of Psychoanalysis*.

Esposito, Roberto. 2020b. "The Twofold Face of Immunity". Translated by Arbër Zaimi *Crisis and Critique* 7 (3), 73–79.

Esposito, Roberto. 2021. *Istituzione*. Bologna: Mulino.

Foucault, Michel. 1998. *The Will to Knowledge: The History of Sexuality* (vol. 1). Translated by R. Hurley. London: Penguin.

Green, Toby. 2021. *The Covid Consensus: The New Politics of Global Inequality*. London: Hurst.

Han, Byung-Chul. 2021a. *Capitalism and the Death Drive*. Translated by D. Steuer. Cambridge: Polity.

Han, Byung-Chul. 2021b. *The Palliative Society: Pain Today*. Translated by D. Steuer. Cambridge: Polity.

Lévy, Bernard-Henri. 2020. *The Virus in the Age of Madness*. Translated by Steven B. Kennedy. New Haven: Yale UP.

Lewis, Michael. 2015. "Of (Auto-)Immune Life: Derrida, Esposito, Agamben". In Darian Meacham (ed.), *Medicine and Society: New Perspectives in Continental Philosophy*. Dordrecht: Springer.

Lewis, Michael. 2022. "Review-Essay: Giorgio Agamben, *Where are we now?* & Other Writings". Journal of Italian Philosophy 5.

Mitropoulos, Angela. 2020. *Pandemonium: Proliferating Borders of Capital and the Pandemic Swerve*. London: Pluto Press.

Penzin, Alexei. 2020. "Pandemic Suspension". *Radical Philosophy* 2 (8).

Rayner, Gordon. 2021. "Use of fear to control behaviour in Covid crisis was 'totalitarian', admit scientists". *Daily Telegraph*, 14 May, www.telegraph.co.uk/news/2021/05/14/sci entists-admit-totalitarian-use-fear-control-behaviour-covid/

Ronchi, Rocco. 2020. "The Virtues of the Virus". *European Journal of Psychoanalysis*, 14 March, www.journal-psychoanalysis.eu/on-pandemics-nancy-esposito-nancy/

Sloterdijk, Peter. 2021. *Der Staat streift seine Samthandschuhe ab: Ausgewählte Gespräche und Beiträge 2020–2021*. Berlin: Suhrkamp.

Smith, Daniel J. 2020. "On the Viral Event". *European Journal of Psychoanalysis*, 25 June, www. journal-psychoanalysis.eu/on-the-viral-event/?fbclid=IwAR08av4U3cjesCLk38RDm AL6Za91F576Dfb2amK541QS_luQLY0ZTAbmpRw

Žižek, Slavoj. 2020. *Pan(dem)ic! COVID-19 Shakes the World*. Cambridge: Polity.

SECTION 2

Pandemic Policy and the Global South

If key concepts are subject to alternative interpretations even within the same context – as the chapters in the previous section have shown – how much more complex does their meaning and impact on policy formation become in diverse contexts? Perhaps the most troublesome aspect of the global response to COVID-19 was precisely that it was "global" – that is, that agenda and policies hastily imported from China to Europe in the early months of 2020 were then thoughtlessly exported to much of the rest of the world, with little or no consideration for the vastly different physical, social, political, economic, and cultural conditions that apply between and within the world's continents. The essays in this section show that the failure to allow for alternative perspectives that emerge from alternative contexts is devastating for the preventable loss of life and welfare that has ensued from the blanket application of one-size-fits-all policies on a global scale; it is also hugely problematic in its reprising of the most regrettable aspects of what has historically been the over-dominance of the Global North.

DOI: 10.4324/9781003259336-8

6

HOW THE WORLD'S HARSHEST LOCKDOWN UNLEASHED A HUMANITARIAN CRISIS

Kunal R. Purohit

Introduction

By the end of February 2020, countries across the globe were moving towards the "new normal" – cancellation of large gatherings, shutting down of schools, travel bans, and even localised lockdowns. By 27 February, the virus had spread from China to 44 countries and caused 2801 deaths, prompting the World Health Organisation (WHO) to warn countries against complacency (UN News, 2020). By 11 March, the WHO had declared the disease a pandemic and said the virus had reached 100 countries across the globe (WHO, 2020).

India recorded its first COVID-19 infection on 30 January 2020 (CNBC, 2020). By 13 March, infections rose to 81, even as the government insisted the coronavirus was not a health emergency (Business Standard, 2020). However, on 24 March, the Indian prime minister, Narendra Modi, announced a 21-day complete lockdown without a warning, coming into effect within four hours of the announcement.

The version of lockdown imposed was one of the sternest in the world and ranked highest in the stringency index developed by the University of Oxford's Blavatnik School of Government (Blavatnik School of Government, 2020). It involved the complete suspension of nearly all economic activity, with strict curfew orders in place for 1.3 billion Indians and penal provisions in place for violators. Public transport was ordered shut, no movement was possible without special permits from police authorities, and only businesses stocking food items and medicines were allowed to function.

The ensuing insecurity and precarity have disproportionately affected the country's most marginalised groups, perhaps irreversibly. Surveys conducted after the lockdown was lifted reveal that incomes, especially for casual workers, have fallen by as much as 62 percent (Mohan et al., 2021) in some urban areas, and workers' bargaining power with employers has reduced drastically. The lockdown

DOI: 10.4324/9781003259336-9

impacted female participation in the labour force, 94 percent of which is in the informal economy (SEWA, 2020), as women who lost their jobs had 20 percent less chances of being re-employed compared to male labourers (Deshpande, 2020).

Families were forced to borrow to get through the lockdown, increasing their indebtedness and resulting in their having to make compromises by cutting down their nutrition intake (SEWA, 2020). A nationwide survey found that nearly a third of 5162 sample households reported a possibility of pulling out children from schools in order to stay afloat (CSO, 2020).

The country's 65-million-strong domestic migrant community (Singh, 2020), most of them wage workers in the country's informal sector, experienced a sudden loss of income and livelihood resulting in widespread hunger and deprivation and triggering a mass exodus of over 11 million workers back to their hometowns and villages (Hindu Business Line, 2021). Disallowing stranded migrant workers to travel home resulted in an uncontrolled exodus, leading to the spread of COVID-19 in the country's hinterlands (Pradhan, 2020). Daily infections had increased to nearly ten thousand when the lockdown was lifted, from 657 total infections in India when the lockdown was imposed (COVID-19 India, 2020). India's devastating second wave of infections, a year after the lockdown, demonstrated that the lockdown period was not optimally utilised to bolster India's weak healthcare systems adequately.

Beyond the immediate dangers of COVID-19, there is a significant danger of a looming health crisis. Lockdown led to the suspension of general healthcare services in the country, disrupting preventive medical care and leading to an estimated 560,000 surgeries being cancelled (Article-14, 2020a), while thousands of patients could not access care for critical illnesses like cancer (Ghosh, 2020).

This chapter highlights how India's sudden lockdown unleashed a humanitarian crisis, unprecedented in post-colonial Indian history, exposing the country's social and economic fault lines while reinforcing pre-existing structural inequalities in the country. It begins by highlighting the politics that shaped the decision to adopt such a lockdown policy. The chapter then traces the lockdown's effects to demonstrate how the country's poor and marginalised suffered disproportionately and were rendered further economically and socially insecure due to the scale and the nature of the lockdown, as it triggered mass unemployment, with the country's joblessness rate reaching a high of 26 percent (Ethiraj, 2020). Lastly, it examines how people from traditionally excluded Dalit communities, at the bottom of India's social hierarchies of caste, were three times more likely to lose their jobs than those from "upper" caste communities (Deshpande and Ramachandran, 2021).

The politics behind the lockdown

The sudden nature of the lockdown announcement by the government was not unprecedented. In 2016, Prime Minister Modi made a similar televised appearance at 8:00 p.m. on 8 November to announce that 86 percent of the Indian currency would no longer be in operation from midnight, sparking massive panic and disruption for months (BBC, 2016). In announcing such decisions, Modi's appearances are always solo, as he prefers not to be in the company of his advisors or ministers, thereby accentuating the personality cult that he has assiduously tried to cultivate around him. The sudden lockdown announcement, after the initial dithering over pandemic-control measures, reflected a calculated political move to burnish Modi's credentials as a strongman who was a bold protector, unafraid of taking swift action against incoming dangers (Nilsen, 2021).

The lockdown imposed in India restricted nearly all economic and social activity. Citizens were required to stay at home at all times, except when they needed to buy essential items. Public transportation was ordered to shut, while private transportation was also prohibited except for medical reasons. Markets and shops were ordered to close, except those which sold groceries and medicines. Routine medical services were disrupted, and the ban on transportation meant many who had non-COVID-19 medical ailments struggled to reach hospitals and clinics. Therefore, overnight, without any warning, livelihoods were lost and freedoms were denied. This pronouncement emerged without consultations with elected public representatives or regional governments. Such a move, in the world's largest democracy, signalled that the lockdown was non-negotiable and so was the unquestioned adherence to rules around it.

Such framing of the lockdown, mathematician Murad Banaji argued, "simplified" the relationship between people and power, with authorities enforcing rules and people merely expected to comply (Banaji, 2020). Furthermore, it also "reframed" disease control measures to imply the enforcement of lockdown, instead of health measures, thus ensuring that "messy narratives about health infrastructure, testing, tracing, monitoring, probabilities, education, research and so forth, are replaced with a list of rules, responsibilities and consequences" (Banaji, 2020). This was reflected in Modi's speech that accompanied the lockdown declaration, wherein he highlighted the danger the country faced and emphasised citizens' duties in fighting the pandemic, but made merely a passing mention of the government's efforts, announcing the allotment of INR 150 billion towards strengthening the country's medical infrastructure, but failing to offer specific details on what that would entail.

The national public healthcare system had been underfunded and, as a result, under-resourced. Compared to the global average of countries' spending on healthcare (9.8 percent of GDP), India spends only 3.5 percent (World Bank, 2021). As a result, there is roughly one hospital bed for every 2,000 people, whereas the global average is three times higher. Similarly, the nation has only half the doctors per 1,000 people compared to the global average (World Bank, 2021).

The prime minister's speech, days after his government underplayed the threat the disease posed, signalled a clear shift in the government's outlook towards the situation, from underestimation to panic. However, the undertone of this shift was also clear – the onus of preventing an outbreak of the disease was on citizens and not the state. That the announcement was made via a televised appearance, and not a press conference where the press could interrogate the move and push the government to give an explanation, was symbolic of an administration that did not believe it was accountable to the citizenry. Consequently, it was met with criticism, with rival political leaders (Pandey, 2020) warning of the economic consequences of such a lockdown, while health and social sector experts urged the government to consider the fate of migrants who might be stranded in their workplaces (Al Jazeera, 2020).

The lockdown also invited scrutiny for possible constitutional overreaches. The Indian constitution places public health and sanitation as subjects firmly in the list of responsibilities of regional governments (Daniyal, 2020). Many of these governments had already started placing restrictions on gatherings weeks before the national lockdown. However, by taking over this role without a minimum level of dialogue with regional governments, the Modi government overstepped constitutional separations between the federal and regional authorities (Daniyal, 2020). This was only made worse by the fact that these regional governments were not consulted before the federal government took over their powers (BBC, 2021). Instead, the sudden announcement meant that local authorities were, overnight, saddled with more responsibilities since they were meant to implement lockdown provisions while simultaneously carrying out measures to fight the pandemic medically (The Hindu, 2020).

The reluctance to conduct wider consultations with authorities and elected representatives indicated an unwillingness to pre-empt and plan to mitigate the ways in which lives, health, and livelihoods were likely to be indelibly altered. The administration believed it could impose such a sudden lockdown, with four hours notice, without even attempting to put in place contingency provisions on the ground. This was revealing of the denial of the spirit of citizenship of ordinary citizens in the world's largest democracy, and was a repudiation of the "deliberative democracy" that Modi has hailed in the past (India Today, 2017). Such a top-down approach to lockdown passed on responsibilities to less powerful stakeholders, while offering them no say in the decision-making process – local authorities were supposed to merely enforce the lockdown, even when they lacked the capacity to do so, while citizens were supposed to unquestioningly accept it.

A humanitarian crisis unfolds

In ordering immediate, sudden, and complete curbs on the mobility of 1.3 billion Indians, the Indian government chose to overlook the interests of some of the most marginalised communities in the country. Of the 470-million-strong labour force in the country, over 88 percent, or 413 million – more than the total population of the United States – are employed in the informal sector (ILO, 2018). These workers lack social protection, employment benefits, and job security (ILO, 2021), and at least 120 million are wage earners, thereby often leading a hand-to-mouth existence (ILO, 2018).

The rural Indian economy, a source of livelihood for nearly two-thirds of the labour force, is predominantly informal in nature, and casual workers form up to 80 percent of its labour market (ILO, 2018). Beyond this, there is also a high level of informality in the formal sector, with much of the regular, salaried employment in India being contractual in nature and thereby lacking job security and social protection (ILO, 2018). The livelihoods of these workers were immediately threatened by the overnight lockdown. From 7 percent before the lockdown, India's unemployment rate climbed to 23.8 percent a week into the lockdown and continued to rise as the lockdown remained in place (Ethiraj, 2020). By April, the rate reached 30 percent, and an estimated 122 million were believed to have suffered job losses (Vyas, 2020).

The overnight lockdown created an immediate financial crisis for workers in informal industries, as these mostly offer daily wages, instead of monthly payments, and wages are often below the national daily minimum wage (MOSPI, 2012). Many of these industries also work on myriad payment models – seasonal agriculture workers, for instance, are paid in part at the start of the season, and the remaining bulk is paid only at the end of the season (Deshingkar and Start, 2003). Workers often sustain themselves by living in large groups on work sites. For instance, building construction workers live in the plots where the construction is taking place, while agricultural workers often live in the fields they are employed on, thereby, saving rent overheads and minimising food costs (Deshingkar and Start, 200). With the sudden lockdown, employers halted payments to their workers, with many not even being paid for the month of March even though the lockdown was announced only on 24 March.

The Indian Census has pegged the number of migrants within the country at 450 million, corresponding to 37 percent of the country's population (Singh, 2020). The lack of reliable data has meant that not much is known about the reasons behind this migration. As a result, data around the number of migrant workers remains hazy (Paliath, 2021), but one estimate pegs the number at nearly 100 million migrant workers (Tumbe, 2019).

Migrant labourers tend to be locked in precarious, casual jobs in the informal and formal economy in India's urban areas, thousands of kilometres away from their homes. The lockdown led to their livelihoods being lost overnight and their being stranded far away from their homes, with limited savings and food supplies. The government failed to consider these workers' plight and to find ways to mitigate the impact of pandemic control measures on them.

As days went by, migrant workers exhausted their savings and grew desperate, even as they remained shackled in small homes shared with several other fellow migrants – the preferred mode of housing for the migrant community in cities like Mumbai. Eventually, they started posting pleas for food and money on social media (BBC, 2020). Many were forced to rely on community kitchens, and others were compelled to beg (Purohit, 2020). A survey by the Stranded Workers Action Network (SWAN) covering over 11,100 stranded migrant workers revealed that at this time, half had less than a day's food rations left (SWAN, 2020), while 74 percent had less than £2 (equivalent to half a day's wage) left with them. Although their incomes had halted, fixed costs like food and rents remained, and the pandemic induced new costs, from face covers to sanitisers. They also had hefty phone-related costs, since this was a crucial mode of connection with their worried families. In Southern India, some migrant workers did not have money to even buy milk for their children (Narayanan, 2020).

Desperation, hunger and deprivation of basic dignity triggered one of the largest human migrations in recent times. For millions of migrants, many of whom are "seasonal" migrants, cities have remained places of work where they sustain themselves without any social security (John et al., 2020). Most send the bulk of their incomes back to their families in the hinterland (Tumbe, 2011). With the lockdown, their wages stopped and most found themselves with no social security net to fall back on. Hence, millions decided to go back home to their villages with no clarity as to how long the lockdown would last for.

In the absence of public transportation, some workers paid exorbitant rates to truckers who smuggled these workers in the backs of goods-carrying vehicles. Most workers could not afford such exorbitant journeys and had no option but to walk back to their hometowns and villages, often thousands of kilometres away (Economic Times, 2020). Desperate to get home, migrants walked back for days in the scorching summer heat, with temperatures regularly above 40 degrees Celsius, often without adequate food and water supplies. Some swam through rivers, walked through forests, and even cycled for days in order to reach home (Hindustan Times, 2020b). At least 209 people died in accidents while walking back home, and at least 47 people died due to exhaustion in these journeys (Aman et al, 2020).

Migrant journeys were made even more dangerous, by a brute state unleashing violence on the fleeing workers. Choosing to ignore their suffering and desperation, police forces across the country repeatedly rained blows on workers using their batons to warn them against violating the lockdown. Migrant workers were asked to crawl as punishment (The Quint, 2020), were fired upon using tear gas shells by police officials (NDTV, 2020a), and many were arrested for attempting to go back home, with the police erecting makeshift detention camps for migrants. Often, the violence was fatal, with at least 12 recorded deaths of migrant workers in episodes of police brutality (Aman et al., 2020).

Cascading effects that will linger

Nearly 28 percent of India's population (365 million) was found to be living below the poverty line in 2018, a figure that is likely only to have grown during the pandemic (Oxford Poverty and Human Development Initiative, 2018). As a result, the economic distress from this sudden halt in incomes and disruption of livelihoods, coupled with inadequate relief measures by the government (Simrin, 2020), had severe detrimental effects for this population. One immediate fallout was widespread hunger among the poor in the urban and the rural areas of the country. While the Stranded Workers Action Group (SWAG) survey revealed hunger among stranded migrant workers, another survey among rural households showed that food insecurity was common among the broader population as well, days into the lockdown (Agarwal, 2021). One survey showed that 68 percent of households had already reduced the number of items that were part of their meals, while half the households surveyed said they were compelled to cut down the number of meals they were consuming (CSO, 2020).

The lockdown-induced deprivation also had distinct gendered effects. Food insecurity in households was made worse by traditional gendered norms which dictate that women and girls must eat after all the male members of the family have consumed their meals. As a result, a survey among 627 women saw 40 percent respondents reporting that they were eating less than they needed and 12 percent saying they were going hungry (Agarwal, 2021). Besides hunger, women were also adversely affected by the financial crisis that the lockdown brought.

Financial precarity forced women to dip into their own savings, with one survey showing that all the 375 women surveyed had exhausted their savings and were forced to borrow money in order to make ends meet (SEWA, 2020). While 91 percent of them had borrowed from their relatives and friends, 9 percent had been forced to borrow from private moneylenders (SEWA, 2020). The financial distress forced some women to start selling off their assets, with others insisting that they would be forced to follow suit if their situation was not alleviated.

The lack of domestic remittances from migrant family members exacerbated the financial distress faced by women, as domestic remittances can contribute as much as 30 percent of household expenses in remittance-receiving families (Tumbe, 2011). Instead, as migrant family members returned home, the financial and domestic burden on family members only intensified. Women bore the brunt of this burden, with significant increases in the time that women members of the household spent on unpaid domestic labour, from making more trips to fetch water to spending more time collecting firewood (CSO, 2020).

The effects of the stringent lockdown were also felt in the country's medical care systems. With public transportation services completely shut, most patients who sought medical care found it challenging to reach hospitals and clinics. In addition, punitive measures were adopted by various local authorities to shut down or seal private nursing homes and hospitals that were treating non-COVID-19 patients if any of the patients tested positive for the coronavirus (Article-14, 2020b). As a result, private doctors dithered about keeping their medical facilities open, while patients feared contracting the disease at medical facilities and hence avoided visits (Article-14, 2020b). This disrupted preventive care as well as treatment for medical ailments, and an estimated 560,000 surgeries across India were cancelled (Article-14, 2020a). Even treatment for critical ailments like cancer was affected, with one of the country's premier cancer-care centres in Mumbai being forced to shut down palliative care (Pramesh and Badwe, 2020). More than 51,000 cancer surgeries had to be cancelled and doctors estimated that 70 percent of the cancer patients could not access timely care and treatment (Ghosh, 2020).

Disruption was witnessed even in critical services of antenatal care as well as in immunisations. A survey in some of Mumbai's poorest slum communities showed that 6 percent of the women who gave birth during the lockdown were forced to do so in their homes, most of them tiny and congested (Article-14, 2020a). The lockdown also affected the functioning of antenatal clinics, resulting in the non-availability of crucial nutritional supplements for expectant mothers (Article-14, 2020a). Immunisations among infants went down by as much as 70 percent (Ghosh, 2020). Poor nutritional levels among infants and expectant mothers are only likely to worsen the country's already troubling malnutrition levels (Mahapatra, 2021).

The direct and indirect effects of the lockdown have not gone away with the lifting of measures, demonstrating the long-term insecurities that might have set in due to the nature and scale of the shutdown. Casual and wage workers have been impacted severely, with many pushed into debt in order to sustain themselves and their families through the lockdown (FirstPost, 2021). The indebtedness is unlikely to improve, as small and medium businesses are in a crisis of capital (Economic Times, 2020). India's economic recovery continues to be muted, with jobless-ness rates soaring (Mint, 2021) over a year after the lockdown was lifted. A reduc-tion in the number of jobs in the market is likely to lead to depressed bargaining power among workers, raising fears that workers could even be forced to enter into exploitative, precarious jobs (Scroll, 2021) as well as debt slavery (FirstPost, 2021). Workers are likely to be much more dependent on such jobs than before, with fears of succeeding waves of coronavirus infections only heightening this precarious form of employment.

Conclusion

Nearly 18 months after 1.3 billion people experienced the imposition of an arbitrary lockdown, its successes are not very clear. When the country began a gradual process of "unlocking" on 8 June, it was recording nearly ten thousand new COVID-19 infections every day, and it had the seventh-highest number of cases in the world, up from 657 total infections when it locked down in March (COVID-19 India, 2020). By September 2021, it was recording, on average, over forty thousand new infections daily (COVID-19 India, 2020). Arguments around the lockdown period being used to bolster the nation's weak healthcare systems were invalidated when a devastating second wave of infections that hit India exactly a year later showed how poorly prepared the country was. Hospitals were full, ICUs were overflowing, and patients were plagued with a crippling shortage of everything from medicines to oxygen supplies. As a result, crematoriums and graveyards were full, with people forced to cremate and bury their loved ones at odd places, from rivers and river banks to playgrounds and even pavements (Yeung and Ward, 2021).

The costs of lockdown are much clearer than their alleged benefits. The trauma of lockdown lingers on in the minds of workers, as many refuse to go back to Indian cities as the economy opens. Even when the nation saw record food-grain production, migrants continued to sleep hungry through most of 2020, having lost their jobs to the shock of the sudden lockdown (Mahapatra, 2021). The economic devastation caused by an overnight lockdown meant that the Indian economy shrank by nearly 24 percent in the financial quarter between April and June, when the lockdown was imposed (Yasir and Gettleman, 2020). The disruption, while benefitting major e-commerce giants and retail corporations, left the country's micro-, small, and medium industries in acute financial distress, with more than half wanting to shut down or sell off the business (Sachin, 2021). Millions of children risked malnourishment due to disruptions in the school food-distribution system during the lockdown (Saha, 2021a). The unplanned lockdown and closure of education institutes has impacted children in rural areas disproportionately, with only 8 percent of them regularly attending online classes (Road Scholarz, 2021).

The trauma revealed itself in an uptick in mental health issues – in a survey reported of migrant workers, more than two-thirds recorded a disturbed mental state due to financial stresses, while nearly two-thirds of the participants said they were suffering from anxiety and depression (Adridi, Dhillon, and Roy, 2020). India's middle class has shrunk by 32 million in a year (Pew Research Center, 2021), even as 230 million Indians have been pushed deeper into poverty (Economic Times, 2021a). Nonetheless, amid a year of horrific struggles and catastrophic deprivation, the country's elite continued to smile their way to the banks, as by the end of the year India's stock market had risen by 75 percent and the country had added 38 new billionaires (Karmali, 2021). It has thus been a "tale of two cities".

References

Afridi, Farzana, Amrita Dhillon, and Sanchari Roy. 2020. "Lockdown Survey: 85% of Respondents Among Delhi's Poor Earned Zero Wages From Main Job". *The Wire*, 11 May, https://thewire.in/rights/urban-poor-lockdown-phone-survey

Agarwal, Bina. 2021. Reflections on the Less Visible and Less Measured: Gender and COVID-19 in India. *Gender & Society* 35(2): 244–255. doi:10.1177/08912432211001299.

Aman, Kanika Sharma, R. Krushna, and G.N. Thejesh. 2020. "India NonVirus Deaths During lockdown" *Zenodo*, 4 July, https://zenodo.org/record/4630198#.YqigQHbMLIU

Banaji, Murad. 2020. "What Effects Has the Lockdown Had on the Evolution of COVID-19 in India?" *Scroll*, 27 May, https://scroll.in/article/962992/what-effects-has-the-lockd own-had-on-the-evolution-of-covid-19-in-india

BBC. 2016. "*Why India Wiped out 86% of Its Cash Overnight*". *BBC News*, 14 November, www.bbc.com/news/world-asia-india-37974423

BBC. 2020. "India COVID-19 Migrants: 'Lockdown Will Make Us Beg for Food Again'". *BBC News*, 13 April, www.bbc.com/news/world-asia-india-56711150.

BBC. 2021. India COVID-19: PM Modi 'did not consult' before lockdown. British Broadcasting Corporation. www.bbc.co.uk/news/world-asia-india-56561095

Blavatnik School of Government. 2020. "*COVID-19 Government Response Tracker*". *Blavatnik School of Government*, www.bsg.ox.ac.uk/research/research-projects/covid-19-governm ent-response-tracker

Business Standard. 2020. "Coronavirus Not Health Emergency, Total 81 Cases in India: Health Ministry". *Business Standard India*, 13 March, www.business-standard.com/article/pti-stor ies/coronavirus-cases-rise-to-81-in-india-officials-120031301149_1.html

CNBC. 2020. "*India Confirms Its First Coronavirus Case*". *CNBC*, www.cnbc.com/2020/01/ 30/india-confirms-first-case-of-the-coronavirus.html

Covid 19 India. 2020. "*Coronavirus in India: Latest Map and Case Count*". *Covid 19 India*, 1 November, www.covid19india.org

CSO. 2020. COVID-19 Induced Lockdown – How Is the Hinterland Coping?. Maharashtra: Vikasanvesh Foundation: www.vikasanvesh.in/wp-content/uploads/2020/06/Presentation-based-on-CSO-consortium-survey.pdf

Daniyal, Shoaib. 2020. "Can the Centre Bypass the States and Declare a Lockdown?". *Scroll*, 26 March, https://scroll.in/article/957239/can-the-union-government-bypass-the-states-and-declare-a-lockdown

Deshingkar, Priya, and Daniel Start. 2003. *Seasonal Migration for Livelihoods in India: Coping, Accumulation and Exclusion.* London: Overseas Development Institute, 2003.

Deshpande, Ashwini, 2020. "The COVID-19 Lockdown in India: Gender and Caste Dimensions of the First Job Losses". Working Papers. eSocialSciences,. https://ideas.repec.org/p/ess/wpaper/id13085.html.

Deshpande, Ashwini, and Ramachandran, Rajesh. 2021. "Is Covid-19 'The Great Leveler'? The Critical Role of Social Identity in Lockdown-Induced Job Losses". GLO Discussion Paper Series 622, Global Labor Organization (GLO).

Economic Times. 2020. "Migrant Workers Walk Thousands of Kms in Scorching Heat to Reach Their Native Places". *The Economic Times*, 15 May, https://economictimes.indiatimes.com/news/politics-and-nation/migrant-workers-walk-thousands-of-kms-in-scorching-heat-to-reach-their-native-places-in-up/articleshow/75760045.cms?from=mdr

Economic Times. 2021a; "One Year of Covid Pushed 230 Million Indians into Poverty: Azim Premji University - The Economic Times." Accessed September 21, 2021. https://economictimes.indiatimes.com/news/economy/indicators/one-year-of-covid-pushed-230-million-indians-into-poverty-azim-premji-university/articleshow/82408369.cms?from=mdr

Ethiraj, Govindraj. 2020. "100-120 Million Jobs Lost Due to COVID-19 Lockdown". *IndiaSpend*, 20 April, www.indiaspend.com/100-120-million-jobs-lost-due-to-covid-19-lockdown/

FirstPost, 2021. "80% of India's Informal Workers Lost Jobs during COVID Lockdown, 63% Survived on Two Meals a Day, Shows Data-India News , Firstpost," February 2, 2021. www.firstpost.com/india/80-of-indias-informal-workers-lost-jobs-during-covid-lockdown-63-survived-on-two-meals-a-day-shows-data-9264141.html.)

Ghosh, Abantika. 2020. "70% of India's Cancer Patients Couldn't Access Care during Lockdown, Experts Say". *The Print* [blog], 27 November, https://theprint.in/health/70-of-indias-cancer-patients-couldnt-access-care-during-lockdown-experts-say/552529/

Hindu Business Line. 2021. "Over 1.14 Crore Migrants Went Back Home: Centre". *The Hindu Business Line*. 10 March, www.thehindubusinessline.com/news/national/over-114-crore-migrants-went-back-home-centre/article34038392.ece

Hindustan Times. 2020a. "1,000 from outside Mumbai stuck at Tata Memorial Hospital due to lockdown". *Hindustan Times*, 30 March, www.hindustantimes.com/mumbai-news/700-cancer-patients-kin-stranded-in-mumbai/story-YzOstmFSWTNr5ie6wMBbWL.html

Hindustan Times. 2020b. "Through Sea and Forests: How Workers Are Trying to Reach Home amid Lockdown". *Hindustan* Times, 21 April, www.hindustantimes.com/india-news/on-foot-on-cycles-in-a-boat-how-desperate-people-are-trying-to-reach-home-amid-lockdown/story-srfOdlp47tnvazxAH3tHLM.html

ILO. 2018. India Wage Report, ILO 2018. Geneva: ILO: www.ilo.org/wcmsp5/groups/public/---asia/---ro-bangkok/---sro-new_delhi/documents/publication/wcms_638305.pdf

ILO. 2021. *Statistical Glossary.* www.ilo.org/ilostat-files/Documents/Statistical%20Glossary.pdf

India Today. 2017. "India Today Conclave 2017: PM Modi Presents Report Card, Calls GST an Example of Deliberative Democracy". India Today. 18 March, www.indiatoday. in/india-today-conclave-2017/story/india-today-conclave-2017-narendra-modi-966 336-2017-03-18

John, J. Jacob, Naveen Joseph Thomas, Megha Jacob, and Neha Jacob . 2020. "A Study on Social Security and Health Rights of Migrant Workers in India". Kerala Development Society, New Delhi, India. https://nhrc.nic.in/sites/default/files/Approved_Health%20 and%20social%20security%20ISMW_KDS-NHRC.pdf.

Karmali, Naazneen. 2021. "India's 10 Richest Billionaires 2021". *Forbes*, 6 April, www.for bes.com/sites/naazneenkarmali/2021/04/06/indias-10-richest-billionaires-2021/?sh= 1c05415159b7

Kochhar, Rakesh. 2021. "India's Middle Class Shrinks amid COVID-19 as China Sees Less Change". *Pew Research Center*, 18 March, www.pewresearch.org/fact-tank/2021/03/18/ in-the-pandemic-indias-middle-class-shrinks-and-poverty-spreads-while-china-sees-smaller-changes/

Mahapatra, Richard. 2021; "Mass Poverty Is Back in India". *Down to Earth*, 7 April, www. downtoearth.org.in/blog/governance/mass-poverty-is-back-in-india-76348

Mohan, Deepanshu, Jignesh Mistry. Advaita Singh, and Snehal Sreedar. 2021. "How Daily Wage Workers in India Suffered in the Lockdown – and Continue to Struggle Months Later". *Scroll*, 26 March, https://scroll.in/article/989258/how-daily-wage-workers-in-india-suffered-in-the-lockdown-and-continue-to-struggle-months-later

Mohan Depanshu, Richa Sekhani, Jignesh Mistry, Advaita Singh, Snehal Sreedhar, and shivani agarwal. 2021. "Narratives of Daily Wage Workers Across Mazdoor Mandis (Labor Markets) of India During a Pandemic: Observations from an Ethnographic Survey in Cities of Lucknow and Pune" (March 24, 2021). SSRN: https://ssrn.com/abstract=3811 208 or http://dx.doi.org/10.2139/ssrn.3811208

MOSPI. 2012. "*Informal Sector and Conditions of Employment in India*". http://mospi.nic.in/ sites/default/files/publication_reports/nss_rep_539.pdf

Narayanan, Rajendran. 2020. "What Migrant Workers Are Revealing In SOS Calls To Us". *NDTV*, 12 April, www.ndtv.com/opinion/what-migrant-workers-are-revealing-in-sos-calls-to-us-2209556

Nilsen, Alf Gunvald. 2021. "India's Pandemic: Spectacle, Social Murder and Authoritarian Politics in a Lockdown Nation". Globalizations 19 (3): 1–21.

NDTV. 2020. "Migrants Clash With Police in Ahmedabad, Stones Thrown, Tear Gas Fired". *NDTV*, 18 May, www.ndtv.com/ahmedabad-news/migrants-clash-with-police-in-ahmedabad-stones-thrown-tear-gas-fired-2231068

Oxford Poverty and Human Development Initiative. 2018. "Global MPI 2018". OPHI, https://ophi.org.uk/multidimensional-poverty-index/global-mpi-2018/

Paliath, Shreehari . 2021. "A Year After Exodus, No Reliable Data Or Policy On Migrant Workers". *India Spend*, 24 March, www.indiaspend.com/governance/migrant-workers-no-reliable-data-or-policy-737499

Pandey, Neelam. 2020. "Rahul Gandhi Questions Lockdown Impact on Economy, but Expresses Solidarity with PM Modi". *The Print* [blog], 29 March, https://theprint.in/ politics/rahul-gandhi-questions-lockdown-impact-on-economy-but-expresses-solidar ity-with-pm-modi/390791/

Pew Research Center. 2021; "India's Middle Class Shrinks amid COVID-19 as China Sees Less Change | | *Pew Research Center*." Accessed September 2, 2021. www.pewresearch. org/fact-tank/2021/03/18/in-the-pandemic-indias-middle-class-shrinks-and-poverty-spreads-while-china-sees-smaller-changes/.

Pramesh, C.S., and Rajendra A. Badwe. 2020. "Cancer Management in India during COVID-19". *New England Journal of Medicine* 382 (20): e61.

Pradhan, Bibhudatta. 2020. "New Covid Hotspots Are Emerging in Villages after Migrants Returned, Govt Estimates Show". *The Print* [blog], 22 June, https://theprint.in/health/new-covid-hotspots-are-emerging-in-villages-after-migrants-returned-govt-estimates-show/446219/

Purohit, Kunal. 2020. "Meraj Shaikh's Lost Body & Other Non-Covid Victims". *Article 14*, 14 August, www.article-14.com/post/meraj-shaikh-s-lost-body-mumbai-s-non-covid-victims

Sachin, Dave. 2021. "MSME: 59% of Startups and MSMEs May Shut Shop, Sell off or Scale down: Survey". *The Economic Times*, 27 May, https://economictimes.indiatimes.com/small-biz/sme-sector/covid-second-wave-59-of-startups-and-msmes-may-shut-shops-sell-off-or-scale-down-localcircles-survey/articleshow/82974477.cms?from=mdr

Saha, Subhamoy, and Rashi Singh. 2021. "Child Malnutrition in India: A Systemic Failure". *Down to Earth*, 15 April, www.downtoearth.org.in/blog/health/child-malnutrition-in-india-a-systemic-failure-76507

Scholarz, Road. 2021. "Road Scholarz – Freelance Scholars Doing Action-Oriented Research". *Road Scholarz*, https://roadscholarz.net/

SEWA. 2020. Gendered Precarity in the Lockdown. Bharat: SEWA: www.sewabharatresearch.org/wp-content/uploads/2020/05/Gendered_Precarity_SB_Lockdown-1.pdf

Simrin, Mediratta. 2020. "Garib Kalyan Yojna: Is the Relief Package Relief Enough?". *ORF*. 26 June, www.orfonline.org/expert-speak/garib-kalyan-yojna-68561/

Singh, Sushant. 2020. "Explained: Indian migrants, across India". *Indian Express*, 6 April https://indianexpress.com/article/explained/coronavirus-india-lockdown-migran-workers-mass-exodus-6348834/

SCMP. 2020a; Purohit, Kunal. "*Coronavirus: How Mumbai's Sprawling Slums Threaten to Become a Covid-19 Breeding Ground*| South China Morning Post." Accessed September 21, 2021. www.scmp.com/week-asia/health-environment/article/3080925/coronavirus-how-mumbais-sprawling-slums-threaten?fbclid=IwAR19x3K4lKNbDMfSLsuTVHFD1G8A9chcMKjyVGL2-ZqzpGQrXJUg-JXEuns.

SWAN. 2020. Lockdown and Distress Report by Stranded Workers Action Network. SWAN: www.thehindu.com/news/resources/article31442220.ece/binary/Lockdown-and-Distress_Report-by-Stranded-Workers-Action-Network.pdf

The Hindu. 2020; "Malkangiri Tribal Migrant Worker Dies Of Exhaustion," May 14, 2020. www.thehindu.com/news/national/other-states/coronavirus-lockdown-malkangiri-tribal-migrant-worker-dies-of-exhaustion/article31584759.ece

The Quint. 2020. "Migrants Made to Crawl as Punishment for Violating Lockdown in UP". *ThevQuint*, 27 March, www.thequint.com/news/india/migrants-made-to-crawl-as-punishment-for-violating-lockdown-in-up

Tumbe, Chinmay. 2011. Migration and Remittances in India. Exim Bank India: Accessed September 21, 2021. www.eximbankindia.in/Assets/Dynamic/PDF/Publication-Resources/ResearchPapers/54file.pdf

Tumbe, Chinmay . 2019. "A Million Migrations: Journeys in Search of Jobs". *Mint*, 16 January, www.livemint.com/Politics/8WPPsZygqR7Mu6e3Fgy55N/A-million-migrations-Journeys-in-search-of-jobs.html

UN News. 2020. "No country should make 'fatal' mistake of ignoring COVID-19: Tedros". *UN News*, 27 February, https://news.un.org/en/story/2020/02/1058221

Vyas, Mahesh . 2020. "*The Jobs Bloodbath of April 2020*". *CMIE*, 5 May, www.cmie.com/kommon/bin/sr.php?kall=warticle&dt=2020-05-05%2008:22:21&msec=776&ver=pf

WHO. 2020. Director-General's Opening Remarks at the Media Briefing on COVID-19. World Health Organisation. Geneva. Switzerland. www.who.int/director-gene ral/speeches/detail/who-director-general-s-opening-remarks-at-the-media-brief ing-on-covid-19---16-march-2020

World Bank. 2021. "Current Health Expenditure (% of GDP) ". *World Bank*, 30 January, https://data.worldbank.org/indicator/SH.XPD.CHEX.GD.ZS?contextual=defa ult&locations=IN

Yasir, Sameer, and Jeffrey Gettleman . 2020. "India's Economy Shrank Nearly 24 Percent Last Quarter". *The New York Times*, 31 August, www.nytimes.com/2020/08/31/world/asia/ india-economy-gdp.html

Yeung, Jessie, and Clarissa Ward. 2021; "'They Keep Coming': India's Second Wave Sees Crematoriums Overflow with Covid Victims". 7 *News*, 1 May. https://7news.com.au/ lifestyle/health-wellbeing/indias-devastating-second-wave-decimates-the-country-with-crematoriums-overflowing-with-covid-victims-c-2730907

7

COVID-19 IN ANGOLA

Militarization of Lockdown Language and State Policy in Angola

Fernandes Wanda

Introduction

The coordination and overall leadership of the state response to the current SARS-CoV-2 pandemic in Angola was handed to the military. This in turn has led to a problematic militarisation of lockdown language and state policy implementation. Thus, despite the republican nature of the security and military forces, the current sanitary crisis has shown that the military class in Angola still holds significant power and that they will do anything to undermine any non-military actor attempting to constrain this status quo.

This chapter starts by examining how the reconfiguration of the initial government's COVID-19 response team was meant to meet the country's macro-balance of power whereby those in the military (or with a military background) have the upper hand over non-military actors. This change was followed by a critical shift in the way COVID-19 was addressed, first as a sanitary crisis and then with a discourse about the need to "fight" SARS-CoV-2. Subsequently, the chapter analyses the perceived impacts of the militarisation of the language on the population and more specifically on how the management of the crisis impacted people's lives and livelihoods.

Bitter "sweets and chocolate": From sanitary crisis to "fight" against SARS-CoV-2

As the news started to spread about an unknown infectious disease in China, in Angola the state was quick to act by creating an Inter-ministerial Commission for Emergencies to strengthen its monitoring capacity, particularly at the borders (LUSA, 2020a), a day before the World Health Organization (WHO) declared the coronavirus outbreak a public health emergency of international concern on the 30

DOI: 10.4324/9781003259336-10

January 2020 (WHO, 2020a). This commission was diverse in its composition as it included the ministers of culture, education, higher education, science, technology and innovation, social communication, as well as representatives from the private sector and UN agencies in Angola (Comissão Interministerial para as Emergências, 2020: 17).

The emergency was treated as a sanitary crisis, therefore, demanding the expertise of both those within the medical sciences and public health. As such, the newly created commission was initially led by the minister of health, as the coordinator, and the minister of interior, as the deputy coordinator (Comissão Interministerial para as Emergências, 2020).

Under the Ministry of Health's leadership, the inter-ministerial commission focused mostly on preventive measures in order to avert the local transmission of the disease. For instance, on 14 March, days before President Lourenço declared a state of emergency that was followed by a nationwide lockdown, the Ministry of Health issued a set of guidelines and recommendations for the population, in line with international health regulations ratified by the Angolan state through Resolution n° 32/08 of 1 September (Government of Angola, Ministry of Health, 2020). There was no intention to restrict people's freedoms. Subsequently when the president addressed the nation in a televised speech on 18 March 2020 to explain Angola's adoption of exceptional measures to handle the pandemic, he also emphasised that the measures taken were meant to save lives (Angola Press, 2020a).

The commission also had the mandate to draft the "National Contingency Plan for the Control of the Coronavirus Epidemic", which aimed at "minimizing the risk of introduction and spread of the new Coronavirus (2019-nCoV) in Angola and the negative impact of an epidemic on the health of the population and on the socioeconomic prospects of the country" (Comissão Interministerial para as Emergências, 2020: 4). One of the key measures taken by this commission was to establish institutional quarantine for anyone (nationals and foreign residents) returning from China in February (LUSA, 2020b). Later in March, following the WHO reassessment of COVID-19 as a global pandemic (WHO, 2020b), this was extended to any passenger coming from abroad. The policy decision to impose institutional quarantine was crucial due to the existing vulnerabilities within the nation's health system following years of underfunding. Indeed, the state has systematically failed to meet its international commitment, under the 2001 Abuja Declaration,[1] to spend at least 15 percent of the national budget on the health sector. Instead, in the five years prior to the crisis, the state spent on average 4.65 percent.[2]

An incident prompted a shift in the official discourse from regarding COVID-19 as a sanitary crisis to placing a stronger emphasis on the need to wage "war" on COVID-19, as the pandemic was regarded as the worst threat to the country in peace time (Aresta, 2021). When the nation was preparing for its first lockdown in March 2020, the commission instructed passengers coming from Europe – particularly from Portugal, which at the time (16 March) had 1,111 confirmed cases[3] – to undergo institutional quarantine at a government-run facility. However, there were claims that the minister of interior defied this directive and took his daughter for home quarantine (Jornal de Angola, 2020). This led to a leadership crisis, and following popular outcry, President Lourenço was forced to release the minister of interior from his duty as the deputy coordinator and instruct him to undergo a 14-day home quarantine for exposing himself to a passenger who had arrived from a high-risk country (Club-K, 2020).

The minister's defiance of the established rules needs to be understood beyond the context of a dispute for influence within the commission. In fact, it is one example of a way for those who join public administration with a military background to assert their power over those who do not. This is a trend[4] that can be traced back to the fact that the post-colonial state in Angola emerged through a civil-war (1975–2002) in which those in uniform played a dominant role. It was also during this period that those at the top of the hierarchy (mostly generals) started to consolidate their political and economic influence within the state. This dominance was enabled particularly in the 1980s, when President dos Santos (in office from 1979 to 2017) requested extraordinary powers to face the continuing threat posed by UNITA's[5] rebellion backed by apartheid South Africa.[6]

In 1984, the People's Assembly created the *Conselho da Defesa e Segurança* (Defence and Security Council). This council was "a restricted collegial body to run State affairs and direct the war, to support the Head of State and Commander-in-Chief of FAPLA (People's Armed Forces of Liberation of Angola)"[7] (MPLA, 1985: 28). This war council placed President dos Santos in a privileged position to control the country's resources and allocate them to key allies with no supervision from party structures.[8] Through this special arrangement the country was divided into military regions, and the president appointed military commanders to not only oversee the military and security aspects of their regions but to actually rule and control those regions.

Moving forward to the present day, people with a military background still occupy key influential positions not limited to the defence and security sectors. The current president, vice president, and attorney general all have a military background (general ranking), and the president of the supreme court (a retired lieutenant colonel) was recently promoted to the rank of brigadier general (Club-K, 2021a) by President Lourenço as the commander-in-chief. All this ensures that the military class supports the current president to retain power and influence in the current affairs of the country, and at the same time it allows them to constrain civilian influence and leadership, particularly in times of crisis.

Therefore, it makes sense to argue that the subsequent changes enacted by the president – such as (1) the rebranding of the commission to focus on the "fight and prevention" of COVID-19, and (2) the appointment of the state minister and head of the president's security house as the coordinator, and of the state minister for the social sector as the deputy coordinator – constitute an adjustment of the government's COVID-19 response team to align it to the prevailing balance of power in Angola, thus ensuring that those within the military and/or with a military background take control of the state policy response and the enforcement of lockdown measures. Moreover, the new coordinator and his deputy are also members of the MPLA (People's Movement for the Liberation of Angola) central committee and its political bureau, which makes them influential within both the ruling party and the cabinet.

Following a global trend as well as WHO recommendations (WHO, 2018: 146), on 25 March the president declared a state of emergency for 15 days. In the absence of proven pharmaceutical measures, this was seen as the only way to delay the spread of such an infectious disease among the population. However, when the state of emergency was subsequently extended on 9 April 2020, there was a shift towards the militarisation of state policy, reflected by the greater involvement of defence and security forces.

Apart from extending the state of emergency, the presidential decree introduced in its Article 4, the possibility for authorities to invade people's homes to enforce the rules. This strategy of expanding the involvement of the defence and security forces in the management of the pandemic was later adopted and incorporated in the revised Civil Protection Law, which took place in May 2020. As a result of this shift, according to the minister of interior and cited in the local press (Folha 8, 2021), 15,658 people were detained by the defence and security forces and 1,606 people were put to trial between 27 March and 25 May for disrespecting COVID-19 restrictions during the state of emergency.

As soon as the military took over the management of the crisis, it became evident that the focus, moved from handling a sanitary crisis to "fighting" COVID-19. Similar to other contexts (as illustrated by Purohit in Chapter 6), the authorities in Angola did not prioritise keeping the population informed about changes and how adopting lockdown measures would impact their livelihoods. Instead, the communication was patronising and unhelpful for the general population. For instance, on 3 April the minister of interior stated in a formal press conference that in cases of violation of the lockdown rules the police would take action, as they were not out there to "distribute sweets and chocolate" (Amnesty International and OMUNGA, 2020; Folha 8, 2021).

It thus became apparent that the authorities were so invested in the application of the rules that they disregarded their impact on the population's ability to simply make ends meet. This constitutes further evidence that the political elite was somehow out of touch with the needs of the population that they are meant to serve. One widely circulated photograph on social media provided a glimpse of the level of violence imposed upon the population. It depicted a group of police personnel in uniform holding the following message: "For you to sit in your house, is it necessary to beat you? Stay home". Indeed, cases of police brutality increased in the region, with protests during the lockdown reported on in Nigeria (Akinwotu, 2020) and South Africa (Trippe, 2020).

Despite these developments, health experts and opinion makers in Angola mostly agree that measures such as the establishment of institutional quarantine, in the context of a fragile health system, as well as the creation of an inter-ministerial commission contributed to the relative low number of cases in Angola. Indeed, as of 26 August 2021, the WHO COVID-19 Dashboard[9] indicated that the country registered 46,539 cumulative total cases and 1,176 deaths, significantly lower than neighbouring countries such as Zambia (205,107 cases and 3,506 deaths), Namibia (124,032 cases and 3,346 deaths), and the Democratic Republic of Congo (54,226 cases and 1,057 deaths).

The shift from tackling a sanitary emergency to focusing on "preventing and fighting COVID-19" remains, however, an important consideration in the state management of the COVID-19 pandemic in Angola. Given that the discourse came to be about a "fight" against COVID-19 (the enemy), it has become clear that the state in Angola believes that those with military background should take leadership roles, to the detriment of much-needed epidemiological and medical expertise. This approach has resulted in the militarisation of lockdown language and state policy. Moreover, the military nature of this leadership led to the adoption of a stricter version of lockdown, which in turn has resulted in the loss of lives and livelihoods.

Lives over livelihoods: Imposing a strict lockdown and its consequences

The composition of the new Multisector Commission to Prevent and Fight COVID-19 was more restricted compared to the previous Inter-ministerial Commission for Emergencies. It prioritised the involvement of all the governmental defence and security departments while leaving aside social communication (critical to keep the population informed of key safety measures), education, culture, as well as representatives from the private sector, who needed to assess how state measures would impact their businesses. At the operational level, the commission established a centre responsible for the "management, treatment, organizational, technical and operational coordination of the epidemiological situation, public safety and any actions to be taken to contain the COVID-19 pandemic" (Comissão Multissectorial para Prevenção e Combate á COVID-19, 2020). Further evidence of the prominence of those in uniform in the fight against COVID-19 is the fact that the centre is coordinated by a lieutenant-general, with a police commissar as his deputy, and it is staffed with military and police personnel.

The involvement of the defence and security forces, and the exclusion of key ministries such as education and culture, meant that the enforcement of lockdown rules did not take into consideration the cultural habits of the population. Furthermore, it disregarded the fact that the Angolan economy had been in recession since 2016.[10] This meant that, prior to the ongoing COVID-19 crisis, a majority of the population was already struggling to make a living, with inflation averaging 25 percent between 2016 and 2019 (INE, 2017b; 2021b). According to the central bank, the high inflation has been driven by increases in the price of food and non-alcoholic beverages (BNA, 2021). The unemployment rate increased to 28.8 percent in 2019 (INE, 2019: 12) from 20 percent between 2015 and 2016

(INE, 2017a). This was further exacerbated by the central bank's depreciation of the local currency, the Kwanza, in order to preserve the country's reserves in foreign currency (Silva, 2018). This resulted, for instance, in a drastic decrease in the agriculture minimum wage of AOA 21,454 (the lowest in the country), which went from the equivalent of USD 129.31 in 2017, to only USD 32.69 in 2020.

The enforcement of such a strict version of lockdown negatively impacted people's capacity to make a living, particularly in the cities. Indeed, official statistics indicate that the overall unemployment rate in the country is now significantly high at 32.3 percent (versus 28.8 percent in between 2018 and 2019), while the urban unemployment rate reached 44.5 percent (versus 36.5 percent between 2018 and 2019) (INE, 2019: 13; 2021a: 25). Furthermore (and similar to what Cook and Borges present in Chapter 15), the female unemployment rate in Angola increased from 30.9 percent between 2018 and 2019 (INE, 2019: 13) to 34 percent in 2020 (INE, 2021a: 25). While the overall data shows that the informal employment rate reached 57,5 percent in 2020, the rate for female employment in the non-agricultural informal sector was 76.9 percent, compared to 41.9 percent for men (INE, 2021a: 21).

Prior to the pandemic, the economic empowerment of women was already a cause of major concern, as most women and young girls were employed in the informal sector of the economy due to lower barrier to entry (Government of Angola, Ministry of Family and Women Empowerment, 2017: 68). The initial state-of-emergency rules dictated that informal markets operate only three days a week (Tuesday, Thursday, and Saturday) instead of the usual seven days, and that they only open for essential goods. Thus, 8,013 informal markets were closed by local authorities (Folha 8, 2021) to enforce lockdown measures. This meant that those who sold non-essential goods in informal markets were prevented from earning a living from March to May 2020, when Presidential Decree N° 128/20 of 8 May was issued, extending the working days from three to five days a week and allowing the sale of all goods and services. This policy decision inadvertently hurt those employed in the informal sector of the economy who lacked an appropriate social safety net. The majority were women.

Despite the improvement brought by Presidential Decree N° 128/20, sellers in the informal markets were still prohibited to work on Sundays and Mondays, as markets were closed on these days, and the decree regarded the violation of this rule as a crime of disobedience. This measure, combined with the already mentioned adverse macroeconomic situation, may have exacerbated poverty, which was already at 40.6 percent between 2018 and 2019 (INE, 2019: 16), and reached 54 percent in 2020 (INE, 2020a: 28). This deterioration of the socioeconomic conditions of families in Angola seems to explain the increase in domestic violence against women and children. Indeed, reports indicate that under lockdown, as well as beyond it (between March and November 2020), authorities reported 19 cases of homicide, an average of 11 cases of domestic violence per day against women, and 103,140 cases of child violence, which represents an increase compared to the same period in the previous year (LUSA, 2020d).

The loss of livelihoods due to this strict version of lockdown, and the subsequent increase of the poverty level, also led to an increase in people's dissatisfaction, and despite the limitation to their freedoms of assembly, they took to the streets to protest, leading to further violence (Amnesty International and OMUNGA, 2020). This in fact meant that those at risk were also more susceptible to experiencing violence from the defence and security forces in Angola, something that was also seen in South Africa (Trippe, 2020).

Between March 2020, when the lockdown was first introduced, and September 2020, after the state of emergency had been lifted and some measures relaxed, particularly outside the capital city Luanda, Amnesty International and OMUNGA[11] (2020: 2) identified the occurrence of "ten killings by the Angolan security forces, including officers of the Angolan National Police (Polícia Nacional de Angola – PNA) and of the Angolan Armed Forces (Forças Armadas Angolanas – FAA)". The victims were aged between 14 and 35 (Amnesty International and OMUNGA, 2020: 2). This level of violence later led to a civil society outcry, particularly when a medical doctor was reported dead after being taken into police custody while driving alone without a mask (Luamba, 2020), which clearly was a consequence of the strict interpretation of the mask mandate by the defence and security forces. The general condemnation of the use of excessive force by the police impelled the authorities, particularly the general commander of the police force, to issue a public apology (Angola Press, 2020b; Kapapelo, 2020). However, a recent report by Human Rights Watch indicates that this gesture has not stopped the killing of innocent people, particularly when they try to exercise their right of assembly and protest against poor social service provision by the state in Angola (Human Rights Watch, 2021).

Undermining the democratic process

The authorities have also seized this pandemic crisis to undermine the democratic process in Angola. The ruling party has been accused of undermining and/or delaying the implementation of local elections as a way to avoid sharing power with the opposition (Sousa. 2014). In 2017, President Lourenço promised, in his first State of the Nation address, to "enact [local elections] from the constitutional text to the reality" (Lourenço, 2017: para. 23).

Due to growing popular dissatisfaction with the government's policies, which failed to tackle the already examined high inflation and unemployment rate, President Lourenço ignored calls for local elections, which would enable the localisation of the COVID-19 response, on the grounds that elections would bring large crowds together and there was a need to keep social distance to save lives (LUSA, 2020c). Yet, parliamentary, presidential, and local elections were held elsewhere in Africa in 2020 (Annor, 2020; Ribeiro, 2020; Kuwonu, 2021). For instance, Benin and Cabo Verde elected their local representatives, and in Ghana, president Nana Akufo-Addo was re-elected. All these examples contradict the argument put forward by the authorities in Angola. Ultimately, President Lourenço emphasised in his

2020 State of the Nation address that, contrary to what members of the opposition parties and civil society organisations argued, local elections in Angola were not delayed *sine die* as they had never been scheduled in the first place (Lourenço, 2020).

In sum, the militarisation of lockdown language and state policy in Angola is a manifestation of a broader problem linked to the military's omnipresence in state institutions undermining any non-military actor's attempt to constrain their entrenched holding power. The current crisis provides a perfect platform for their continuing control and domination, now under the guise of saving lives. However, as examined in this section, in the process there has been substantial loss of lives: victims of the security forces' brutality as people try to maintain their livelihoods.

Conclusion

The deployment of the defence and security forces has led to the adoption of a strict version of lockdown and the subsequent loss of lives and livelihoods, with little regard to the fact that people were already living in dire socioeconomic conditions prior to the COVID-19 pandemic. This chapter has illustrated that due to pre-existing inequalities in labour-market participation, in Angola lockdown measures have disproportionately impacted women, leading to higher unemployment rates. This rightfully calls for specific measures targeted at women if the nation is to meet its international commitments such as the UN Sustainable Development Goal 5 (to achieve gender equality and empower all women and girls), Goal 8 (to promote sustained, inclusive, and sustainable economic growth, full and productive employment, and decent work for all) and Goal 10 (to reduce inequality within and among countries).

The ruling party and its leadership were quick to use this context of crisis, and lockdown, to undermine the democratic process in Angola, for instance by limiting civil liberties (allowing defence and security forces to conduct home violations to enforce the rules) and delaying the implementation of local elections, while allowing President Lourenço to increase and consolidate his political power through changes in the civil protection law.

Ultimately, the militarisation of lockdown language and state policy in Angola has enabled the military class (active and retired) to consolidate its holding power over the civilian population in times of peace. In the debate of lives over livelihoods, the state in Angola, rather than striving for balance, has chosen to side with lives. However, in the process, there has been significant loss of both lives and livelihoods.

Notes

1 www.who.int/healthsystems/publications/Abuja10.pdf
2 Author's own calculations based on national budget data available from the Government of Angola, Ministry of Finance website: www.minfin.gov.ao/PortalMinfin/#!/materias-de-realce/orcamento-geral-do-estado/oge-passados
3 Data available at https://covid19.who.int/region/euro/country/pt

4 In politics there is the recent case of former governor of Luanda province, Bento Bento, and general José Tavares Ferreira (mayor of the city of Luanda), who had a showdown during their time in office between 2011 and 2014 (Club-K, 2021b).

5 The acronym for the National Union for the Total Independence of Angola, one of the three main liberation movements in Angola. The other two being the MPLA – the People's Movement for the Liberation of Angola MPLA (the ruling party in Angola since independence in 1975), and the FNLA – the National Front of Liberation of Angola. Following independence, UNITA's leadership decided to fight a guerrilla war, from the countryside, claiming to be fighting against the spread of socialism and on behalf of "those who did not feel represented by the MPLA" (Chabal, 2007: 7).

6 In this period, South Africa's apartheid regime was waging an undeclared war against Angola, targeting mainly its economic and social infrastructure (Bhagavan, 1986: 18).

7 FAPLA was created in 1974 and it was essentially the MPLA military wing turned into the national army after independence (MPLA, 1979).

8 This status of affairs allowed for the emergence of a centralised presidential clientelism system (Vidal, 2016).

9 Data available at https://covid19.who.int/table

10 According to official statistics, in 2016 Angola's GDP was -2.6 percent, but it recovered slightly in 2018 to -2 percent and -0.5 percent in 2019 before plummeting to -5.4 percent in 2020 (Instituto Nacional de Estatística, 2021c: 12), leading to the deterioration of the macroeconomic situation of the country.

11 An Angolan human rights NGO. Further information can be found here: www.omu nga.org/

References

Akinwotu, E. 2020. "Nigeria Cracks down on "end Sars" Protesters, Alleging Terrorism". *The Guardian UK Edition*, 13 November, www.theguardian.com/world/2020/nov/13/nige ria-cracks-down-on-end-sars-protesters-alleging-terrorism

Amnesty International, and OMUNGA. 2020. *ANGOLA: THE POLICE ARE NOT ON THE GROUND TO DISTRIBUTE SWEETS: SECURITY FORCES' VIOLENCE IN ANGOLA*. London: Amnesty International Ltd: www.amnesty.org/en/documents/ afr12/3424/2020/en/.

Angola Press. 2020a. "COVID-19: Governo Angolano Toma Medidas Excepcionais". Youtube, uploaded by Angola Press, 18 March: www.youtube.com/watch?v=IU2ls6d7q1g

Angola Press. 2020b. "COVID-19: Polícia Nacional Pede Desculpa à População". Youtube, uploaded by Angola Press. 10 June: www.youtube.com/watch?v=YBH3D56Gg0s

Annor, I. 2020. "Year in Review: Africa's 2020 Elections". *Africanews*, 24 December, www.afr icanews.com/2020/12/24/year-in-review-africa-s-2020-elections/.

Aresta, L. 2021. "Depois Da Guerra, a COVID-19 é o Pior Inimigo de Angola". *Radio Renascença*, 20 March, https://rr.sapo.pt/2020/03/20/mundo/depois-da-guerra-a-covid-19-e-o-pior-inimigo-de-angola/noticia/186000/

Bhagavan, M.R. 1986. *Angola's Political Economy 1975-1985*. Research Report No. 75. Uppsala: Scandinavian Institute of African Studies.

BNA. 2021. "Comité de Política Monetária - Notas de Imprensa". www.bna.ao/Conteu dos/Artigos/detalhe_artigo.aspx?idc=139&idsc=266&idi=17639&idl=1

Chabal, P. 2007. "E Pluribus Unum: Transitions in Angola". In *Angola: The Weight of History*, edited by P. Chabal and N. Vidal. London: Hurst & Company: 1–19

Club-K. 2020. "Presidente Suspende Ministro Do Interior". *CLUB-K,* 25 March https://club-k.net/index.php?option=com_content&view=article&id=39882:presidente-suspe nde-ministro-do-interior&catid=8&lang=pt&Itemid=1071

Club-K. 2021a. 'Presidente Do Supremo Promovido a Brigadeiro'. *CLUB-K,* 28 January, www.club-k.net/index.php?option=com_content&view=article&id=43422:preside nte-do-supremo-promovido-a-brigadeiro&catid=8:bastidores&lang=pt&Itemid=1071

Club-K. 2021b. "JL Medeia Reconciliação Entre General Tavares e Bento Bento". *CLUB-K,* 3 May, www.club-k.net/index.php?option=com_content&view=article&id=44285:jl-medeia-reconciliacao-entre-general-tavares-e-bento-bento&catid=8:bastidores&lang=pt&Itemid=1071

Comissão Interministerial para as Emergências. 2020. *Plano Nacional de Contingência Para o Controlo Da Epidemia Por Coronavírus (2019-NCoV).* Ministry of Health: http://alime ntacplp.com/wp-content/uploads/2020/05/Angola_PlanoNacionaldeContingenciae EmergenciaCOVID-19.pdf

Comissão Multissectorial para Prevenção e Combate á COVID-19. 2020. "Comissão Multissectorial Para Prevenção e Combate á COVID-19 - Centro de Direcção". https://cdircovid19.gov.ao/index.php?secao=home

Folha 8. 2021. "'Operação Laborinho', Êxito Total!' *Jornal Folha 8,* 6 February, https://jorna lf8.net/2021/operacao-laborinho-exito-total-2/

Government of Angola, Ministry of Family and Women Empowerment. 2017. *Relatório Analítico de Género de Angola'. 1º.* Luanda: Ministry of Family and Women Empowerment.

Government of Angola, Ministry of Health. 2020. "Comunicado". Comissão Interministerial de Angola. www.covid19.gov.ao/assets/arq_pdf/COMUNICADOCOVID19ALE RTAPOPGERAL_versao2.pdf

Human Rights Watch. 2021. "Angola: Policia Mata Manifestantes Na Província de Lunda Norte". *Human Rights Watch,* 4 February, www.hrw.org/pt/news/2021/02/04/377768

INE. 2017a. *Relatório Sobre Emprego: Inquérito de Indicadores Múltiplos e de Saúde, 2015–2016.* Luanda: Instituto Nacional de Estatística.

INE. 2017b. "Índice de Preços No Consumidor Nacional". Folha de Informação Rápida. Instituto Nacional de Estatística. www.ine.gov.ao/

INE. 2019. 'Indicadores de Emprego e Desemprego: Inquérito Sobre Despesas, Receitas e Emprego Em Angola, IDREA 2018–2019'. Luanda: Instituto Nacional de Estatística.

INE. 2020a. *Índice de Pobreza Multidimensional de Angola.* Luanda: Instituto Nacional de Estatística.

INE. 2020b. *Relatório de Pobreza Para Angola: Inquérito Sobre Despesas e Receitas.* Luanda: Instituto Nacional de Estatística.

INE. 2021a. *Relatório Anual 2020: Inquérito Ao Emprego Em Angola.* Luanda: Instituto Nacional de Estatística.

INE. 2021b. 'Índice de Preços No Consumidor Nacional'. Folha de Informação Rápida. Instituto Nacional de Estatística. https://www.ine.gov.ao/

INE. 2021c. 'Contas Nacionais Trimestrais Ajustado Sazonalmente'. 1o Trimestre. Luanda.

Jornal de Angola. 2020. "Chegada de Passageiros de Lisboa e Porto é Marcada Por Confusão e Horas de Espera". *Jornal de Angola,* 13 March, www.jornaldeangola.ao/ao/noticias/chegada-de-passageiros-de-lisboa-e-porto-e-marcada-por-confusao-e-horas-de-espera/

Kapapelo, D. 2020. "Excesso Policial: Comandante-Geral Pede Desculpas à População e Assegura Responsabilização Criminal Dos Efectivos Envolvidos". *Portal de Angola,* 12 September, www.portaldeangola.com/2020/09/12/excesso-policial-comandante-geral-pede-desculpas-a-populacao-e-assegura-responsabilizacao-criminal-dos-efectivos-envolvidos/

Kuwonu, F. 2021. "Elections in Africa Go on amid COVID-19". Africa Renewal. 4 January, www.un.org/africarenewal/magazine/january-2021/elections-africa-amid-covid

Lourenço, J. 2017. "Mensagem Sobre o Estado da Nação, Pronunciado Pelo PR João Lourenço". *CLUB-K*, 16 October, www.club-k.net/index.php?option=com_cont ent&view=article&id=29716:mensagem-sobre-o-estado-da-nacao-pronunciado-pelo-pr-joao-lourenco&catid=11&Itemid=1072&lang=pt

Lourenço, J . 2020. "Mensagem Sobre o Estado da Nação". www.missionangola.ch/discou rs_du_president/Estado_Nacao15102020.pdf.pdf

Luamba, M. 2020. "'Eu Sou Sílvio Dala': Sociedade Civil Angolana Protesta Contra a Morte Do Médico". *Deutsche Welle Notícias*, 12 September, www.dw.com/pt-002/ eu-sou-s%C3%ADlvio-dala-sociedade-civil-angolana-protesta-contra-a-morte-do-m%C3%A9dico/a-54908113

LUSA. 2020a. "Angola Cria Comissão Multissetorial Para Reforçar Medidas de Vigilância". *RTP Notícias*, 30 January, www.rtp.pt/noticias/mundo/angola-cria-comissao-multissetor ial-para-reforcar-medidas-de-vigilancia_n1201752

LUSA. 2020b. "Angola Impõe Quarentena e Reforça Prevenção Do Coronavírus". *Deutsche Welle Notícias*, 6 February www.dw.com/pt-002/angola-imp%C3%B5e-quarentena-e-refor%C3%A7a-preven%C3%A7%C3%A3o-do-coronav%C3%ADrus/a-52278972

LUSA. 2020c. "Primeiras Autárquicas Em Angola Adiadas - UNITA Fala Em Falta de Vontade Política". *Público*, 10 September, www.publico.pt/2020/09/10/mundo/noticia/ primeiras-autarquicas-angola-adiadas-unita-fala-falta-vontade-politica-1931052

LUSA. 2020d. "Angola Regista 'Considerável Aumento' de Crimes Contra Mulheres". *Deutsche Welle Notícias*, 25 November, www.dw.com/pt-002/angola-regista-consi der%C3%A1vel-aumento-de-crimes-contra-mulheres/a-55728807

MPLA. 1979. "First Congress of MPLA, Luanda, 4-10 December 1977: Report of the Central Committee: Theses on Education". *State Papers and Party Proceedings* 2 (11).

MPLA. 1985. *Second Congress of the MPLA-Workers' Party, Luanda, 2-9 December 1985.* London: Agência Angola Press.

Ribeiro, S. 2020. "Autárquicas 2020: MpD Vence, Mas Resultados Dão Novo Fôlego Ao PAICV". *Expresso Das Ilhas*, 28 October, https://expressodasilhas.cv/politica/2020/10/ 28/autarquicas-2020-mpd-vence-mas-resultados-dao-novo-folego-ao-paicv/71931

Silva, P. 2018. *Evolução do Mercado Cambial em Angola'. Presented at the VIII FÓRUM BANCA, Hotel EPIC SANA*, Luanda.

Sousa, G. 2014. "Oposição Acusa Governo de Angola de Falta de Vontade Para Realizar Autárquicas". *Deutsche Welle Notícias*, 2 April, www.dw.com/pt-002/ oposi%C3%A7%C3%A3o-acusa-governo-de-angola-de-falta-de-vontade-para-realizar-aut%C3%A1rquicas/a-17537763

Trippe, K. 2020. "Pandemic Policing: South Africa's Most Vulnerable Face a Sharp Increase in Police-Related Brutality". *Atlantic Council*, 24 June, www.atlanticcouncil.org/blogs/afric asource/pandemic-policing-south-africas-most-vulnerable-face-a-sharp-increase-in-pol ice-related-brutality/

Vidal, N. 2016. "O MPLA e a Governação: Entre Internacionalismo Progressista Marxista e Pragmatismo Liberal-Nacionalista". *Estudos Ibero-Americanos* 42 (3): 815–54.

WHO. 2018. "Managing Epidemics: Key Facts about Major Deadly Diseases". *World Health Organisation*, www.who.int/emergencies/diseases/managing-epidemics-interactive.pdf

WHO . 2020a. "Statement on the Second Meeting of the International Health Regulations (2005) Emergency Committee Regarding the Outbreak of Novel Coronavirus

(2019-NCoV)". *World Health Organisation*, 30 January, www.who.int/news/item/30-01-2020-statement-on-the-second-meeting-of-the-international-health-regulations-(2005)-emergency-committee-regarding-the-outbreak-of-novel-coronavirus-(2019-ncov)

WHO. 2020b. "WHO Director-General's Opening Remarks at the Media Briefing on COVID-19 - 11 March 2020". *World Health Organisation*, 11 March, www.who.int/director-general/speeches/detail/who-director-general-s-opening-remarks-at-the-media-briefing-on-covid-19---11-march-2020

8

THE ECONOMIC IMPACT OF COVID-19 LOCKDOWN POLICIES IN ARGENTINA

Maddalena Cevese

Introduction

On 11 March 2020, the World Health Organisation (WHO) officially declared the COVID-19 outbreak an epidemic turned pandemic (WHO, 2020). As of 6 September 2021, Argentina had recorded 5,203,802 confirmed cases of COVID-19 and 112,444 deaths, the second-highest rates in South America after Brazil. Almost a million people have died across 12 countries in South America. Although the region is home to 5 percent of the global population, it has experienced peaks of COVID-19-related deaths amounting to a quarter of deaths globally. The underlying reasons for such high rates are mainly linked to the steep rise of infectious SARS-CoV-2 variants in the region, overburdened and/or underfunded public healthcare systems, crowded neighbourhoods, and entrenched poverty exacerbated by rising levels of "pandemic fatigue" (WHO, 2020).

In Argentina, the COVID-19 pandemic has become a serious public health and economic challenge, particularly in urban areas where the majority of the population lives. Most cases were registered in the Metropolitan Area of Buenos Aires (AMBA), home to 15 million inhabitants, about one-third of the total population (45,479,118).

Following the WHO pandemic announcement, Argentina introduced a nationwide mandatory lockdown from 19 March to 10 May 2020, later extended until 17 July in AMBA. The Ministry of Health extended the health emergency for a year, introducing a variety of preventive restrictions as well as imposing a ban on flights from the most affected countries in order to curb the epidemiological spread. Despite these restrictions, however, a second wave was recorded in April–May 2021, leading to the imposition of a second nationwide lockdown lasting until the end of May.

According to the Government Response Stringency Index (Hale et al., 2020), Argentina not only imposed the highest number of lockdowns as well as the longest

DOI: 10.4324/9781003259336-11

lockdowns across Latin America, its measures were also among the strictest. The preventive and mandatory social-isolation measures (*Decree 297/2020*) entailed the closure of all non-essential businesses, schools, universities, and parks, suspension of outdoor activities, as well as national nighttime curfews and border controls. Law enforcement officers were stationed across the country and individuals who could not justify their transit were fined according to the penal code. Citizens were expected to refrain from leaving their homes except for essential shopping limited to groceries and medication. Interestingly, banks were not considered essential businesses at first, and remained closed for most of the first lockdown (Alzúa and Gosis, 2020). Essential workers were exempt from most restrictions and there was limited public transportation available exclusively for them.

Overall, the general public supported the measures in the early stages of the pandemic but became more critical with the increased severity of the impacts of lockdown policies (Busso et al., 2020). The economy was already in a fragile state marked by a history of perpetual economic crisis and systemic inequalities (Ocampo, 2015; Judzik, Trujillo, and Villafañe, 2017). As the lockdown was prolonged multiple times during the first wave, there was mounting concern about how long the measures could be sustained before people started to suffer from severe income loss, unemployment, and increased indebtedness, coupled with rising concerns for the mental health of both essential and non-essential workers (Abeldaño Zuñiga et al. 2021; Steinmetz et al. 2021). Lockdowns had different outcomes in different social segments (Busso and Messina, 2020; Furceri et al., 2020), and the *essential worker* became a newly created social subject, exposing a variety of class-based inequalities intrinsic to the employment market (Diaz, 2020). Furthermore, as expected, households with fewer economic resources were hit the hardest in the immediacy of the crisis and are also expected to take the longest to recover (Busso and Messina, 2020).

This chapter examines the impact of COVID-19 lockdown policies in Argentina. It starts by analysing some of the impacts on the national economy, highlighting how the current crisis exacerbated a history of perpetual recessionary crisis in Argentina. Indeed, lockdowns have aggravated historic economic hardships and contributed to unsustainable volumes of indebtedness that were already stifling the country's economic capacity. The magnitude of impacts of COVID-19 lockdowns is so extensive, it compares to the 2001 crisis that led to the biggest sovereign default in global modern economic history. Subsequently, the paper discusses socio-economic impacts on employment and social assistance in Buenos Aires, illustrating how the social benefit schemes introduced during the pandemic were insufficient for many households, forcing individuals to resort to other means in order to compensate for large reductions in incomes.

Arguably, the government of Argentina did not sufficiently account for the losses and risks that lengthy lockdowns entailed. They were all ill-equipped to deal with the precarious economic situation' and extended lockdowns over a period of more than a year were simply not a measure the economy could afford. There is a possibility that Argentina reacted rather impulsively to international pressures, following suit with global trends in the fight against COVID-19. The first lockdown may have made sense at the time of introduction as the pandemic was a novel scenario and yet required an exhaustive understanding of the epidemiological spread and harm. In hindsight, acknowledging what we know about the virus today and the aggravated economic hardships and social costs caused by lockdowns, the decision to extend and reintroduce the lockdowns at several intervals is met with consternation.

Macroeconomic impact and mounting indebtedness

The first lockdowns were introduced in South America in March 2020. In comparison to many other "emerging markets" across Asia, Eastern Europe, the Middle East, and Africa (Cottani, 2020), the regional economy of South America has contracted more drastically. The following numbers give a concrete picture: across South America in 2020, the regional real gross domestic product (GDP) fell by 7.4 percent (Werner et al., 2021). While it grew again by 6.5 percent in 2021 (BBVA research, 2021) with an additional expected growth of 3.5 percent in 2022 (BBVA Research, 2021), the overall real GDP has, at the time of writing in November 2021, plummeted by 8.7 percent below the pre-pandemic forecasts by the International Monetary Fund (IMF) for that period (IMF, 2021; Werner e. al., 2021). On top of this, post-lockdown recovery is estimated to be fairly weak and uneven (IMF, 2021) due to pre-existing economic conditions that threaten to exacerbate the sharp human and social costs of lockdowns, and associated policies with severe consequences for poverty rates and living standards that are already entrenched in systemic levels of inequality in the region.

Argentina is the third-largest economy in South America, with a real GDP of $445.5 billion USD (Romo and Ojeda-Galaviz, 2020) yet large levels of inequality and indebtedness. The health crisis hit the country at a time when economic activity had already suffered significantly. The inflation rate had risen from 48 percent in 2018 to 54 percent in 2019 (Cottani, 2020), unemployment rates were in double digits, poverty levels neared 40 percent, and the sovereign debt increased to $311 billion USD, including a $57 billion USD loan by the IMF (INDEC, 2020). This picture worsened significantly during the lockdowns in 2020, with the seasonally adjusted real GDP decreasing to $383 billion USD by the second quarter of the year (Bronstein, 2020). In order to avoid a run on the Argentinian peso, the country entered its ninth sovereign debt restructuring with private creditors and opened new negotiations with the IMF, which eventually led to a loan reduction to $44 billion USD (Bronstein, 2020). This measure was needed to alleviate the increased pressures coming with the introduction of lockdowns. At the same time, other measures that could have helped further financial adjustments were blocked, such as a wealth tax reform.

In order to bolster state income, a wealth tax proposal was passed in congress on 20 April 2020 to deduct 2–3.5 percent from capital reserves of over $3 million USD, targeting 11,000 eligible payees (Barlow, 2020). However, on the same day this proposal was introduced, international creditors rejected another outstanding government proposal to renegotiate $66.6 billion USD of debt, and dropped other debt renegotiations as well, resulting in further augmentation of the fiscal pressure. This indicates the manner in which Argentina is subject to continuous financial and international pressures that limit the government's ability to act in the country's best interest, and shows how the majority of the population has little room to manoeuvre under these conditions.

A month into the first lockdown, pressure on the fiscal space increased so considerably that a $10 billion USD debt repayment had to be deferred, resulting in the Standard and Poor's (S&P) immediate downgrading of the Argentine credit level. This rendered future borrowing considerably more expensive than it already was (Barlow, 2020). Argentina was the only one of the six biggest economies in the region that required emergency assistance during the crisis. Instead of emergency instruments, other countries had access to voluntary lending from both domestic and external private sources, with low interest rates due to their favourable local capital market conditions, strong policy frameworks, solid track records, and stable current balance of payments. This meant that they were able to resort to precautionary financial assistance from the IMF, such as the rapid credit facility (RCF), the rapid financing instrument (RFI), and flexible credit lines (FLCs) (ECLAC, 2021), to cover any eventual crisis emerging from the pandemic. Thus, although the IMF approved FCLs worth $23.9 billion USD for Chile, $16.9 billion USD for Colombia, and $11 billion USD for Peru (Cottani, 2020), Argentina was ineligible as it was already tied by the aforementioned $44 billion USD IMF loan.

There was no alternative for Argentina other than to react to the costs of the pandemic by taking on increased amounts of debts; thus, by the end of 2020, its sovereign debt increased to $335 billion USD (CEIC Data, 2020). Considering that Argentina defaulted on $97.6 billion USD of sovereign debt in December 2001 (Hornbeck, 2013; Guzman, 2016), the sharp rise in indebtedness that came with extended lockdowns brought forth critical concerns over the preparedness and resilience of its economy. The longer this trend continues, the greater the risk for another serious sovereign default. Even though the IMF forecasts a solid real GDP surge by 2022, the risk of default remains as the accumulated permanent real GDP loss since 2019 amounts to 8.7 percent (IMF, 2021). This all took place in the context of an economic depression that for the last seven years has been marked by consistent economic stagnation, a fiscal deficit that increased by 8–10 percent of GDP, and very high exchange-rate volatility as a result of depleted levels of foreign reserves (Cottani, 2020).

Not only does this growing financial precarity reveal the extent to which lockdowns are not affordable in Argentina, it also remains unclear how debt incurred from the impact of COVID-19 lockdown policies will be paid back. This is a serious matter for any country, but particularly for economies already facing large pre-pandemic repayment obligations. Indeed, countries around the world have seen lockdowns contribute to a so-called "debt pandemic" on top of the ongoing health emergency (Bulow et al., 2020). Furthermore, low- and middle-income economies tend to collect low tax revenues, which results in a slow repayment rate.

If lockdowns generate even more debt through increased borrowing, this sets the condition for a vicious cycle of economic setbacks. In fact, in a previous study from 2018 the IMF estimated that 40 percent of low-income countries (LICs) were on the verge of defaulting on debt liabilities, an increase from 21 percent in 2013, the figure doubling in just five years (IMF, 2020). Following such trends, the long-term costs of added indebtedness as a result COVID-19 lockdowns can be envisioned quite tangibly.

In the context of the argument that the government gave insufficient consideration to the increased social costs of lockdowns for an already precarious, debt-burdened economy, it is clear that the lockdowns moved Argentina further down the path toward long-term normalisation of crises. In other words, "economic emergency measures are so normalised because of past crises that their effectiveness is diminished, if not exhausted" (Barlow, 2020: 1). Although there is hope that conversations between the Argentine government and the IMF may help to extend the maturity of the country's significant existing debt, as occurred previously, this option cannot be the long-term solution. There is an urgent need for structural alternatives to indebtedness in order to alleviate the effects of the crisis. The most sustainable approach to mitigate the impacts of the current emergency cannot rely on the accumulation of more debt (Graeber, 2011). It is also contrary to the attainability of the's UN Sustainable Development Goals by 2030, as debt-sustainability is deemed a crucial feature of a sustainable economy (Prizzon, 2019).

Socioeconomic impacts on employment and social assistance

As the pandemic began to unfold worldwide in March 2020, the state implemented a wide range of policies to minimise the social costs of the pandemic (Blofield, Giambruno, and Filgueira, 2020). Considering the state of emergency, most measures were introduced by presidential decrees rather than passed as laws of the national congress in order to expedite a quickened response and at the same time concentrate decision-making in the national executive power (Arza, 2021). In this way, decrees were the fastest tool with which to address the immediate international pressures posed by this crisis and dominate the national lockdown narrative.

The Preventive and Compulsory Social Isolation Decree (ASPO, Decree 297/ 2020) placed the economy at a significant standstill as it covered all sectors of the economy and the state. Article 2 of this decree established that all residents, including temporary visitors to the country, and with the exception of essential workers, were required to refrain from attending their workplaces and travelling along routes, roads, and public spaces. This measure was justified as part of the effort to prevent the circulation and contagion of the SARS-CoV-2 virus and the consequent impact on public health and on the civic rights of individuals. Essentially, individuals were restricted to minimal and essential trips to stock up on food, medication, and cleaning supplies.

Large numbers of workers were compelled to stay at home. While around 27 percent of the total workforce (Albrieu, 2020) were able to transition fairly directly to working remotely during the lockdown, many more were not, imposing the need for immediate adjustment among the majority of the population. The National Institute of Statistics lists a broad range of occupations that were far less able to transition to teleworking, particularly in the sectors of construction, manufacturing, sales, services, gastronomy, and domestic care (Diaz, 2020). The industrial sector was adversely impacted due to the drop in demand for final products, hardship in delivering merchandise, and the large-scale disruption in global value chains (Sturzenegger, 2020). In total, about 35 percent of economic activity was completely shut down, an unprecedented scale in Argentina's economic history, which was estimated to cost the economy US$500 million a day (Sturzenegger, 2020). While the employment rate dropped from 53.1 percent to 42.8 percent (INDEC, 2020), the rate of unemployment within the economically active population reached the highest level of the last decade, increasing from 11.3 percent in 2019 to 13.9 percent in 2020 (Donza and Poy, 2021), and under-employment was at 13 percent, both figures illustrating that a good quarter of the labour force was struggling (Alzúa and Gosis, 2020).

In order to mitigate the loss of income due to the total or partial standstill of economic activities, the government introduced a series of packages tailored to both individuals and companies. These support measures were intended to protect workers and families across social strata and included key policy provisions to safeguard employment and the living conditions of families, such as regulations to control the prices of essential goods and services, rent, employment, and access to credit (Lustig and Tommasi, 2020). To cushion livelihoods, price controls were introduced on essential consumption goods, basic public utilities for households were protected from suspension, and certain mortgage payments were frozen. Furthermore, the issuing of loans provided by the National Social Security Administration (ANSES) was also suspended, and a subsidised credit-for-consumption programme with credit card instalments was introduced (Arza, 2021). Lastly, all domestic rental contracts were placed under a price freeze and subject to automatic extension, with rents suspended for a period of six months, later extended until 31 January 2021.

To safeguard employment, the government strengthened the legal framework to limit the ability of companies to lay off workers for unjustified reasons. These decrees, first introduced on 31 March 2020 and subsequently extended several times, prohibited the dismissal and suspension of employees for lack or reduction of economic activity or due to force majeure for an initial period of 60 days. Nonetheless, many companies found it impossible to guarantee full salaries during lockdowns, which led to the introduction of an exception for simplified lay-offs. Suspensions or terminations of employment contracts by dismissal were only allowed if compliant with the guidelines issued by the Ministry of Work, Employment and Social Security and agreed to by both employers and workers. In cases where there was evidence of unfair dismissal, these could be suspended (Linklaters, 2021). In addition, workers' salaries in the formal sector were subsidised by the government until December 2020, and as of November 2020, more than 1.7 million workers were found to have benefited from this package (Arza, 2021). It shows that the government was heavily invested in finding the right measures of compensation for the major losses and strains placed on society. However, a deeper look into the packages reveals socioeconomic biases which would come to leave out many people and companies in need.

One such example is a formulation in the lockdown policy that disproportionately addressed the protection of the private sector; as important as it is, other areas seem to fall short in comparison or have been completely left out.

In the terms established by the regulations of the Ministry of Labour, Employment and Social Security, workers in the formal private sector would be entitled to their full income. These wages were protected by two major packages: the Programa de Recuperación Productiva 2 (REPRO 2) and the Programa de Asistencia de Emergencia al Trabajo y la Producción (ATP). REPRO 2 offered grants to the most affected industries across all sectors, with special bonuses for health and security personnel. While sectors that weren't critically affected were entitled to receive up to 9,000 pesos, critically affected sectors as well as health sectors could receive up to 22,000 pesos.

ATP was a wage-support programme guaranteeing 50 percent of salary liabilities for workers in critically affected economic sectors who could no longer perform their activities due to the lockdown. Interest-free loans were made available for the self-employed in the formal sector covering up to 25 percent of the gross income limit of their tax category (and a maximum of 150,000 ARS/$2,041 USD) (Ernst et al., 2020). The ATP also deferred and reduced up to 95 percent of employer contributions for companies, awarding a higher reduction for the most affected sectors and securing loans with subsidised interest rates (Arza, 2021). In May 2020, the programme was found to have benefited 230,000 firms and 2.3 million workers (ANSES, 2020). However, there was evidence that biases in the implementation of the ATP led to the exclusion of many workers, as banks applied preferential treatment to clients with previous positive credit scores and a favourable credit history (Arza 2021).

Importantly, despite government measures trying to limit the impact of lockdowns, many workers across non-essential sectors experienced income reductions or complete losses. Workers who were not entitled to either REPRO 2 or ATP had no choice but to resort to other financial means in order to meet their expenses. A study found that in Buenos Aires, almost four in ten households used savings or sold belongings during lockdowns, and more than 40 percent went into debt to meet their expenses (INDEC, 2020). A further 11 percent requested loans from banks and state agencies such as ANSES or AFIP (INDEC, 2020). As much as the government is bound by international financial pressures, the extent to which lockdowns were introduced during the COVID-19 emergency meant that the internal pressures were to increase consistently throughout the pandemic.

It is helpful to look at sectors individually to illustrate the mounting inability of citizens to carry the financial burdens of the lockdown. The cultural sector, for instance, was one of the most severely impacted during the lockdowns. All cultural, recreational, sporting, and religious events, or any other events involving the coming together of people, had to be cancelled. In addition, theatres, cinemas, cultural and artistic venues, shopping centres, and wholesale and retail establishments were all required to close. A survey by the Cultural Information System of Argentina (SInCA, 2020) found that after three months of lockdown measures, 44 percent of workers in the cultural sector had to cancel their activities. This in turn meant that these workers experienced a variety of salary suspensions: 35 percent did not receive any income for their ongoing remote cultural activities, and 32 percent found themselves incapable of covering their rents and/or household utility bills (Serafini and Novosel, 2021). At the same time, many companies in the sector (similar to other non-essential sectors) which were yet to become fully operational when the lockdown started had to close or lost production capacity due to their inability to survive in light of lockdown restrictions (Lustig et al., 2021).

When it comes to support for informal workers, the unemployed, and vulnerable families, three main social packages were introduced. Emergency Family Income (IFE), a bonus for pensioners and social welfare recipients, and food stamps (*Tarjeta Alimentar*). These complemented existing cash-transfer programmes, such as the Universal Child Allowance (AUH), the Universal Allowance for Pregnancy (AUE), pension benefits, and other government grants (Progresar). Considering that higher degrees of vulnerability are associated with income loss, the social aid package was intended to guarantee a basic source of income for households that were already facing economic difficulties before the pandemic and those whose opportunities to secure an income and employment were severely affected by the economic lockdown.

The IFE provided by ANSES was paid to vulnerable citizens between the ages of 18 and 65 $ARS10k ($) up to three times. It reached nine million individuals across Argentina, from the unemployed to informal workers, small contributors under the simplified tax scheme (*monotributistas*), beneficiaries of AUH or Progresar, as well as domestic workers (ANSES, 2021). The Tarjeta Alimentar was selectively directed at pregnant women and children up to the age of six or those with a disability. About 1.5 million families and 2.8 million individuals received the benefit, ranging from ARS 4,000 to 6,000 per month ($61–91 USD) to spend on food (Arza, 2021).

The implementation of IFE was fairly complex as it required eligible applicants to substantiate their asset and employment status by proving that they were not recipients of other income sources (such as from a dependency relationship, self-employment with a higher scheme of single tax contribution, or complementary social salary plans) and that they were not dependent on more than one income per household unit. As such, the processing times and confirmation of status, particularly for informal workers, required long waiting periods. The efficiency of the package was further compromised by the unprecedentedly large volume of incoming applications from vulnerable citizens, resulting in many more requests pending for long periods of time (Ernst et al., 2020) and many being left unsupported (Arza, 2021). The same happened in relation to the unemployment benefit, which was also only paid to a small share of the eligible unemployed population as individuals were required to provide proof of contribution for at least six months from the three years prior to the end of the contract, and that they were not receiving any other social insurance benefit (Arza, 2021). In this way, many social packages were inaccessible for many individuals and households.

Although it was important for the government to introduce social policies to minimise the impact of the crisis, these measures also proved relatively insufficient for many workers and households as they could still not cover the incumbent costs created by the lockdowns despite being recipients of emergency support (Busso et al., 2020). This increase in precarity and insufficient social-protection coverage was one of the main problems encountered during this pandemic. In fact, in order to make ends meet or counter the losses, many workers from both the formal and informal sectors complemented pandemic emergency measures with pre-pandemic social support (World Bank, 2021). After the first lockdown, 21 percent of households in Buenos Aires requested social protection for the first time, while 27 percent complemented pandemic social benefits with pre-pandemic support. A further 25 percent remained with pre-pandemic social benefits (INDEC, 2020).

On the other side of the spectrum, many others, particularly informal workers, were excluded from key labour rights within the current policy framework, with limited monetary protection, no access to formal health insurance, no paid holidays, no sick leave or coverage for professional absence, as well as no pay record and pension provision (CEPA, 2020; Suaya and Gross, 2021). As such, only 12 percent of informal workers in Buenos Aires benefited from state subsidies, the majority of whom were women. Furthermore, 31 percent of informal workers made out-of-pocket retirement contributions in the form of a social monotax (INDEC, 2020). These different biases in the implementation of lockdown policies led to a considerable escalation in poverty levels despite the government's attempt to address increased vulnerability (McWilliams, 2020). The poverty rate increased from 35.5 percent in the second half of 2019 to 40.5 percent in the first half of 2020, and extreme poverty rose from 8 percent to 10.5 percent (INDEC, 2020).

Additionally, important gender-based asymmetries have been observed in the impact of lockdowns, as women were the most adversely affected due to their over-representation in the informal economy (Esquivel, 2010) as well as in low-paid roles on the frontline of emergency duties (as nurses, caregivers, cleaners, and other domestic employees). Among informal workers in Buenos Aires, only 31 percent of female informal workers receive a salary, compared to 73 percent of the male informal workforce, while only 10 percent and 24 percent respectively have registered jobs (UN Argentina, 2020).

From a poll of 1,250,000 domestic and care workers in Argentina, 97 percent were women. This number represents about 17 percent of the total female labour force, with an over-representation of migrant women as no formal training or legal residency is required (Diaz, 2020). Despite legal improvements (Labour Contract Law 26844, March 2013) to end the historical discrimination suffered by workers in private homes that saw the rate of informal work reduced from 90 percent to 74 percent, many domestic employees continue to see their labour rights infringed upon (Diaz, 2020).

During the pandemic, women were more likely to work second shifts, as they disproportionately carried growing burdens of care due to school closures and the lack of household support (Arza, 2021). The "double shift" meant that in addition to the responsibilities at their paid jobs, women faced a second shift of unpaid labour in the home (Hochschild and Machung, 2012). Lastly, in Buenos Aires, 19.6 percent of active women were unemployed during the lockdown, in contrast to 9.9 percent of active men (Alzúa and Gosis, 2020). Evidence showed that this was due to the over-representation of women in temporary, part-time, and agency work, which is usually lower paid and less stable and has a higher likelihood of redundancies (Esquivel, 2020).

Conclusion

The extension of lockdowns for a prolonged period resulted in an increased risk of worsening vulnerabilities, as both companies and individuals struggled to cope with the crisis. This in turn led to increased poverty, labour inactivity, unemployment, and wealth gaps, resulting in the most regressive policy interventions since the Argentinian dictatorship in the late 1970s.

The difficulty of implementing mandatory social-distancing measures, securing employment, and managing indebtedness have added to the fragility of society to a great degree. Thus, the COVID-19 crisis engendered significant health and economic challenges in the context of an economy that was already struggling with unsustainable levels of debt. The support packages introduced by the state were insufficient to cover basic expenses for many workers and households. Thus, while the risks of the pandemic affected everyone, emerging data confirms a more acute impact on the poor (Furceri et al., 2020), the vulnerable, and those in the informal sector as lockdown policies have deepened pre-existing urban inequalities in a variety of ways, particularly in terms of access to shelter, health, and job security. Furthermore, the move to teleworking and overreliance on the internet for basic e-services and education deepened pre-existing digital divides and heightened the lived marginalisation experienced by many during successive lockdowns.

In conclusion, Argentina could not afford such extended lockdowns and the government has not accounted for the increased social costs that arose despite different pandemic support packages as they do not sustainably respond to the needs of society to get out of the "normalisation of crisis".

References

Abeldaño Zuñiga, R. A., Juanillo-Maluenda, H., Sánchez-Bandala, M. A., Burgos, G. V., Müller, S. A., & Rodríguez López, J. R. 2021. Mental Health Burden of the COVID-19 Pandemic in Healthcare Workers in Four Latin American Countries. *Inquiry : A Journal of Medical Care Organization, Provision and Financing* 58. https://doi.org/10.1177/004695 80211061059

Albrieu, R. 2020. "Evaluando las oportunidades y los límites del teletrabajo en Argentina en tiempos del COVID-19". Argentina: CIPPEC, Buenos Aires.

Alzúa, M.L. and Gosis, P. 2020. "Social and Economic Impact of COVID-19 and Policy Options in Argentina". Center for Distributional, Labor and Social Studies, Universidad Nacional de La Plata and Partnership for Economic Policy (PEP). UNDP LAC C19 PDS No.6.

ANSES. 2020. "Boletin IFE I-2020: Caracterización de la población beneficiaria". Administración Nacional de la Seguridad Social. Dirección General de Planeamiento, Buenos Aires, Argentina.

ANSES. 2021. "Ingreso Familiar de Emergencia". Administración Nacional de la Seguridad Social. Buenos Aires, Argentina. www.anses.gob.ar/informacion/ingreso-familiar-de-emergencia

Arza, C. 2021. "Argentina's Social Policy Response to COVID-19: Protecting Income and Employment". *Global Dynamics of Social Policy*. CRC 1342 COVID-19 Social Policy Response Series 17. University of Bremen, Germany.

Barlow, M. 2020. "Blog: Debt and more debt: The cost of the response to COVID-19 in Argentina". *University of York*, 12 May, www.york.ac.uk/igdc/news/news/cost-of-the-response-to-covid-19-argentina/

BBVA Research. 2021. "Argentina Economic Outlook. Third Quarter 2021". *BBVA Research*, 27 July, www.bbvaresearch.com/en/publicaciones/argentina-economic-outlook-third-quarter-2021/

Blofield, M., C. Giambruno, and F. Filgueira. 2020. "Policy expansion in compressed time: assessing the speed, breadth and sufficiency of post-COVID-19 social protection measures in 10 Latin American countries". *Social Policy series* 235. Economic Commission for Latin America and the Caribbean (ECLAC).

Bronstein, H. 2020. "New Argentine IMF deal 'solely' to repay $44 bln already owed to fund -country rep". *Reuters*, 27 August, www.reuters.com/article/argentina-imf-idUSL1N2FT1A2

Busso, M., and J. Messina. 2020. "The Inequality Crisis. Latin America and the Caribbean at the Crossroads". Inter-American Development Bank (IDB), Washington D.C., USA.

Busso, M., J. Camacho, J. Messina, and G. Montenegro. 2020. "The Challenge of Protecting Informal Households during the COVID-19 Pandemic: Evidence from Latin America". *Covid Economics: Vetted and Real Time Papers* 27: 48–73.

CEIC Data. 2020. "Argentina Government Debt: % of GDP". *CEIC Data*, www.ceicdata.com/en/indicator/argentina/government-debt--of-nominal-gdp

CEPA. 2020. *Pandemia y crisis económica: análisis del paquete económico impulsado por el gobierno.* Buenos Aires: Centro Economía Política Argentina.

Cottani, J. 2020. *The Effects of COVID-19 on Latin America's Economy.* Washington: Center for Strategic and International Studies: www.csis.org/analysis/effects-covid-19-latin-americas-economy

Davis, M.F. 2021. "The Human (Rights) Costs of Inequality: Snapshots from a pandemic". In *COVID-19 and Human Rights.* Abingdon: Routledge.

Diaz, M.L. 2020. "Essential workers, caring, space and COVID-19 in Buenos Aires, Argentina". *Urban Transcripts The Journal*, http://journal.urbantranscripts.org/article/essential-workers-caring-space-and-covid-19-in-buenos-aires-argentina-mayra-luciana-diaz/

Donza, E. and S. Poy. 2021. *Efectos de la pandemia COVID-19 sobre la dinámica del trabajo en la argentina urbana. Una mirada crítica sobre el impacto heterogéneo del actual escenario tras una década de estancamiento económico (2010-2020).* Observatorio de la Deuda Social Argentina. Educa: http://wadmin.uca.edu.ar/public/ckeditor/Observatorio%20Deuda%20Social/Documentos/2021/2021-OBSERVATORIO-Documento-Estadistico-Trabajo.pdf

ECLAC. 2021. "Financing for development in the era of COVID-19 and beyond". COVID-19 Special Report 10. Economic Coommission for Latin America and the Caribbean (ECLAC), https://repositorio.cepal.org/bitstream/handle/11362/46711/1/S2100063_en.pdf

Ernst, C. E.L. Mourelo, M. Pizzicannella, S. Rojo. and C. Romero. 2020. *COVID-19 and the Labour Market in Argentina: The challenge of fighting the pandemic and its socio-economic impact at a time of severe difficulty.* Geneva: International Labour Organisation (ILO).

Esquivel,V. 2010. "The informal economy in greater Buenos Aires: a statistical profile". *Women in Informal Employment: Globalizing and Organizing* 8. Working Paper (Urban Policies) No. 8. Cambridge, MA, USA. ISBN 978-92-95095-10-6. www.wiego.org/publications/informal-economy-greater-buenos-aires-statistical-profile

Esquivel, V. 2020. "Put gender equality at the heart of the post-COVID-19 economic recovery". *ILO* [blog], 20 August, https://iloblog.org/2020/08/20/put-gender-equality-at-the-heart-of-the-post-covid-19-economic-recovery/

Furceri, D., Prakash Loungani,, and Jonathan D. Ostry. 2020. "How Pandemics Leave the Poor Even Farther Behind". *IMF* [blog], 11 May, https://blogs. imf.org/2020/05/11/how-pandemics-leave-the-poor-even-farther-behind/

Graeber, D. 2011. *Debt: The First 5,000 Years.* Brooklyn, NY: Melville House.

Guzman, M. 2016. "An Analysis of Argentina's 2001 Default Resolution". Centre for International Governance Innovation (CIGI) Papers 110, www.cigionline.org/sites/defa ult/files/documents/CIGI%20Paper%20No.110WEB_0.pdf

Hale, T., S. Webster, A. Petherick, T. Phillips, B. Kira. 2020. "Oxford COVID-19 Government Response Tracker". Blavatnik School of Government: Oxford, UK. Accessed July 30, 2021. https://covidtracker.bsg.ox.ac.uk/stringency-scatter

Hochschild, A., and A. Machung. 2012. *The Second Shift: Working Families and the Revolution at Home.* New York: Penguin Books.

Hornbeck, J. F. 2013. "Argentina's Defaulted Sovereign Debt: Dealing with the "Holdouts"." Congressional Research Service Reports and Issue Briefs . https://sgp.fas.org/crs/row/R41029.pdf

IMF. 2020. "The evolution of public debt vulnerabilities in lower-income economies". *IMF Policy Paper.* International Monetary Fund (IMF), Washington D.C.

IMF. 2021. "World Economic Outlook. Managing Divergent Recoveries". *Semiannual Occasional Papers* 001: 37,132, 147. International Monetary Fund. Washington, DC.

INDEC. 2020. "Study on the impact of COVID-19 in the homes of Greater Buenos Aires First report of results August–October 2020". [Estudio sobre el impacto de la COVID-19 en los hogares del Gran Buenos Aires Primer informe de resultados Agosto-octubre de 2020.] Instituto Nacional de Estadística y Censos (INDEC). Republic of Argentina, www.indec.gob.ar/ftp/cuadros/sociedad/EICOVID_primer_informe.pdf

Judzik, D., L. Trujillo., and S. Villafañe. 2017. "A Tale of two decades: Income inequality and public policy in Argentina (1996-2014)". Cuadernos de Economía 36 (72): 233–264.

Linklaters. 2021. "COVID-19 second lockdown. Frequently Asked Questions". *Linklaters,* www.linklaters.com/en/insights/publications/2021/february/covid-19-second-lockdown

Lustig, N. and M. Tommasi. 2020. "COVID-19 and Social Protection of Poor and Vulnerable Groups in Latin America: A Conceptual Framework". In *The Economics of the COVID Pandemic in Latin America and the Caribbean: Ideas for Policy Action.* Policy Document Series. United Nations Development Program (UNDP).

Lustig, N., V.M. Pabon, G. Neidhöfer, and M. Tommasi. 2021. "Short and Long-Run Distributional Impacts of COVID-19 in Latin America". *Working Papers* 153. Departamento de Economia, Universidad de San Andres, Argentina.

McWilliams, S. 2020. " El Ingreso Familiar de Emergencia en Argentina: una exploración cualitativa preliminar de la suficiencia relativa y el acceso". *Independent Study Project (ISP) Collection.* 3303. https://digitalcollections.sit.edu/isp_collection/3303

Ocampo, E. 2015. "Commodity price booms and populist cycles: An explanation of Argentina's decline in the 20th Century". Working Paper Series 562. Universidad del Centro de Estudios Macroeconómicos de Argentina (UCEMA). Buenos Aires, Argentina.

Prizzon, A. 2019. "Long-term debt sustainability and the Sustainable Development Goals: Beyond the short-term prioritization of creditor interests". Paper presented at the 12th UNCTAD Debt Development Conference, 18–20 November, Geneva, Switzerland. Available at: https://unctad.org/system/files/non-official-document/2019_panel4_priz zon.pdf

Romo, A. and C. Ojeda-Galaviz. 2020. "It Takes More than Two to Tango with COVID-19: Analyzing Argentina's Early Pandemic Response (Jan 2020-April 2020)". *International Journal of Environmental Research and Public Health* 18 (1): 73.

Serafini, P. and N. Novosel. 2021. "Culture as care: Argentina's cultural policy response to COVID-19". *Cultural Trends* 30 (1): 52–62.

SInCA. 2020. Encuesta Nacional de Cultura. Caracterización de personas y organizaciones de la cultura en el contexto de COVID-19. [National Survey on Culture. Characterisation of people and cultural organisations in the context of Covid-19]. Retrieved July 23, 2020. www.sinca.gob.ar/VerNoticia.aspx?Id=58

Steinmetz, L.C.L., Leyes, C.A., Florio, M.A.D., Fong, S.B., Steinmetz, R.L.L., and Godoy, J.C. 2021. "Mental Health Impacts in Argentinean College Students During COVID-19 Quarantine". *Front. Psychiatry* 12: 557880. https://doi.org/10.3389/fpsyt.2021.557880

Sturzenegger. 2020. "Thoughts from a total lockdown in Argentina". VoxEu CEPR, 9 April, https://voxeu.org/article/regressive-covid-policies-argentina

Suaya, A. and Gross, M. 2021. "Misma crisis, ¿mismos efectos? La pandemia y el mercado de trabajo en asentamientos informales". *CIPPEC.* February, www.cippec.org/wp-content/ uploads/2021/05/INF-MyE-Misma-crisis-mismos-efectos-Suaya-Gross-mayo-2021.pdf

UN Argentina. 2020. *Analisis incial de las Naciones Unidas COVID-19 en Argentina: Impactio Socioeconomico y Ambiental.* New York: United Nations: https://argentina.un.org/sites/ default/files/2020-10/Informe-COVID-19-Argentina.pdf

Werner, A., A. Ivanova, and T. Komatsuzaki. 2021. "Latin America and Caribbean's Winding Road to Recovery". *IMF* [blog], 8 February, https://blogs.imf.org/2021/02/08/latin-america-and-caribbeans-winding-road-to-recovery/

WHO. 2020. Pandemic fatigue – reinvigorating the public to prevent COVID-19. Policy framework for supporting pandemic prevention and management. Copenhagen: WHO Regional Office for Europe: https://apps.who.int/iris/bitstream/handle/10665/335 820/WHO-EURO-2020-1160-40906-55390-eng.pdf

World Bank 2021. "The World Bank in Argentina". *World Bank*, 13 April, www.worldbank. org/en/country/argentina/overview

9

AN ANALYSIS OF THE SOCIOECONOMIC IMPACTS OF THE LOCKDOWN POLICY IN GHANA

Samuel Adu-Gyamfi

Introduction

The beginning of the year 2020 took an unexpected turn from what many people had anticipated. A new viral disease of the coronavirus virus family, initially known as the 2019 novel coronavirus and later renamed COVID-19 by the World Health Organisation (WHO), erupted in the Wuhan province of China in December 2019 (WHO, 2020; Green, 2021). In January 2020, the WHO declared COVID-19 a public health emergency of international concern (PHEIC), and a pandemic in March 2020.

Countries around the world responded by imposing stringent measures, including mandatory nationwide lockdowns (Green, 2021), with significant socioeconomic impacts for local communities. As such, by the end of March 2020, the United Nations (UN) was already warning that almost half of Africa's jobs were at risk (UN, 2020). There was, therefore, awareness within the international community that the pandemic and its responses threatened to devastate economies and potentially deepen global inequality (Ibn-Mohammed, 2020). Given the pre-existing vulnerabilities faced by many communities in Africa, there were warnings about the negative impacts of one-size-fits-all approaches to pandemic management, which disregard the local context (Green, 2021).

In Ghana, the government's imposition of a partial lockdown in March 2020 triggered a massive recession, resulting in major disruptions in the food value chain (Asante and Mills, 2020). This in turn meant that the lockdown policy became very unpopular, particularly among the poor and vulnerable, who were hit hard economically, and yet there was limited support offered to mitigate their loss of earnings (Swinnen and McDermott, 2020; Adom, Adu-Mensah, and Sekyere, 2020; Adom, Adu-Mensah, and Kquofi, 2021).

DOI: 10.4324/9781003259336-12

This chapter explores Ghana's lockdown policy to stem the tide of COVID-19 and its impacts on the broader society, including women, children, and other vulnerable groups. It starts by analysing the implementation of the lockdown policy, then it examines the socioeconomic ramifications of the policy, with particular emphasis on how it disproportionately impacted the most vulnerable, including women and children. The chapter also studies the traditional and local dynamics in pandemic management. Lastly, it concludes with an analysis of the discourse on lockdowns in relation to Ghana.

Ghana's COVID-19 response and the lockdown policy

Ghana confirmed its first two cases of COVID-19 on 12 March 2020: two people returning from Norway and Turkey (Ghana Health Service, 2020). On 15 March 2020, the president, Nana Addo Dankwa Akufo-Addo addressed the nation on the measures taken to combat the spread of the pandemic. He directed the attorney general to submit immediately to parliament emergency legislation in accordance with Article 21 (4) (c) and (d) of the 1992 Constitution. The government further directed the minister of health to declare a public health emergency pursuant to section 169 of the Public Health Act, 2012 (Act 851) to govern the relevant measures taken up against the pandemic (Communications Bureau, 2020). The attorney general developed and delivered the Imposition of Restrictions Bill, 2020, to parliament under a certificate of urgency within five days following the president's address, and parliament approved the Restrictions Bill into law (Communications Bureau, 2020; Ghana News Agency, 2020).

Following these ensuing legal processes regarding the imposition of restrictions in the country, the president, on 30 March 2020, imposed partial restrictions on the movement of persons in the Greater Accra Metropolitan Area (GAMA, which included Awutu Senya East), the Greater Kumasi Metropolitan Area, and contiguous districts, for a period of two weeks. The partial lockdown required that residents of the affected districts stayed home but allowed them to go outside to access essential services. All passenger travel between the restricted districts and other parts of the country was prohibited. The prime objective was to contain the spread of the virus, ensure adequate care for the sick, and limit the impact of the virus on social and economic life (Communications Bureau, 2020).

The government adapted the recommendations of the WHO to fit the country's particular circumstances. The local strategy included measures such as the suspension of public meetings, the disinfection of market facilities, severe enforcement of social distancing and personal hygiene, closure of all land, sea, and air borders to human travel, and the lockdown of disease epicentres (Asante and Mills, 2020). Enhanced surveillance in the form of active case search and contact-tracing procedures were also launched to find, isolate, and treat all confirmed cases early. With funding from the Ghana Field Epidemiology and Laboratory Training Programme (GFELTP), the National Health Service mapped out existing cases, conducted risk assessments, and sampled members of households within a 1–2 km radius of the cluster of cases based on the setting. The increased surveillance and contact-tracing techniques assisted in identifying a large number of cases, with 93 percent of them being asymptomatic (Odikro et al., 2020).

The government provided households with free piped water and subsidised electricity bills for three months, from April to June 2020. Water tankers, publicly and privately owned, were mobilised to ensure a constant supply of water to poor communities (Antwi-Boasiako et al., 2021). The government also implemented other measures to support poor households and small and medium-sized enterprises. A GH₵1.2 billion (US$200 million) Coronavirus Alleviation Programme was introduced to assist affected homes and businesses, supplemented by donations from both private sector corporations and civil society organisations. Even though the lockdown was lifted after three weeks, post-lockdown procedures continued to be implemented to keep the disease from escalating. Personal hygiene measures, mask wearing, restrictions on social gatherings, social distancing, and humanitarian aid were maintained to curb the pandemic.

Socioeconomic ramifications of the lockdown policy for Ghana

The social and economic implications of the COVID-19 pandemic and the lockdown policy for vulnerable populations in Ghana cannot be overstated. There are questions pertaining to heightened economic and social challenges for vulnerable individuals and groups who were subjected to domestic and sexual abuse, arbitrary arrests, healthcare inaccessibility, and educational challenges throughout the pandemic. Additionally, food insecurity and poverty were cross-cutting effects of the pandemic on vulnerable populations (Naami and Mfoafo-M'Carthy, 2020).

While some measures were necessary to curb the spread of the virus following standard epidemiological protocols, the imposition of strict lockdowns in African countries had widespread negative impacts on their economies (Lakemann, Lay, and Tafese, 2020). Restrictions on movement led to a general halt in economic activities and a disruption in the income of workers in the predominantly informal sector, amounting to about 66 percent of the total employment in sub-Saharan Africa, who rely on small daily earnings (Onyekwema, 2020). These workers in the African labour market, which is largely characterised by chronic short-term contracts and freelance work as opposed to permanent jobs (Onyekwema, 2020), have very limited savings to ease the burden of expenditure (including consumption). In Ghana, such economic disruptions necessitated a quick turn to find ways of easing the lockdown to curtail the economic gloom that could have been devastating.

On a macroeconomic level, the impact of COVID-19 on the economy of Ghana has been both direct and indirect. Directly, lockdown policies adversely impacted production, investment, and trade within the country and with the rest of the world, especially with China, Europe, and the United States (Green, 2021). On a global scale, it witnessed adverse impacts on commodities like crude oil, gold, and cocoa, which experienced a dip in prices (Green, 2021).

The implementation of lockdown policies led to massive hoarding of essential commodities including food and medical supplies, which caused a spike in demand for these commodities (Swinnen and McDermott, 2020). Businesses also shut down and economic activities continued to shrink as a result of the pandemic and its related lockdowns, resulting in significant unemployment and a drop in demand for domestic commodities (World Bank, 2020). A joint survey by the Ghana Statistical Service, the United Nations Development Programme, and the World Bank in 2020 indicated that COVID-19 caused a reduction of wages among 25.7 percent of the total workforce and further caused about 42,000 lay-offs in the country (World Bank, 2020). The socioeconomic impacts of the lockdown, especially in the marketplaces, were evident in increased food prices, which led to serious economic hardships among the already poor and vulnerable groups like women and children. Essentially, the prices of both imported and locally manufactured food items doubled, and in some cases tripled (Asante and Mills, 2020).

Some businesses saw demand drop dramatically, and employees' jobs and incomes were at risk. Big companies drilling Ghana's oil offshore, farmers and the street hawkers who sold finished products on the streets of big cities, the self-employed, including hairdressers, barbers, carpenters, traders, builders, dressmakers, musicians, "trotro" or taxi drivers, and the "kayayie",[1] among others in the informal economy, were pinned down due to the global pandemic (MoF, 2020).

Women were more likely to lose their jobs, and working mothers struggled with increased childcare demands (Kotlar et al., 2021) as facilities like daycares were closed and mothers had to fully care for their children. This was particularly prevalent in urban areas, where many women are employed in the informal and private sector (Fawole, Okedare, and Reed, 2021), resulting in a higher degree of insecurity in the labour market. This was further exacerbated by pre-existing gendered income differentials, which have been persistent worldwide, including the advanced economies of the world (World Economic Forum, 2021).

A sector which was adversely affected by the lockdown policy in Ghana was agriculture. The lockdown affected how people accessed food and disrupted the production of certain food products (Onyeaka et al., 2021). Human and vehicular movement restrictions resulted in the disruption of food supply chains. Movements along roads connecting major food production communities were curtailed, which led to shortage of essential commodities in the Ghanaian market. Such a situation brought economic losses for traders and producers, and there was a slowdown in the importation of essential goods as a result of the disruptions. This quandary hampered farmers' access to inputs, such as seeds, fertilisers, and insecticides. The ensuing uncertainty and fear impacted planting decisions and reduced the volume of the main agricultural exports in Ghana (Hodey, Asante, and Dzanku, 2020).

Generally, the lockdown policy caused private-sector workers, mostly traders in the informal sector, artisans, and entrepreneurs, who were concerned about their economic upkeep in these difficult times, to oppose the idea of closing the economy. Pockets of protests erupted just a few days after the first lockdown was enforced at the end of March 2020. Resistance came from informal workers, who found themselves unable to guarantee their livelihoods (Akinwotu and Asiedu, 2020). Traders protesting in Kasoa, which is part of Awutu Senya East and joins Accra from the west, highlighted that even though it was clear that the lockdown was necessary to stop the virus from spreading, the government ought to have recognised that the adverse impact of the burden of fighting the disease ought not to have fallen on them (Akinwotu and Asiedu, 2020). These traders were driven by their loss of earnings, which could threaten their livelihoods and that of their families the longer the lockdown was kept in place. The Ghana Union Traders Association (GUTA) also mounted pressure on the government to ease the lockdown restrictions, because the impact of the lockdown was unbearable for its members.

Parliamentarians from the main opposition political parties were also among those who resisted the imposition of lockdowns. This had the propensity to score political points for the main opposition party, leading up to the December 2020 elections in Ghana. Among the minority caucus of Ghana's parliament, the National Democratic Congress (NDC) accused the government of not taking pro-active measures and establishing policies to protect the borderlands at the initial spark of the pandemic as the former president, Mahama, did during the Ebola crisis in West Africa. They argued that if the government had done so, it would have made the lockdown an unnecessary policy to deploy (Oxford Analytica, 2020). The parliamentarians accused the Nana Addo–led government of not replicating or drawing lessons from the past.

The government responded to the criticisms by reaffirming that the lockdown enabled officials to analyse the country's needs and gave them time to improve the health infrastructure, test its capacity, and target outbreak locations (Akinwotu and Asiedu, 2020). The central question is whether lockdowns by themselves had the propensity to solve the spread of the pandemic without exacerbating the already ailing social and economic conditions in poor jurisdictions or communities across the world, and Africa in particular. Indeed, in West Africa (and Ghana in particular) there is a body of experience concerning the management of pandemics to draw from. Drawing on the experience of the Ebola outbreak, the president could have made efforts to incorporate local context into their response to the COVID-19 pandemic rather than merely mimicking global responses that did not necessarily reflect local peculiarities.

Impacts on women, children, and other vulnerable groups

The focus of the pandemic-management policies was on preventive measures, which would ensure the protection of public health and the basic functionality of hospitals and other national health services. In the process, however, there was little concern for other socioeconomic outcomes (Rahman et al., 2020; Boateng et al., 2021) and how isolation and social-distancing measures would impact individuals.

The closing of primary and senior high schools and universities, both public and private, was ordered by the government on 15 March 2020. These were only reopened in January 2021 (UNICEF, 2021). This meant that although the primary effects of the pandemic on children appeared to be limited, children were highly susceptible to the indirect secondary effects of the pandemic. This was due to strained service systems, limited household income, and disruptions to social services. These impacts, however, built on pre-existing vulnerabilities, as prior to the pandemic about one in three children in Ghana lived in monetary poor households, and two in three children could not realise their full rights, lacking access to essential goods and services and consequently to their ability to maximise their developmental potential (UNICEF Ghana, 2021).

It is thus unsurprising that the effects of school closures were more severe among underprivileged children and their families, resulting in disruptions in schooling, poor nutrition, and extra financial costs to families who were unable to work due to the lack of childcare provision (UNICEF, 2021a). School closures also meant that children were increasingly confined at home, spending less time with their friends and classmates, resulting in limited opportunities to socialise with other children. Children who live in violent or stressful environments were more likely to suffer negative mental health consequences, and thus faced numerous violations of their rights (UNICEF, 2021a).

The Mastercard Foundation COVID-19 Recovery and Resilience Programme was an interesting initiative introduced to support the implementation of virtual and distance learning through radio, SMS, and online learning platforms, and was made available to children across the country. To ensure equitable access for all, children in remote locations or without access to smart devices benefited from lessons via community radio stations and text messaging (UNICEF, 2021a). However, for disadvantaged children in rural and poor urban communities, there were the usual disruptions in electricity and sometimes the absence of same, which hindered their ability to benefit from the initiative.

Human-rights violations of marginalised groups, particularly women and children, were also a cause of concern during lockdowns (Fawole, Okedare, and Reed, 2021). For instance, the deployment of the military, instead of the police, to enforce the lockdown policy exacerbated the level of human-rights infractions. The harsh enforcement of lockdown policies imposed by the military and the police service, compelling and sanctioning market women and households who wittingly or unwittingly breached the lockdown protocols, were not warranted (Asante and Mills, 2020). Asante and Mills (2020) have reported that there were instances when women who were purchasing affordable foodstuffs were brutalised for flouting social-distancing protocols. Similarly, some traders who were permitted to trade under the lockdown directive were brutalised by security personnel (Asante and Mills, 2020).

Lockdowns also sparked serious domestic violence cases in many communities and households. Particularly, changes in the unemployment rate, the gender income disparity, and access to money or employment prospects affected household incomes, resulting in an increase in domestic violence (Fawole, Okedare, and Reed, 2021). Both unemployment and the lockdown lengthened people's time at home, thereby increasing their vulnerability to domestic violence. A key aspect of this was intimate-partner violence (IPV). There was an increase in violence against women and girls in Ghana since the COVID-19 pandemic started, due to lockdowns, social isolation measures, and school closures (Usher et al., 2020). In support of this claim, Raghavendran et al. (2021) have indicated that 35 percent of the total women surveyed in Ghana suffered some form of violence during the COVID-19 outbreak.

In areas where there are slums and highly impoverished communities, restrictions or withdrawal of relief services exacerbated the situation (Asante and Mills, 2020). It is possible that the lockdown contributed to further COVID-19 transmissions in Ghana's large and overcrowded informal settlements, especially in Accra and Kumase. Considering that roughly 53 percent of households were living in single rooms, and many individuals relied on public bathrooms and toilets, for many home confinement was almost impossible to follow during the lockdown (Haider et al., 2020). This led to overcrowding among certain households. People found it diffi-cult to adhere to the lockdown protocols; thus, while the lockdown policy aimed at reducing and preventing the spread of COVID-19, the housing deficit, the exist-ence of large, overcrowded slums, and increasing rural-urban migration made the implementation of the policy more problematic.

In addition, social isolation led to increased anxiety, stress, boredom, negative religious coping, extreme hopelessness, and suicidal ideation (Adu et al., 2021). Considering the extent to which social interactions take place outdoors in Ghanaian society, it was particularly challenging for individuals to keep indoors. Individuals also experienced increased anxiety and depression during the lockdown, driven by the fear of contracting the virus or dying, as reports of the shortage of essen-tial supplies and the uncertainty of the pandemic led to feelings of helplessness (Boateng et al., 2021).

Traditional and local dynamics in pandemic management

Lockdowns and quarantine are not new concepts within Ghanaian society. As part of administering traditional medical therapies among the Asante of Ghana within traditional communities, the sick were temporarily exempted from performing normal social roles such as going to work or housekeeping (Twumasi, 1975: 34). If the sick person was a father, he was not obliged to attend work to support his family or take part in decision-making processes within various social groups. The traditional sick-role theory permitted quarantine, as it was an adjuration from the indigenous priest healer (IPH) which was further supported by the head of the family. It was intended to allow the sick breadwinner to be properly taken care of and to allow for some time of recuperation within the family home or the "trad-itional clinic" of the healer before joining the workforce (Adu-Gyamfi, 2013). It also prevented the spread of diseases if they were known to be contagious.

The practice subsisted within pre-colonial cultures in African societies (Adu-Gyamfi and Anderson, 2019). This in turn should mean that government's efforts to impose the lockdown ought to have been embraced by communities in the strictest sense. However, the traditional notions of quarantine and lockdown operated within the context of high levels of trust among communities. In present day Ghanaian society this trust has disappeared, and the lack of faith in government precluded the government from gaining the full support of the people. This was in part due to the fact that economic disruptions, general anxiety, and the lack of adequate housing meant that people did not feel that they had the material conditions necessary to stay home.

Another important question was the burial of the dead. The ban on social gatherings limited the number of funeral and burial attendees to 25 persons. Considering the general cultural attachment Ghanaians have with the dead, the lockdown rendered inactive practices such as burial customs, mortuary rites, feastings, flashy displays of family riches, singing, and dancing (Oliveira-Cardoso et al., 2020). The majority of Ghanaians objected to private burials; as for locals, it breached their custom and represented a social mockery of the dead and the bereaved family (Adom, Adu-Mensah, and Kquofi, 2021). Proper customary burial meant the dead would be more acceptable in the ancestral world (Ademiluka, 2009).

At the time of the upsurge in the Ebola crisis in Guinea, Liberia, and Sierra Leone, it became necessary for policymakers and international organisations to revert to finding common pathways with local authorities and communities, who found it nauseating for their chiefs and prominent members of society to be buried in mass graves. It was realised that building consensus with the traditional authorities and the local people in Sierra Leone and Liberia produced some incredible success stories in the fight against Ebola (Adu-Gyamfi, 2019). There was scope for similar strategies to be deployed, at least to engage local communities through the traditional authority concerning the proper interpretation and implementation of COVID-19 burial protocols and the lockdown policy, especially concerning the number of persons who could be in attendance from time to time to honour the passing of a youth,[2] as distinct from the family heads, linguists, queen mothers, and chiefs, among others, who are the rulers of the people and highly revered in their respective local communities.

Even during earlier epidemics in the Gold Coast (Ghana), local action involved chiefs and native authorities leading the charge to fight against diseases. Among the Asante of Ghana, where leprosy was at its peak during the colonial period, the *Asantehene* (king of Asante) restricted lepers to the Kumase leprosarium. The ongoing COVID-19 crisis, however, saw government authorities preclude chiefs, who are traditional custodians of the local communities, from pandemic management. Though the Asantehene engaged in food distribution to support some members of the local communities in Asante during the lockdown, other divisional chiefs did not emulate this.

The government's approach shows that the current democratic governance apparatus has a general disregard for traditional authority, even though a 2019 survey by Afrobarometer found that 55 percent of Ghanaians trust traditional leaders "somewhat" or "a lot" (Logan and Katenda, 2021). The survey also found that across 22 countries in Africa, traditional leaders obtain significantly more positive ratings on "trust", "performance", "listening", and "lack of corruption" than their elected counterparts (presidents, members of parliament, and local councillors) (Logan and Katenda, 2021).Therefore, greater synergy between traditional authority and the government could have potentially increased the efficiency of pandemic management.

At the local level, earlier pandemics were associated with varied interpretations, including accusations of witchcraft and sorcery (Ellison, 2003). From that perspective, some religious individuals considered lockdown policies, especially concerning COVID-19, to be useless. The Ghanaian cosmology of witches and malevolent spirits as disease-causative agents found a place in the social discourse, resulting in some Ga traditional priests in the Greater Accra Region reaffirming their power and influence through their deities, often defying lockdown policies.They believed that such prayers would deal with COVID-19 and render the lockdown policy useless.

Significantly, in the early days of the pandemic, the president held a national prayer breakfast meeting with Christian pastors at Flagstaff House, the seat of government, for spiritual intervention (Communications Bureau, 2020). Ghana, being a multi-religious country, witnessed different forms or expressions of prayer during the outbreak of COVID-19.This was not dissimilar from the well-attended open-air crusades which were held in the Gold Coast (Ghana) during the 1918–19 influenza pandemic (Patterson, 1983). Although people continued to die, Ghanaians drew inspiration from their "religious capital" to seek emotional, psychological, and social cohesion through prayer. Religion and prayer have long been part of Ghana's social capital (Prempeh, 2021), irrespective of the visible flaws that are found in the character of some of the spiritual leaders and their devotees. It was believed that prayers would at least ease the burden of COVID-19 and the concomitant lockdown policy.

The structure of the Ghana Health Service (GHS), which is highly centralised, deepened the challenges in implementing the lockdown policy.This in turn beats the imagination of proponents of decentralisation and devolution of power, who often highlight the benefits for improving development at the local level: metropolitan, municipal, and district.Therefore, instead of a one-size-fits-all model, there was scope to develop an approach that prioritises home-grown strategies and education on lockdowns within the traditional notion of quarantining, as well as the involvement of chiefs and other key actors at the local level. This could potentially yield better dividends in terms of pandemic management.

Conclusion

The overall efficacy of lockdown policies is debatable (Greenberger, 2018). Some empirical studies have suggested that from a public health perspective, lockdown had a positive effect on the pandemic (Meo et al., 2020), as the implementation of lockdown policies decreased the rate at which COVID-19 cases were increasing across all regions in the world. Thus, lockdowns were considered to be effective in reducing incidence and mortality rates of COVID-19 (Nussbaumer-Streit et al., 2020).

In Ghana, lockdown measures were not sufficient to slowdown the spread of the pandemic, as their success was hindered by the lack of basic infrastructure in the form of adequate housing, the possibility of delivering remote learning, and support for vulnerable households. Decentralising pandemic responses at the local level and adjusting them to the local needs of the population would help with the containment of pandemics and support efforts in the procurement and distribution of necessary medical equipment.

The failure of the lockdown agenda reached its peak in the lack of faith in government due to implementation challenges as well as the country's fragile economy. The critical challenge was to support vulnerable individuals with no sustained income or adequate housing. As their survival was based on daily and consistent engagements in the informal economy, namely subsistence farming, petty trading, driving, fitting, blacksmithing, and masonry, among others roles, the halt of these critical activities resulted in starvation and suffering. The imposition of the lockdown left the poor and the vulnerable with no option and in abject poverty, associated with emotional and psychological stress. The already impoverished were left to rest on some non-existent magic wand to curtail the pressure from their nuclear and extended families, who relied on them even in normal times.

Could lockdowns have been avoided? The available evidence demonstrates that the government could have applied lockdown measures with a greater degree of understanding of the societal context, instead of using a one-size-fits-all approach. A more holistic policy would ensure the safeguarding of the social and economic interests and well-being of the overall population.

Notes

1 Kayayie refers to head porters. They carry items in pans or directly for individuals who go to markets in Ghana to purchase items including foodstuffs for a fee. Several of these people are from the Northern and Upper Regions of Ghana who travel to big cities like Accra and Kumase to carve-out a living for themselves.
2 Local reference to all members of the local community including the elderly who are not title holders.

References

Ademiluka, Solomon Olusola. 2009. "The sociological functions of funeral mourning: Illustrations from the old testament and Africa". *Old Testament Essays* 22 (1): 9–20.

Adom, Dickson, Jephtar Adu-Mensah, and Steve Kquofi. 2021. "COVID-19 private burial with 25 persons in the lens of the mortuary rites culture in Ghana". *African Identities*: 1–16.

Adom, Dickson, Jephthar Adu-Mensah, and Paul Appiah Sekyere. 2020. "Hand-to-mouth work culture and the COVID-19 lockdown restrictions: experiences of selected informal sector workers in Kumasi, Ghana". *Research Journal in Advanced Humanities* 1 (2): 45–63.

Adu, M.K., L.J. Wallace, K.F. Lartey, J. Arthur, K.F. Oteng, S. Dwomoh, and V.I. Agyapong. 2021. "Prevalence and correlates of likely major depressive disorder among the adult population in Ghana during the COVID-19 pandemic". *International journal of environmental research and public health* 18 (13): 7106.

Adu-Gyamfi, Samuel. 2019. "Ebola haemorrhagic fever in Africa: A necessary highlight". *International Journal of Public Health* 8 (1): 1–13.

Adu-Gyamfi, Samuel, and Eugenia Anderson. 2019. "Indigenous Medicine and Traditional Healing in Africa: A Systematic Synthesis of the Literature". *Philosophy, Social and Human Disciplines* 1: 69–100.

Adu-Gyamfi, Samuel, Prince Osei-Wusu Adjei, and Daniel Owusu-Ansah. 2013. "Preventive Healthcare Strategies and Impact among the Asante People of the Early Twentieth Century Gold Coast: A Historical Narrative and Lessons for the Present Sanitation Challenge in Kumase". *Journal of Studies in Social Sciences* 5 (2): 214–238.

Akinwotu, E., and Kwasi Asiedu. 2020. "Easing of lockdown a relief to Ghana's poor– despite fears it is premature". *The Guardian*, 3 May, www.theguardian.com/global-development/2020/may/03/coronavirus-easing-of-lockdown-a-relief-to-ghanas-poor-despite-fears-it-is-premature

Antwi-Boasiako, Joseph, Charles Othniel A. Abbey, Patrick Ogbey, and Rita Amponsah Ofori. 2021. "Policy Responses to fight COVID-19: the case of Ghana". *Revista de Administração Pública* 55: 122–139.

Asante, Lewis Abedi, and Richael Odarko Mills. 2020. "Exploring the socio-economic impact of COVID-19 pandemic in marketplaces in urban Ghana". *Africa Spectrum* 55(2): 170–181.

Boateng, G.O., D.T. Doku, N.I.E. Enyan, et al. 2021. "Prevalence and changes in boredom, anxiety and well-being among Ghanaians during the COVID-19 pandemic: a population-based study". *BMC Public Health* 21 (985): 1–13.

Communications Bureau. 2020. "President Akufo-Addo Addresses Nation on Measures Taken by Gov't to Combat the Coronavirus Pandemic". The Presidency, 15 March. https://presidency.gov.gh/index.php/briefing-room/speeches/1535-president-akufo-addo-addresses-nation-on-measures-taken-by-gov-t-to-combat-the-coronavirus-pandemic

Ellison, James G. 2003. "'A Fierce Hunger': Tracing the Impacts of the 1918-1919 Influenza Pandemic in Southwest Tanzania". In *The Spanish Influenza Pandemic of 1918-1919: New Perspectives* edited by David Killingray, and Phillips Howard. Abingdon: Routledge, pp. 221–229.

Fawole, Olufunmilayo I., Omowumi O. Okedare, and Elizabeth Reed. 2021. "Home was not a safe haven: women's experiences of intimate partner violence during the COVID-19 lockdown in Nigeria". *BMC Women's Health* 21(1): 1–7.

Ghana Health Service. 2020. "For Immediate Release: Ghana Confirms Two Cases of COVID-19". *Ghana Health Service*, 12 March, https://ghanahealthservice.org/covid19/downloads/covid_19_first_confirmed_GH.pdf

Ghana News Agency. 2020. "Parliament passes Imposition of Restrictions Bill". *FAAPA*, 21 March, www.faapa.info/en/2020/03/21/parliament-passes-imposition-of-restrictions-bill-2020/

Green, T. 2021. *The Covid Consensus: The New Politics of Global Inequality*. London: Hurst & Company.

Greenberger, Michael. 2018. "Better prepare than react: reordering public health priorities 100 years after the Spanish flu epidemic". *American Journal of Public Health* 108 (11): 1465–1468.

Haider, Najmul, Abdinasir Yusuf Osman, Audrey Gadzekpo, George O. Akipede, Danny Asogun, Rashid Ansumana, Richard John Lessells, et al. 2020. "Lockdown measures in response to COVID-19 in nine sub-Saharan African countries". *BMJ Global Health* 5 (10): e003319.

Hodey, Louis, Kofi Asante, and Fred Dzanku. 2020. "Agricultural-based livelihood implications of COVID-19 in Ghana". *Future Agricultures*, 28 September, www.future-agricultures.org/blog/agricultural-based-livelihood-implications-of-covid-19-in-ghana-1/

Ibn-Mohammed, T., K.B. Mustapha, J.M. Godsell, Z. Adamu, K.A. Babatunde, D.D. Akintade, Adolf Acquaye, et al. 2020. "A critical review of the impacts of COVID-19 on the global economy and ecosystems and opportunities for circular economy strategies". *Resources, Conservation and Recycling* 164: 105–169.

Kotlar, Bethany, Emily Gerson, Sophia Petrillo, Ana Langer, and Henning Tiemeier. 2021. "The impact of the COVID-19 pandemic on maternal and perinatal health: a scoping review". *Reproductive Health* 18 (1): 1–39.

Lakemann, Tabea, Jann Lay, and Tevin Tafese. 2020. "Africa after the COVID-19 lockdowns: economic impacts and prospects". *GIGA*, 6 November, www.giga-hamburg.de/en/publications/giga-focus/africa-after-the-covid-19-lockdowns-economic-impacts-and-prospects

Logan, C., and Katenda, L.M. 2021. "African citizens' message to traditional leaders: Stay in development, stay out of politics". *Afrobarometer Dispatch* 443: 1-16.

Meo, Sultan Ayoub, Abdulelah Adnan Abukhalaf, Ali Abdullah Alomar, Faris Jamal AlMutairi, Adnan Mahmood Usmani, and David C. Klonoff. 2020. "Impact of lockdown on COVID-19 prevalence and mortality during 2020 pandemic: observational analysis of 27 countries". *European Journal of Medical Research* 25(1): 1–7.

Naami, Augustina, and Magnus Mfoafo-M'Carthy. 2020. "COVID-19: Vulnerabilities of persons with disabilities in Ghana". *African Journal of Social Work* 10 (3): 9–17.

Nussbaumer-Streit, Barbara, Verena Mayr, Andreea Iulia Dobrescu, Andrea Chapman, Emma Persad, Irma Klerings, Gernot Wagner, et al. 2020. "Quarantine alone or in combination with other public health measures to control COVID-19: A Rapid Review". *Cochrane Database of Systematic Reviews* (9): 1–78.

Odikro, Magdalene A., Ernest Kenu, Keziah L. Malm, Franklin Asiedu-Bekoe, Charles L. Noora, Joseph Frimpong, Benedict Calys-Tagoe, and Kwadwo A. Koram. 2020. "Epidemiology of COVID-19 outbreak in Ghana, 2020". *Ghana Medical Journal* 54 (S4): 5–15.

Oliveira-Cardoso, E.A., B.C.A. Silva, J.H. Santos, L.S. Lotério, A.G. Accoroni, and M.A. Santos. 2020. "The effect of suppressing funeral rituals during the COVID-19 pandemic on bereaved families". *Rev. Latino-Am. Enfermagem* 28: e3361.

Onyeaka, Helen, Christian K. Anumudu, Zainab T. Al-Sharify, Esther Egele-Godswill, and Paul Mbaegbu. 2021. "COVID-19 pandemic: A review of the global lockdown and its far-reaching effects". *Science Progress* 104 (2): 1–18.

Onyekwema, Chukwuka. 2020. "The Impact of COVID-19 on Africa's Pre-Existing Vulnerabilities". ISPI, 12 June 12, www.ispionline.it/en/pubblicazione/impact-covid-19-africas-pre-existing-vulnerabilities-26480

Patterson, K. David. 1983. "The Influenza Epidemic of 1918–19 in the Gold Coast". *The Journal of African History* 24 (4): 485–502.

Prempeh, C. 2021. "Religion and the state in an episodic moment of COVID-19 in Ghana". *Social Sciences & Humanities Open,* 4 (1), 100-141.

Raghavendran, Srinivasan, Kijong Kim, Sinéad Ashe, Mrinal Chadha, Felix Asante, Petri T. Piiroinen, and Nata Duvvury. 2021. "Violence against women and the macroeconomy: The case of Ghana". *Journal of International Development,* 34 (2), 239–258.

Rahman, Muhammad, Rabab Ahmed, Modhurima Moitra, Laura Damschroder, Ross Brownson, Bruce Chorpita, Priscilla Idele, et al. 2020. "Mental distress and human rights violations during COVID-19: a rapid review of the evidence informing rights, mental health needs, and public policy around vulnerable populations". *Frontiers in Psychiatry* 11: e603875.

Swinnen, Johan, and John McDermott. 2020. "COVID-19 and global food security". *EuroChoices* 19 (3): 26–33.

Twumasi, P.A. 1975. *Medicinal Systems in Ghana: A Study in Medicinal Sociology.* Tema: Ghana Publishing Corporation.

UNICEF Ghana. 2021. *Primary and Secondary Impacts of the COVID-19 Pandemic on Children in Ghana.* Accra: UNICEF.

United Nations (UN). 2020. "What happened after COVID-19 hit Ghana". *Un Women*, 9 December, www.unwomen.org/en/news/stories/2020/12/what-happe ned-after-covid-19-hit-ghana

Usher, K., N. Bhullar, J. Durkin, N. Gyamfi, and D. Jackson. 2020. "Family violence and COVID-19: Increased vulnerability and reduced options for support". *International Journal of Mental Health Nursing.* Advance online publication.

World Bank. 2020. "COVID-19 forced businesses in Ghana to reduce wages for over 770,000 workers, and caused about 42,000 layoffs - research reveals". *World Bank*, 3 August, www.worldbank.org/en/news/press-release/2020/08/03/covid-19-forced-bus inesses-in-ghana-to-reduce-wages-for-over-770000-workers-and-caused-about-42000-layoffs-research-reveals

World Economic Forum. 2021. "Global Gender Gap Report 2021: Insight Report". *World Economic Forum*, 30 March, www.weforum.org/reports/global-gender-gap-report-2021

World Health Organisation (WHO). 2020. "Q&A on coronaviruses (COVID-19)". *World Health Organisation*, April 17, www.who.int/emergencies/diseases/novelcoronavirus-2019/question-and-answershub/q-a-detail/q-a-coronaviruses

10

THE COVID-19 SYNDEMIC AND LESSONS (NOT) LEARNED FROM PAST EPIDEMICS

One Size Doesn't Fit All

Llanos Ortiz-Montero

Introduction

I have spent half my life working in so-called Global Health programmes, responding to international humanitarian emergencies, including many epidemics, contributing to providing healthcare for the most vulnerable, but also confronting dilemmas as to whether Non-Governmental Organisations (NGOs) are part of the solution or part of a wider problem. I have felt conflicted between a public's praise for my work, sometimes with an idealised vision of humanitarianism associated with religious charity, and another perception that accuses it of being a form of neo-colonialism, even of being instrumentalised for biopolitical objectives.

This tension underpins the reflections on the global response to COVID-19 that I offer in this chapter. Throughout the text, I use the term "syndemic" rather than "pandemic" to refer to the situation that has unfolded across the world in the wake of the virus's spread. By pairing the concepts of "synergy" and "epidemic", I highlight the social aspects that shape the disease pattern and its prognosis, shifting the focus away from the virus's biological side and acknowledging that diseases do not occur independently of social, economic, cultural, or environmental conditions, all of which shape not only the impact of a pathogen on a society but also the way a society responds to the pathogen's spread (Singer and Scott, 2008; Singer and Rylko-Bauer, 2020: 8).

We can appreciate the synergistic effects of biological and non-biological factors by considering the history of pandemics. There is, indeed, an overwhelming resemblance between past pandemics – including the plague from the Middle Ages, nineteenth-century cholera, or the so-called 1918–20 Spanish flu – and the current syndemic. History shows how some pandemics produced important social and cultural changes: the high mortality during the Black Death in medieval feudal Europe led to a huge drop in the number of workers available, creating more job

DOI: 10.4324/9781003259336-13

opportunities in the cities, which coincided with agrarian innovations and hastened the end of feudalism (Garcia Luaces, 2015). In the nineteenth century, cholera ripped through parts of European industrial cities, bringing reforms in the provision of water and sanitation (Zarzoso, 2000). It is argued that the high male mortality during the Spanish flu pandemic resulted in the definitive inclusion of women in the labour market in roles that had been seen as being exclusively for men until then (Crudo Blackburn, Parker, and Wendelbo, 2018). In all these cases, the pandemics interacted in complex ways with the social, cultural, political, and economic landscapes of societies.

In the case of COVID-19, some of the control measures that have been introduced bring to mind Foucault's reflection on a sixteenth-century "plague model" which shows how such measures can be used to control and segregate society, modifying life after a pandemic (Sánchez, 2020: 160). Foucault writes: "On the designated day, each one is ordered to lockup himself in his house, with the prohibition to leave the house .... Each family would already have accumulated its provisions. When it is absolutely necessary to leave the houses, it is done in turns, avoiding any encounters" (Foucault, 1975: 217). Unlike the previous leprosy model, which secluded only those who were infected, the plague model included the entire population, in which subjects were isolated in a fixed, interior place, and even the smallest movements were controlled.

The syndemic has dramatically altered our social fabric, exposing inequalities, adding new layers of vulnerability, imposing changes in our daily lives, and highlighting failures of our hegemonic biomedical health model.

Some high-income countries that claimed to have "the best healthcare in the world", have been humbled by COVID-19, having missed the opportunity to put aside their pride and look to other countries with fewer economic resources but more experience fighting epidemics, to learn from their experiences, and to dust off historic strategies to use against epidemics.

Aligned with the study on preparedness by Lakoff, a reality I have experienced in my work is the inadequacy of epidemic preparedness plans in most countries, even though, for years, there has been speculation about emerging pathogens capable of causing a pandemic (Lakoff, 2017). In fact, many organisations, including the World Health Organisation (WHO), acknowledging some flaws in emergency preparedness, worked on contingency plans for novel virus scenarios (WHO, 2019). Similarly, several gaps in their response capacity were identified in almost all participating countries in a coronavirus-pandemic-simulation exercise, called "Event 201", held in New York at the end of 2019 (Pearce, 2019).[1] Was, then, the COVID-19 syndemic a disaster waiting to happen?

The COVID-19 syndemic has raised many questions that remain unanswered: Why have lessons from past epidemics been widely overlooked? To what extent have international organisations been able to contribute their experience to the global response? Have the voices of the most vulnerable populations been heard? How are societies' (and individuals') subjectivities reshaping in the current context of uncertainty and socioeconomic constraints (Avalos, 2020)? Why are we still denying the impact of some of the syndemic control measures? Are we writing a new social contract (UN, 2020)?

I do not pretend that I can answer all these questions, but I offer my reflections on some of the enabling factors of the current situation and point to the shortcomings of a top-down, standardised model of public health for all. In the first part of this chapter, I reflect on the history and governance of "Global Health". I argue that this concept is rooted in an imbalance of power between the Global North and South. In the following section, I reflect on the lessons we could have learned from previous epidemics, drawing particularly on my experience of working on the response to Ebola and other epidemics. I suggest that the power imbalances underpinning our understanding of Global Health identified in the first section help explain the lack of learning from previous epidemics. In the third part of the chapter, I discuss how this systemic amnesia helped enable the "lockdown consensus" (a phenomenon discussed in more detail by Anthony Mckeown in Chapter 1 this book) in the global response to COVID-19 and the devastating consequences this has had on economic and social inequality. Ultimately, I argue that the syndemic has been a missed opportunity to re-imagine 'Global Health' in a highly globalised world; instead of grappling with complexity, we have re-enacted "simplistic" one-size-fits-all approaches, with devastating consequences.

Global Health: Power, biopolitics, and the relationship between the Global North and South

Some key elements of power and dependence underlying our Global Health model have conditioned the management of the syndemic.

Global Health's relevance in the international agenda doesn't begin or end with COVID-19, but it has magnified many existing problems and fuelled unresolved conflicts, generating a perfect storm of economic, health, and social crises. This has shown us the hegemony that a small group of wealthy individuals and countries have over the world population, and the relationship of dependence and power between the Global North and Global South, reflecting an underlying ideology of biopolitics. Here, I understand biopolitics beyond Foucault's view (Foucault, 2007) not only as a relationship of power and dominance over populations but also between communities, ubiquitous and replicated in all areas of society as a model of governance that standardises life but also produces inequalities and normalises precarity. It is a notion that invites rethinking the meaning of vulnerability (Fassin, 2009).

The very division in our discourse between a Global North and a Global South can be seen as an expression of global biopolitics, which goes beyond a geographical notion to become a paradigm of poverty,[2] asymmetric living conditions, and subordinated relationships, as described by Balandier (1973). It could be understood as "a project", as Prashad sustains, referring to the "Third World" (Prashad, 2008), or a political and socio-cultural "space-time" of submission/domination as expressed by Sousa Santos (2020).

Since decolonisation, many former European colonies have failed to shed a bond of economic dependency with the Global North. Global South economies are reliant on the demand of consumers in the more affluent North, and many of their basic public services, such as health services, depend on external support, being often financed by philanthropic or aid organisations based in the North.

With COVID-19, we have been witnessing echoes of an approach to Global Health reminiscent of the colonial model of the nineteenth century (Bell and Green, 2021), when international sanitation measures were designed to protect the rich in the European colonial metropole. It seems to be a reconstitution of neo-colonial societies within the new global (dis)order triggered by the spread of COVID-19.

This has occurred against the backdrop of a supposed transformation of the notion of Global Health. Since the 1990s this was assumed to reconceptualise international health and adapt health policies to the phenomenon of globalisation (Brown, Cueto, and Fee, 2006; Arrizabalaga, 2021: 275). Arguably, such a transformation has never transpired. The COVID-19 syndemic could have been the perfect opportunity to seek changes towards a true Global Health; however, so far it has only exacerbated inequalities.

The Global Health Summit held in Rome on 21 May 2021 represented, according to the host government, an opportunity for "all world leaders" to adopt a declaration as a "point of reference to prevent future global health crises" (EFE, 2021), emphasising a clear "no" to health nationalism. However, the enormous underrepresentation of low-income countries at the summit shows the reality of what is considered Global Health, whereby countries of the Global South are merely objects of discourse but rarely meaningfully participate in decision-making.

History repeats itself: Lessons from past epidemics

Against this backdrop, it is not surprising that we have witnessed the repetition – and sometimes even deepening – of our past mistakes in managing epidemics. In this section, I highlight several lessons that we have failed to learn from the past in our approach to COVID-19. In pointing out these lessons, I draw particularly on my experience working on the Ebola and other epidemic responses.

Global South matters

Sometimes, epidemics – and COVID-19 is an example of this – only seem to trigger global responses when the populations from the richest countries are affected. As Louis Vives' text from the sixteenth century reveals, the health of the poor only attains global socio-political interest once it poses a danger of spreading to the rich or when it involves significant economic loss ([1526] 1997). Nearly five hundred years later, having hardly reacted during the four decades that elapsed since the first

Ebola epidemics in Sudan and the Democratic Republic of Congo (DRC), the Global North finally woke up to the threat posed by this virus when Ebola broke the imaginary barrier that had kept all the previous outbreaks isolated in small rural areas to simultaneously reach urban areas in several countries in West-Africa, and reaching also for first time countries in the Global North, with the first infection outside Africa identified in Spain, and single imported cases reported also in United Kingdom and United States (MSF, 2015: 11).

It was only then that the Global North moved to find a treatment and vaccine, and in just over a year a vaccine was developed. This feat has been repeated with COVID-19, leading to the development of successful vaccines in record time, demonstrating that when there is international political will, translated into resources, great advances can be made. However, this also is evidence of a perverse reality; only diseases affecting high-income countries seems to generate interest from the pharmaceutical companies which have the resources to develop effective treatments.

Disease can easily mask social inequalities. An example of this can also be found in cholera outbreaks. I have worked in many cholera interventions in countries such as Zambia, Guinea Bissau, Yemen, South Sudan, the DRC, Tanzania, Mozambique, and Haiti. Cholera epidemics tend to become highly politicised because they expose the lack of adequate infrastructure for basic provision of water and sanitation in many neighbourhoods. Some governments evaded responsibility by accusing the most-vulnerable people of being responsible for the epidemic through their inappropriate behaviour and lack of hygiene; the victims are blamed. Recognising that cholera is not a disease caused by voluntary bad-hygiene practices, but rather a social disease, would be political suicide for leaders, as it would expose potential negligence relating to the services they are responsible for. Similarly, during the COVID-19 outbreak, many people have been blamed for not complying with the government restrictions, such as by breaking the "stay at home" rule, regardless of their circumstances.

Neglecting other critical problems: The wider impact on health

Fixating solely on the virus means we could leave aside other pressing problems. The Ebola epidemic had serious consequences for the already precarious health services of the affected countries in West Africa. Not only did it lead to many deaths among health personnel and community caregivers, but the local lockdown measures had enormous economic impact that took years to reverse (Rasul et al., 2020). The fear of infection also led to a decrease in the search for medical care and to a lack of medical assistance even for pregnant women giving birth, altering health-seeking behaviour patterns.

In Freetown, where I was during part of the Ebola epidemic, there was a moment when practically the only functional health structures were the Ebola treatment centres, posing a serious risk of exposure to people who had Ebola-like symptoms caused by another health issue and had to go the Ebola centres to seek medical attention. To mitigate this, Médecins Sans Frontières (MSF), together with the ministry of health, organised a challenging but successful mass distribution of malaria prophylaxis (distributing anti-malaria drugs, door to door, with over a thousand community health workers to over two million people in four days) (MSF, 2014a).

This offered a key lesson: other critical diseases cannot be left aside during an outbreak response. This has been dramatically overlooked during the COVID-19 syndemic, with many other pressing health problems left aside, even diseases that are major killers, such as malaria in the case of many sub-Saharan countries.

Movement restrictions and lockdowns of non-infected people

While the self-isolation of contacts and quarantine of the sick has often been generally accepted in many societies, the lockdown of healthy people has been controversial. During the West African Ebola outbreak, several local restrictions were put in place: quarantine in high-risk areas; curfews lasting anywhere from days to several months; closures of schools and markets; the cancellation of all large gatherings including sporting events; and the strengthening of border controls (Coltart et al., 2017: 16).

The quarantine imposed on asymptomatic workers for the mere fact of having worked in the Ebola epidemic, coupled with the suspension of flights to affected countries by some airlines, presented significant operational disruptions for many organisations, leading to a general shortage of much-needed healthcare workers at a crucial time. This is something that has again been a problem during COVID-19, including within Western healthcare systems, where isolation of asymptomatic health workers has caused shortages of staff.

In the case of Ebola, where the case fatality rate ranges from 50 to 90 percent, regardless of age, strong measures were attempted. In Liberia, for example, the government made it illegal to conceal an Ebola-infected patient, an offence punishable by a prison sentence of two years (Coltart et al., 2017: 12). Similarly, fines to coerce people to comply with imposed norms have been broadly used with COVID-19 in several countries. However, where government tried to impose population lockdowns and curfews reinforced by the army, the population often protested, since the controls proved unfeasible for many. In Sierra Leone during the Ebola outbreak, the government announced a three-day lockdown of six million people at least twice, while volunteers went door to door to detect Ebola and take suspected cases to Ebola facilities, often against their will. Organisations, such as the one I was working for, spoke out publicly against this measure (BBC, 2014), claiming: "Large-scale coercive measures, such as forced quarantines and lockdowns, are driving people underground and endangering trust toward health providers" (Ellis and Gigova, 2015). MSF publications claim that their overall experience in West Africa was that top-down forced measures increased mistrust and fear, causing effects that were counterproductive to containing the epidemic (Calain and Poncin, 2015; Pellecchia et al., 2015).[3]

The use of fearmongering measures is another similarity between the Ebola and COVID-19 responses. We saw involvement of the army in reinforcing lockdowns during the West African Ebola outbreak; this has also been done in several regions during the COVID-19 syndemic. In my experience, the involvement of the military in emergency response – beyond logistical support, where it can be helpful – is often counterproductive, because it can be seen by the population as intimidating and disproportionate. In some contexts, it can even "undermine the perceived neutrality of assistance" (Lamoure and Juillard, 2020).

Societies are not homogeneous: One size doesn't fit all

One of the things I have appreciated most during my time with MSF is the organisation's ability to self-reflect. Every major emergency response is followed by an evaluation to learn from mistakes. The fact that a one-size-fits-all model is inadequate due to the specificity of each population is a recurring lesson; a plan to respond to a cholera outbreak developed in Haiti doesn't necessarily work in Yemen. Each society is different. This may sound trivial, but when the emergency strategy doesn't reflect this lesson, it's worth reinforcing the point. In my view, this is the key error in the current COVID-19 response.

This is also one of the reasons I prefer the term "syndemic" to "pandemic". This word helps highlight the ways in which specific interactions of biological and social circumstances in each population have an impact on the shape of the pandemic, which results in COVID-19 affecting different groups very differently.

In my view, the WHO have been progressively distancing themselves from the reality of many people in the Global South, with the Alma-Ata Declaration becoming a faded memory. This disconnect has been noticeable in recent epidemics; particularly 2003's SARS, 2005's avian flu (H5N1), and 2009's swine flu (H1N1). An analysis of the international response to these epidemics is essential to understanding the political and institutional pressures and failures that the current COVID-19 response has exposed (Caduff, 2020; Bell and Green, 2021).

The WHO has been increasingly criticised, since the SARS epidemic, for its overestimated mortality predictions based on mathematical modelling, which tends to overlook differentiating social determinants that are essential for epidemiological analysis. With the avian and swine flu epidemics, the WHO generated a campaign fuelling panic that urged governments to purchase the "miracle" treatment (Tamiflu), which ended up being of little use and a multimillion-dollar waste and which mainly benefited the pharmaceutical industry. This was a turning point for the WHO at which it lost its credibility with many health professionals (Boseley, 2010; Rego, 2010; López, 2011)

Epidemiological prediction models should incorporate social determinants characteristic of each population, and a custom-made strategy should be used for each context. A densely populated urban area or a refugee camp will experience a pandemic very differently from a rural setting. Communities are not homogenous, and responders should understand contextual power relationships between groups to ensure a community-led response that is relevant to each community specifically.

Community engagement: Key for epidemic control

The 1978 Alma-Ata Declaration promoted by the WHO implied a turning point in the Global Health paradigm. It aspired to "health for all by the year 2000" through a comprehensive, community-based primary-healthcare approach.

My experience is that community-based approaches help to identify failures of the measures to control outbreaks, including rumours and fears that could affect the response. Persuading communities and involving them in decisions has been proven more useful than imposing measures.

At the beginning of the Ebola epidemic in West Africa, most responders opted for a centralised model of care, going as far as constructing the largest Ebola treatment centre ever built. But often such an approach was shunned by communities, and outreach teams faced significant challenges in identifying cases in communities and transferring them to centralised isolation facilities (Calain and Poncin, 2015: 126). Shifting to a more decentralised model, with centres built closer to the affected communities and ensuring communication links between patients and families, proved more effective (Ripoll et al., 2018). In contrast, during the current syndemic, many Global North countries have opted for a "Hospital-centric" approach, once again neglecting primary healthcare.

At the same time, the lack of community-based health services has generated social initiatives of solidarity between populations and neighbours for mutual aid and support for vulnerable groups. This has been the case in Brazil during the syndemic, where the large population living overcrowded in favelas, huge numbers of homeless people, and a president denying the COVID-19 threat triggered many people, communities, and institutions to carry out their own "group self-caring" initiatives (Ortega and Orsini, 2020).

In every epidemic there are intersectional factors present specifically for each community. In the case of Ebola in West Africa, vulnerability to contracting the virus was highly correlated with gender, age, and socioeconomic status, as well as with access to health services. The use of an anthropological lens was an essential part of the response and helped identify these factors and their complex interactions. The anthropologist Paul Richards pointed out that the main lesson of Ebola in West Africa for the global response to COVID-19 is to share the learning experiences between communities and medical professionals. Indeed, West Africa's experience of Ebola had a lot to offer the COVID-19 response: communities experiencing Ebola in West Africa in 2014–15 rapidly learnt how to cope with a deadly new infection by understanding infection pathways and implementing domestic precautions. It was clearly recognised that this was a disease requiring families to change their behaviour in major ways, especially in how they cared for the sick (Richards, 2020).

As obvious as many of these lessons learned may seem, it is striking that they were often not considered during the ongoing syndemic of COVID-19.

Hidden impacts of the syndemic: Lockdowns as generators of social inequalities

Although no two societies and governments are the same, during the initial months of the syndemic there was a certain consensus among most governments on the measures imposed on their population, with each adopting a similar sequence of policies (Hale, 2021) and compulsory lockdowns in many countries. This apparent consensus overshadowed significant differences in the way certain measures, such as lockdowns, border closures, health passes and others, affect people in the Global South as compared to people from the North.

The WHO's COVID-19 special envoy, David Nabarro (2020), admitted the damaging effect of lockdowns in an interview (broadly misquoted and generating controversy) in October 2020, saying: "We in the World Health Organization do not advocate lockdowns as the primary means of control of this virus…lockdowns just have one consequence that you must never, ever belittle, and that is making poor people an awful lot poorer."

The motto "The virus doesn't care about social class", so often repeated during the first wave, has lost meaning, because every day it becomes clearer that the virus "knows" about inequalities. After all, "pandemics do not kill as indiscriminately as is believed" (Sousa Santos, 2020: 65).

A large part of the population in the Global South lives in an informal economy, relying on going out daily to find a way to earn an income to buy food and basic subsistence items. For this part of the world's population, lockdown, however short, makes the difference between survival and starvation. Also, for people who already suffer difficulties and depend on the social assistance of relatives and neighbours, lockdowns cut these essential social ties, turning adversity into misery. Not to mention what the slogan "Stay at home" – promoting the lockdown – meant for the homeless population.

COVID-19 particularly affects informal caregivers, a role that often still falls on women that are also poor and immigrant, making them more susceptible to infection. But if there is a particularly vulnerable group which COVID-19 puts at greatest risk, it is the elderly. We were urged by governments to protect them, but above all, surprisingly, to lock them up. Alone, without family or professional support, the situation worsened when the lockdown denied them any possibility of healthcare (Loyola, 2020: 208). We have failed our elders as a society.

This had different impacts in the Global North and the South. The aging of the population in Europe and the associated caregiving crisis have been decisive in the death toll left behind by the progression of the virus in Europe. But other societies with younger populations have faced different impacts; in many countries of the Global South, the COVID-19 impact didn't come directly from the disease itself but rather from the measures imposed by governments to stop it.

Global measures, such as border closures and lockdowns, have caused enormous supply ruptures that have affected the availability of essential items. They have also led to shortages of health workers in the Global South due to a reduction in mobility, making access to health services even more limited for many. These ruptures have forced many health institutions and humanitarian agencies to take difficult decisions about reducing or interrupting health services and programmes at a time when they needed to be expanded.

There have also been disruptions in the supply of some basic medicines and other essentials, such as malaria rapid tests, due to the shift by pharmaceutical companies to producing more lucrative COVID-19 tests (MSF, 2020). The supply-chain rupture for essential drugs was very evident during the wave that hit India last April. This affected many countries, India being the world's leading producer of generic drugs and responsible for a large proportion of global drug manufacturing.

Having a sole focus on COVID-19 and leaving aside other acute health problems can have fatal consequences for populations, overshadowing other medical-humanitarian emergencies. All malaria and malnutrition prevention activities have suffered enormous disruptions, even though these are the main causes of morbidity and mortality among young children in much of sub-Saharan Africa. HIV and TB services have also been affected (The Global Fund, 2021). To this must be added a reduction in community and primary-care services, which are the main gateway to medical care, including malaria diagnosis and treatment.

An internal analysis carried out by MSF of COVID-19's collateral impacts in the countries where they work shows that preventive immunisation activities were heavily affected. This is consistent with the Global Alliance for Vaccines and Immunisation's (GAVI) November 2020 findings, according to which 42 countries were affected due to vaccination activity suspensions or delays during the first year of the syndemic (GAVI, 2020). This has caused a reduction in immunisation coverage that will create dangerous immunity gaps in some countries. An MSF publication estimates that for every COVID-19 death "prevented" by diverting all resources to COVID-19, more than one hundred unvaccinated children could die due to the disruption of other essential activities (West, 2020).

Differential access to COVID-19 vaccination has been another indicator of inequality. While many Low Income Countries (LICs) have barely managed to vaccinate 5 percent of their population, the Global North is debating whether to also vaccinate young children, aiming for the desired herd immunity, and administering a third booster dose.

The uncertainty and pressure of lockdown resulted to the development of stigma around healthcare personnel and mistrust of healthcare services. This had an impact on health-seeking behaviour and practices, partly due to a misinterpretation of the message to "stay at home", resulting in a decrease in demand for primary-care consultations.

In the first months of the syndemic there were even attacks on healthcare personnel in some countries. Lockdowns have also caused an increase in domestic and gender-based violence (The Global Fund, 2021). According to an ACLED (Armed Conflict

Location and Event Data Project) report which monitored changes in patterns of violence since the syndemic began, there has been an increase in violent events globally, although the situation has varied greatly from country to country, largely due to the different reactions to the imposition of lockdown measures (Kishi, 2021).

Conclusion

In July 2020, the UN secretary general, Antonio Guterres, gave a speech at the Nelson Mandela Foundation acknowledging that the legacy of colonialism persists in Global Health and that COVID-19 has laid bare the risks of ignoring structural inequalities, inadequate health systems, and gaps in social protection. He called for a new social contract for a new era which would create equal opportunities and respect the rights and freedoms of all, stating also that a new model for global governance must be based on full, inclusive, and equal participation in global institutions (UN, 2020).

We have failed to protect the most vulnerable with our current Global Health model, particularly in low-income communities. Any future model of response to a pandemic must break the status quo of the current pharmaceutical-commercial model whereby financial profit is what dictates policies. Inequality begins at the top, in global institutions, and addressing it starts with reforming those institutions. It would be useful if an institution like the WHO could recognise the crisis in which it has found itself and reform its governance model. "We need a model of sovereign and global governance evolved from what is today the model we have from WHO" (Martínez-Hernáez, 2020).

If there is one lesson from the syndemic, it is that we must change. Returning to the pre-COVID-19 "normality" should not be the desired goal. We should look for opportunities for change that contribute to more supportive, equitable, and resilient societies. We should rethink the "old normal" rather than rush back to it (Green, 2021). To this end, communities should be allowed to participate in developing response strategies to any future outbreaks, rather than merely being recipients of blueprints imposed from above.

Medical anthropology gives us some of the tools we need to bring about such a change in our collective mindset. This discipline helps us understand that the world is heterogeneous and dynamic in nature. It can also help us make room for a critical debate about replacing our hegemonic, biomedical Global Health model with one in which local knowledge from the Global South is integrated. There is a need for an epistemological shift that can help us see alternative ideas and prospects to the current socio-political model and help us decolonise our thinking about future global emergencies – a new Social Contract to tackle inequities is urgently needed, as Guterres has advised.

> The coronavirus pandemic is one manifestation among many of the model of society that began to be imposed worldwide from the seventeenth century and is now reaching its final stage.
>
> *(Sousa Santos, 2020: 64)*

Notes

1 "Event 201" was a simulation exercise organised by the Johns Hopkins Centre together with the World Economic Forum, the CDC, and the Bill & Melinda Gates Foundation, held in New York on 18 October 2019. The pathogen chosen for the exercise was a coronavirus, which months later, when the pandemic was declared, fed some conspiracy theories. The organisers maintain that the event was only a simulation exercise which didn't include predictions (JHCHS, 2020).

2 The "Global North/South" labels are metaphors for inequality and a corrective attempt to replace the previous terms "first/third world" or "developed/underdeveloped", concepts perceived as controversial (Adams et al., 2019).

3 This is consistent with the wider literature (Coltart et al., 2017: 10; Ripoll et al., 2018: 17; Lamoure and Juillard. 2020: 18).

References

Adams Vincanne, Behague Dominique, Caduff Carlo, Löwy Ilana, and Ortega Francisco. 2019. "Re-Imagining Global Health Through Social Medicine". *Global Public Health* 14 (10): 1383–1400.

Arrizabalaga, Jon. 2021. "El desafío de las enfermedades (re)emergentes, los limits de la respuesta biomedica y el nuevo paradigma de salud global". *Historia, Ciencia, Saude. Manguinhos* 28: 275.

Avalos, Miguel Alejandro. 2020. "#Quédateencasa: medidas de aislamiento social". In *RESET. Reflexiones antropológicas ante la pandemia de COVID-19*, edited by Stella Evangelidou and Angel Martinez-Hernaez. Tarragona: URV: 139.

Balandier, G. 1973. *Teorías de la descolonización. Las dinámicas sociales*. Traslated by Rafael di Muro. [Original title: *Sens et puissance. Les dynamiques sociales*. 1971]. Colección Critica ideológica. Editorial tiempo Contemporáneo. Buenos Aires.

BBC. 2014. "Sierra Leone's Ebola lockdown will not help, says MSF". *BBC*, 6 September, https://www.bbc.com/news/world-africa-29096405

Bell, David and Toby Green. 2021. "The World Health Organization and COVID-19: Re-Stablishing colonialism in Public Health". *Pandata*, June, https://www.pandata.org/wp-content/uploads/PANDA_WHO_ReestablishingColonialism.pdf

Boseley, Sarah. 2010. "WHO accused of losing public confidence over flu pandemic". *The Guardian*, 28 March, https://www.theguardian.com/world/2010/mar/28/who-public-confidence-flu-pandemic

Brown, Theodore M., Marcos Cueto, and Elizabeth Fee. 2006. "The World Health Organization and the Transition From 'International' to 'Global' Public Health". *American Journal of Public Health* 96 (62): 72.

Calain, Philippe, and Marc Poncin. 2015. "Reaching out to Ebola victims: Coercion, persuasion or an appeal for self-sacrifice?". *ELSEVIER. Social Science and Medicine* 147: 126–133.

Caduff, Carlo. 2020. "What Went Wrong: Corona and the World after the Full Stop". Medical Anthropology Quarterly. International Journal for the Analysis of Health 34, (4.467): 487.

Coltart, Cordelia E.M, Benjamin Lindsey, Isaac Ghinai, Anne M. Johnson, and David L. Heymann. 2017. "The Ebola outbreak, 2013–2016: old lessons for new epidemics". *Philos Trans R Soc Lond B Biol Sci*. 372(1721): 1–24.

Crudo Blackburn, Christine, Gerald W. Parker, and Morten Wendelbo. 2018. "How the devastating 1918 flu pandemic helped advance US women's rights". The Conversation, 1 March, https://theconversation.com/how-the-devastating-1918-flu-pandemic-helped-advance-us-womens-rights-91045

EFE. 2021. *El G20 se compromete a cooperar y a combatir la desigualdad en la vacunación.* www. efe.com/efe/espana/sociedad/el-g20-se-compromete-a-cooperar-y-combatir-la-desi gualdad-en-vacunacion/10004-4542314. 21 de May 2021.

Ellis, Ralph, and Radina Gigova. 2015. "Sierra Leone leader orders new national lockdown to battle Ebola". *CNN*, 22 March, https://edition.cnn.com/2015/03/21/africa/sierra-leone-lockdown/index.html.

Fassin, Didier. 2009. "Another Politics of Life is Possible". *Theory, Culture & Society 2009* 26(5): 44–60.

Foucault, Michel. 1975. *Vigilar y Castigar, nacimiento de la prisión.* Translated and edited by Aurelio Garzón. Mexico, Argentina and España: Siglo XXI.

Foucault, Michel. 2007. *Nacimiento de la biopolítica: curso en el Collège de France (1978-1979).* Translated and edited by Horacio Pons. Buenos Aires: Fondo de Cultura Económica.

Garcia Luaces, Pedro. 2015. "La peste negra: Hacia una nueva era". *Historia y Vida* 568: 38-45.

GAVI. 2020. GAVI situation report #20. Geneva: GAVI: https://www.gavi.org/sites/defa ult/files/covid/Gavi-COVID-19-Situation-Report-20-20201118.pdf. https://www. gavi.org/sites/default/files/covid/Gavi-COVID-19-Situation-Report-18-20200924.pdf

Green, Toby. 2021. *The COVID Consensus: The new Politics of Global Inequality.* London: Hurst &Co.

Hale, Thomas. 2021. "What we learned from tracking every COVID policy in the world". *The Conversation*, 24 March, https://theconversation.com/what-we-learned-from-track ing-every-COVID-policy-in-the-world-157721

JHCHS. 2020. "Statement about nCoV and our pandemic exercise". *Center for Health Security*, 24 January, www.centerforhealthsecurity.org/news/center-news/2020/2020-01-24-Statement-of-Clarification-Event201.html

Kishi, Roudabeh. 2021. *A year of COVID-19: The pandemic impact on global conflict and demon-stration trends.* ACLED. https://acleddata.com/acleddatanew/wp-content/uploads/2021/04/ACLED_A-Year-of-COVID19_April2021.pdf

Lakoff, Andrew. 2017. *Unprepared: Global Health In a Time of Emergency.* Los Angeles: University of California Press.

Lamoure, G., and Juillard, H. 2020. *ALNAP Lessons Paper: Responding to Ebola epidemics.* London: ALNAP: www.alnap.org/help-library/alnap-lessons-paper-responding-to-ebola-epidemics

López, María. 2011. "Hasta los médicos han dejado ya de creer en la OMS". *El Confidencial*, 12 June, https://www.elconfidencial.com/sociedad/2011-06-12/hasta-los-medicos-han-dejado-ya-de-creer-en-la-oms_483304/

Loyola, Silvia. 2020. "Paciente 0. La invención del culpable". In *Cuarenta historias para la cuarentena: reflexiones historicas sobre epidemias y salud global*, edited by Perdiguero-Gil y Bueno.. Madrid: Sociedad Española de Historia de la Medicina: 203–209

Martínez-Hernáez, Angel. 2020. "El director del Centro de Antropología Médica pide una gobernanza mundial ante pandemias". Interview by Susana Rodriguez, 28 May.

MSF. 2014a. "Quarantine can undermine efforts to curb epidemic". *MSF*, 28 October, www. msf.org/ebola-quarantine-can-undermine-efforts-curb-epidemic

MSF. 2014b. "Distribución masiva de medicamentos contra la malaria en Sierra Leona". *MSF*, 10 December, www.msf.es/actualidad/distribucion-masiva-medicamentos-la-mala ria-sierra-leona

MSF. 2015. *Pushed to the Limit and Beyond: A year into the largest ever Ebola outbreak.* Barcelona: MSF

MSF. 2020. *Collateral Impacts of COVID-19 on non-COVID health.* Internal organization update. Barcelona: MSF.

Nabarro, David. 2020. The Week in 60 Minutes #6 – with Andrew Neil and WHO Covid-19 envoy David Nabarro. The Spectator TV, interview. (9 October 2020). Retrieved from: https://www.youtube.com/watch?v=x8oH7cBxgwE

Ortega, Francisco and Michael Orsini. 2020. "Governing COVID-19 without Government in Brazil: Ignorance, Neoliberal Authoritarianism, and the Collapse of Public Health Leadership". *Global Public Health* 15: 1257–1277.

Pearce, Katie. 2019. "Pandemic simulation exercise spotlights massive preparedness gap". *Hub*, 6 November. https://hub.jhu.edu/2019/11/06/event-201-health-security/

Pellecchia, Umberto, Rosa Crestani, Tom Decroo, Rafael Van den Bergh, and Yasmine Al-Kourdi. 2015. "Social Consequences of Ebola Containment Measures in Liberia". *Europe PMC* 10 (12): e0143036

Prashad, Vijay. 2008. *The Darker Nations: A people's History of the Third World*. London: The New Press.

Rasul, Imran, Markus Goldstein, Niklas Buehren, Oriana Bandiera, and Andrea Smurra. 2020. "What happens after the lockdown ends? Lessons from the 2015 Ebola epidemic in Sierra Leone". *IGC*, 25 May, https://www.theigc.org/blog/what-happens-after-the-lockdown-ends-lessons-from-the-2015-ebola-epidemic-in-sierra-leone/

Rego, Paco. 2010. "EL CAMELO DE LA GRIPE 'A'". *EL Mundo*, 24 January, https://www.elmundo.es/suplementos/cronica/2010/745/1264287607.html

Richards, Paul. 2020. "What Might Africa Teach the World? COVID-19 and Ebola Virus Disease Compared". *African Arguments*, 17 March, https://africanarguments.org/2020/03/what-might-africa-teach-the-world-covid-19-and-ebola-virus-disease-compared/

Ripoll, S., I. Gercama, T. Jones, and A. Wilkinson. 2018. "Social Science Lessons Learned from Ebola Epidemics. Institutional, SSHAP. Lecciones de ciencias sociales aprendidas de las epidemias de ébola: resumen de evidencia, UNICEF.

Sánchez, Salvador Cayuela. 2020. "Reflexiones biopolíticas en torno a la COVID-19". In *Cuarenta historias para una cuarentena*. Edited by Perdiguero-Gil and Bueno Campos. Sociedad Española de Historia de la Medicina, Madrid: 160.

Singer, Merill, and Clair Scott. 2008. "Syndemics and Public Health: Reconceptualizing Disease in Bio-Social Context". *Medical Anthropology Quarterly*: 423–441. https://doi.org/10.1525/maq.2003.17.4.423

Singer, Merrill, and Barbara Rylko-Bauer. 2020. "The Syndemics and Structural Violence of the COVID Pandemic: Anthropological Insights on a Crisis". *Open Anthropological Research* 17(4):423–444. https://doi.org/10.1525/maq.2003.17.4.423

Sousa Santos, Boaventura. 2020. La cruel pedagogía del virus. Buenos Aires: CLACSO.

The Global Fund. 2021. The impact of COVID-19 on HIV, TB and malaria services and systems for health. A snapshot from 502 health facilities across Africa and Asia. 13th April. www.theglobalfund.org/en/updates/other-updates/2021-04-13-the-impact-of-COVID-19-on-hiv-tb-and-malaria-services-and-systems-for-health/.

UN. 2020. "Tackling Inequality: A New Social Contract for a New Era". *UN*, www.un.org/en/coronavirus/tackling-inequality-new-social-contract-new-era

Vives, Juan Luis. 1997. El socorro de los pobres. Translated by Luis Fraile Delgado. Madrid: Tecnos. (Original work from 1526.)

West, Kim. 2020. "Cuando (solo) miramos a la COVID-19, ¿qué sucede con millones de personas más?". *MSF*, 2 July, www.msf.es/actualidad/cuando-solo-miramos-la-covid-19-que-sucede-millones-personas-mas

WHO. 2019. *Non-Pharmaceutical Public Health Measures for Mitigating the Risk and Impact of Epidemic and Pandemic Influenza*. Geneva: WHO.

Zarzoso, Alfons. 2000. "Los orígenes de la salud pública: ¿una cuestión política y económica? consideraciones historiográficas a propósito del libro de Christopher Hamlin". Asclepio Vol. LII-2: 283–294. https://doi.org/10.3989/asclepio.2000.v52.i2.213

SECTION 3
Alternative Lenses on Pandemic Response

Alternative perspectives on governments' pandemic responses during 2020–22 are not only generated by different interpretations of key COVID-19 concepts and by evidence and analysis from contexts outside of the Global North, as we have seen in the first two parts of this book. They also arise when governments' management of the spread of SARS-CoV-2 is examined through the lens of paradigms that have been overlooked during this crisis. Entire frameworks for identifying possible and appropriate policies for the management of the spread of the virus and of the disease with which it is associated have been missing from the COVID-19 debate, leading to highly truncated intellectual horizons for the proper regulation of that debate. The essays in this final section seek to help expand these horizons—a vital endeavour in the world's effort to make sense of the last two years.

DOI: 10.4324/9781003259336-14

11

THE PROPORTIONALITY OF LOCKDOWNS

Kai Möller[1]

Introduction

Lockdowns are repressive state measures that severely restrict individual freedom and rights and are therefore constitutionally suspect. The legal and constitutional standard that courts around the world rely on to assess the justifiability and legitimacy of such measures is the principle of proportionality. This chapter examines whether the lockdowns imposed in response to the COVID-19 pandemic in 2020 and 2021 were proportionate and therefore legitimate. It points out which questions a court assessing the proportionality of lockdowns would have to ask, and develops normative standards with regard to some of the relevant issues.

At the core of the issue is the question of the acceptable balance between what we might call "the protection of life and health" and "freedom". I will argue that the balance struck by most states was affected by a number of biases in favour of imposing lockdowns. First, by focusing in a one-sided way on the protection of health and lives, the public and political discourse neglected the question of the severity of the restriction on freedom and, relatedly, the costs of lockdowns, in particular their social, medical, psychological, cultural, and economic costs. Second, by *de facto* placing a taboo on the question of the relevance of the age distribution of the people dying from COVID-19, a proper consideration of this relevant factor was prevented. Third, the considerations that were regarded as determinative in striking the balance, namely the protection of the health services from being overburdened and/or the prioritisation of human life as the highest value, were normatively unconvincing. Because of the complexity of, in particular, the empirical questions relating to the costs of lockdowns, this chapter cannot reach a confident conclusion as to the proportionality of the recent lockdowns. It does, however, show that the public and political discourse was biased in favour of lockdowns, and

DOI: 10.4324/9781003259336-15

offers a doctrinal structure as well as normative reflection on how to conduct the proportionality assessment properly.

Proportionality

The standard of review that courts around the world use to assess the justifiability of repressive state measures is called "the principle of proportionality", or simply "proportionality". Proportionality requires the state measures to pursue a legitimate goal, to be a suitable means of achieving the goal, to be necessary in that there must not exist a less restrictive but equally effective alternative, and to be "proportionate in the strict sense", the establishing of which requires a balancing exercise between the severity of the restriction and the importance of the public interest pursued.[2] Proportionality was first developed by the Prussian administrative courts to review the exercise of police powers in the context of administrative law. It has since then quickly spread from administrative to constitutional as well as EU and international law, and from Prussia and Germany to many parts of the liberal democratic world.[3]

There has been a wide-ranging debate about the principle of proportionality in recent years. The view that has emerged from this is that the point of a proportionality review is to ensure that an act which burdens a person is *reasonably justifiable to him or her*; a judicial system that is committed to this idea is sometimes referred to as endorsing a *"culture of justification"*[4] or as giving effect to each person's *"right to justification"*.[5] Thus, if a state imposes a repressive measure such as a lockdown, an affected citizen might ask: "How dare you limit my liberty? What's your justification for this?". And our citizen might not only ask this question but also take the case to court. The court's job will then be to assess whether the lockdown is reasonably justifiable. The test that courts use to establish this is proportionality. If the court reaches the conclusion that the measure is disproportionate – not reasonably justifiable – and therefore in violation of the citizen's right to justification, it will make a declaration to this effect or strike it down (depending on the specifics of the legal system).

For our purposes, it is important to note two points. First, the legitimacy of repressive state measures is not only a *political* and/or *moral* question but also a *legal* and *constitutional* one. A state that restricts our liberty must have a sufficient justification for doing so, and policing this is the proper role of the courts, which apply the principle of proportionality to fulfil their task. Second, the considerations that courts rely on when assessing the proportionality of a repressive measure are not different in character from the considerations that politicians, journalists, or ordinary citizens utilise when assessing various actual or proposed policies. The law does not require any "secret knowledge" accessible only to the initiated in this regard. Proportionality is simply a structure that allows judges to engage in the practical reasoning required to assess the justifiability of a policy. The fact that, as will be shown, we have no, or only clearly deficient, answers to some of the basic questions that proportionality directs us to examine shows that something has gone seriously wrong with our democratic deliberation of this crucially important issue.

Lockdowns and proportionality

Legitimate goal, suitability, and necessity

The recent lockdowns passed the first three stages of the proportionality test relatively smoothly. First, regarding the legitimate goal stage, lockdowns were imposed for a clearly legitimate goal, namely to protect people's lives (preventing death) and health (preventing, in particular, severe cases of COVID-19 and what has come to be called "long Covid").

Second, they were also a suitable means for achieving this goal because they plausibly achieved the reduction of social contacts and therefore opportunities for spreading the virus. There seems to be some disagreement on this point because, in some cases, lockdowns were imposed when infection numbers were already declining; hence the case could be made that any subsequent reduction in infection rates was the result of other factors. This may or may not be empirically true; nevertheless, the link between limiting or reducing the number of social contacts and reducing infections with a virus that is spread through social contact is plausible. Hence, it is also plausible to assume that lockdowns will have led to a reduction in the numbers of people getting infected with the virus and therefore also to a reduction in the numbers of people dying of it or developing long Covid. This is sufficient in the context of this stage of the test.

The third question is whether lockdowns were necessary in that there was no less restrictive but equally effective alternative. Critics of lockdowns often point to the "Swedish way" of dealing with the pandemic, which focused less on legal prohibitions and more on recommendations, or the approach advocated by the "Great Barrington Declaration", which proposed "shielded protection" of those most at risk from the virus but otherwise no restrictions, in order to build up herd immunity which would then also protect the vulnerable.[6] But whether these approaches really are equally effective is empirically unclear. For example, the proponents of the "Swedish way" tend to compare the number of COVID-19 deaths in Sweden with those in other European countries, its opponents with those in the other Scandinavian countries. There are empirical uncertainties here partly because it is difficult to compare the effectiveness of one country's approach with that of another country or a hypothetical alternative. Where there is empirical uncertainty, proportionality grants the original decision maker (the state) a certain margin of appreciation. Note, also, that it would seem that lockdowns work quite well precisely because they are such extreme measures. Connected to this point, the strongest argument in favour of the "Swedish way" and the "Great Barrington Declaration" seems to be not that they are necessarily (or demonstrably) better at protecting lives and health but rather that they strike a more appropriate balance between freedom and protecting lives; this is, however, not a question to be considered at the necessity stage but rather at the balancing stage.

At this point a qualification is in order and a limitation of this paper has to be stated. The real question with regard to how to respond to the COVID-19 pandemic was not a "yes/no" decision as to whether or not to impose lockdowns. Rather, there is a sliding scale of measures reaching from letting the virus rip through society, to an approach broadly following the "Swedish way", to a "soft" lockdown, and then towards a strict lockdown and a "No Covid" policy. A properly conducted proportionality assessment would therefore have to assess the lockdown chosen by the state relative to the other possible responses.[7] Furthermore, the individual measures, which in their totality amount to a lockdown, would have to be examined individually such as school closures, curfews, closure of shops, prohibitions on visiting the inhabitants of care homes, and so on. This paper perhaps crudely, glosses over those questions and chooses a simpler structure in order to focus our attention on the more basic normative questions that proportionality directs us to investigate.

Balancing

This takes us to the fourth stage, the balancing stage, and here the substantive problems lurk. Remember that the proportionality test requires the establishment of three things at this stage: first, the severity of the interference with freedom (thus, in particular, the burdens that the respective lockdown imposes on people's ability to freely live their lives); second, the importance of the competing public interest (the importance of protecting health and lives); third, the relationship between the two (to determine whether the importance of the public interest in protecting health and lives outweighs the severity of the restriction on freedom).[8] Each of these issues raises difficult questions, and none of them was satisfactorily addressed in public and political discourse at the time.

The severity of the restriction

Let us start with the first question. Lockdowns are indisputably extremely severe restrictions on personal freedom. The principle of proportionality as well as common sense require that a government contemplating the imposition of a measure as drastic as a lockdown must assess very carefully not only what the desired and likely positive effects of such a measure might be (more on that below) but also what the likely collateral damage caused by this social intervention for people's freedom – in the terminology of human and constitutional rights law, their ability to "freely develop their personality"[9] – will be. This requires the government to engage in a comprehensive impact assessment before imposing the lockdown, and it further requires that this assessment be kept under review for the duration of the lockdown to ensure that its continuation is justified.

The harms of lockdowns to freedom are considerable. Humans are social beings and social contact is necessary for our flourishing. The limitation of social contact imposes a considerable burden on virtually everyone's ability to flourish and freely develop his or her personality. The outer symptoms of such deprivation will often be loneliness and understimulation, and in more severe cases depression, anxiety, or substance abuse; in the most extreme cases it may lead to suicide. Lockdowns that involve school and university closures place a particularly grave burden on children and students by hindering their education and their ability to develop skills and competence – important both for themselves as well as society – and their broader personal development. The outer symptoms will, again, often be loneliness, isolation, and poor mental health.[10] Lack of in-person contact with, in particular, teachers and physicians makes it harder to spot signs of abuse, the likelihood of which will also be increased during lockdowns in light of the intense stress this creates for many parents and carers; in general, the data suggests that domestic violence has risen during the lockdowns.[11] The restrictions that lockdowns have brought for many old people, and in particular the inhabitants of care homes – who often suffer from isolation and, relatedly, poor mental health even during normal times – are perhaps in the region of what we would ordinarily consider to be inhuman.[12]

Lockdowns further have grave economic consequences, and in particular have led and will lead to the closure of a large number of businesses, imposing severe burdens on their owners and employees, who may face unemployment together with its associated negative consequences for individual well-being (although it will have to be factored in that some of the economic damage may not result from the lockdowns but from the spread of the virus itself, which may lead, for example, to heightened anxiety, less spending, and so on). Similar considerations apply to the lives and careers of artists and others working in the cultural sector. The enormous debts that governments have accumulated to deal with the pandemic and the consequences of the lockdowns will undoubtedly have long-term financial and economic implications affecting many people negatively in the future.

Beyond the above-mentioned, more general harms of lockdowns, they affect specific vulnerable groups particularly severely, in particularly those who rely more than others on personal contact, the existence of some form of social life or interaction, or help from others, such as psychiatric patients, people with severe health problems more generally (who may have avoided or delayed treatment), care home inhabitants (as mentioned), prisoners, and homeless people.

The above list is not meant to be comprehensive. If a court were given the task to assess the proportionality of a lockdown, it would ultimately be the court's task to determine the severity of the restriction. But given that a court does not have the necessary empirical expertise to assess this issue, it would heavily rely on the submission of the respective government that imposed the lockdown and that would ordinarily be expected to have undertaken an assessment of its likely collateral damage – the severity of the restriction – which it would have used for its own decision-making process. On the basis of the political and public discourse since the beginning of the pandemic, it would seem that such a comprehensive assessment has never been undertaken;[13] in any case, its results do not seem to have been communicated to the public. Nor was there much public discussion about the harms of lockdowns, for example in the media. Rather, the focus both on the part of the governments as well as the public was continually on the other side of the balance, namely on questions such as the Sars-Cov-2 incidence rates, hospitalisations, death rates, long Covid, and so forth. This created an imbalanced picture which will have led many to believe that the protection of people from the virus was the only relevant factor in assessing the justification and proportionality of lockdowns.

Needless to say, in the spring of 2020, with no prior experience of lockdowns in the liberal democratic world, the harms of lockdowns might have been very difficult to predict, and there was a great urgency at the time. This, however, does not imply that no attempt to determine them was even necessary. Unless we have some (however uncertain and provisional) understanding of the effects of a proposed lockdown on people's freedom to live their lives, we cannot assess whether their benefits outweigh the harms. This applies even more obviously to the further lockdowns imposed in the autumn and winter of 2020–21, by which time governments surely had had enough time to prepare a comprehensive assessment.

The importance of the public interest

The second question at the balancing stage is the importance of the public interest, that is, the importance of protecting people's health and lives. Indisputably, this is an issue of great public interest that could potentially justify severe measures. There was no shortage of models to calculate the number of people likely to die or develop long Covid if lockdowns were not imposed. But the problem with the public and political discussion of this issue was that a taboo was quickly placed on one of the crucially important questions: the relevance of the age distribution of the people dying of COVID-19. Thus, it became publicly and politically impossible to openly and freely discuss whether the fact that the average age of people dying of COVID-19 was in the low 80s was relevant in deciding what measures were justified. The reason given for this was that all lives are equally valuable and entitled to the same protection.[14]

It seems to me that the age question is clearly a relevant consideration in deciding about the justifiability of lockdowns. To demonstrate this point, let us look at the following example. Imagine that you come to a lake and discover that two people have fallen into it and are about to drown. They are in different parts of the lake and you can only reach and save one of them in time. One of the two is 20 years old, and the other 90. Under the approach that was promoted during the COVID-19 crisis, the age of the person should be irrelevant because the lives of all people are equally valuable and all people are entitled to the same protection. But I think it is quite obvious that in the example the 20-year-old should be saved. Why is this so? One answer might be that what matters is the remaining life span: since it is likely that the 20-year-old will have much longer to live than the 90-year-old, he is the one to be saved.[15] I believe that this is not entirely correct. To demonstrate this, imagine the same scenario, but you know one additional piece of information, namely that the 90-year-old, if saved, would enjoy five more years of life before dying of old age, whereas the 20-year-old has incurable cancer and would also live for five more years if saved, before dying of his illness. I believe that in this case, again, the 20-year-old should be saved. The reason is that he has had less opportunity to live a full life than the 90-year-old. Other things being equal, the more of a full life a person has lived, the less urgent it becomes to save his life. This is also reflected in the insight that it is sad when someone close to us dies of old age, but tragic when a young person dies.

These reflections support the view that the age of the average COVID-19 death matters. One final illustration. Let us imagine that the next pandemic that hits mankind will kill overwhelmingly young adults (as the Spanish flu did). It seems to me that a virus that kills young people justifies stricter measures, including stricter lockdowns, than an otherwise equally dangerous virus that, however, kills mostly very old people. Again, the reason is not that young people's lives are "worth more" than old people's lives, but rather it reflects the simple fact that the older a person is, the closer they have come to living a full life.

Now, the fact that older people are entitled to less protection than younger people in this regard does not imply, of course, that lockdowns to protect mostly older people are disproportionate. The average age of the people dying of COVID-19 is just one consideration among many, and it may well turn out that the COVID-19 lockdowns were justified despite the fact that the average age of the people dying of COVID-19 was in the low 80s. But it is a relevant factor that needs to be considered in the proportionality assessment. The misguided insistence that age is irrelevant distorts the normative picture that needs to be developed at the balancing stage of the proportionality test.

Relating the severity of the restriction to the importance of the public interest

The third and final task at the balancing stage requires placing the benefits and harms of lockdowns into a relation with each other. So we have to ask whether the harms of lockdowns, once they have been established as precisely as possible, are justified in light of the protection that lockdowns offer to the health and lives of mostly older people.

Two ideas featured in the public and political discussions of this topic. The first, which I observed particularly in the German public discourse at the time, is that because of the high importance to be attached to the value of human life, the protection of life must always or usually take precedence over conflicting considerations. The second, which was relied on in the UK, Germany, and other places, is that the balance between freedom and protecting lives must be struck such that the healthcare system is not overburdened. Both approaches are unconvincing and ultimately suffer from the same deficiency: while they present their proposed solution as the outcome of a balancing exercise, in reality they do not engage in balancing at all and instead give categorical preference to one consideration over all others.

Let us first consider the idea that the protection of life always or virtually always outweighs other considerations. The implicit claim here is that it is not necessary to specify the harms of lockdowns because virtually any level of harm will be outweighed by the need to protect lives. This argument fails on a number of grounds.

First, it is not a principle that we have accepted in other parts of life. Thousands of people in the UK and elsewhere die of the flu every year, and until recently, this was not even considered newsworthy let alone regarded as justifying even the mildest measures such as making it compulsory to wear face masks on public transport. Another example is that we allow driving, even though this leads to innocent people, including children, dying without any fault of their own. The bottom line is that we tolerate a certain level of risk in the pursuit of going about our lives, even if this leads to innocent people dying. This means that in practice, we balance what we might call "being physically alive" ("life") against "living one's life" ("freedom"), and we do not give automatic priority to the protection of physical life over living one's life.

This is also normatively appropriate and is captured in the saying "A ship is safe in harbour, but that's not what ships are built for". Just as the point of having a ship is to use it for its purpose – transport of goods or people over water – even though this creates risks for the continued existence of the ship, the point of being physically alive is to live one's life, even though living one's life inevitably creates risks for one's health and survival. Societies develop certain levels of risk to physical life that they are willing to tolerate in the name of protecting people's ability to live their lives.

It is therefore a mistake to give categorical preference to physical life (life) over living one's life (freedom). This applies even to restrictions on freedom that many rightly or wrongly consider trivial, such as mask mandates. Imagine that imposing a national mask mandate in the UK would lead to five fewer persons dying per year. Under the logic that life takes precedence over the avoidance of trivial restrictions, such a mandate would be justified and might indeed be obligatory. But quite obviously in this case, such a mandate would be disproportionate. The lesson is that a small burden imposed on many people may outweigh a grave burden on the few. Thus, what matters for striking the balance between life and freedom is not only, qualitatively, the importance of the respective values but also, quantitatively, the number of people affected.

It follows that the idea that protecting lives takes precedence over other considerations is wrong and what is instead necessary is what the proportionality test instructs us to do, namely to balance the need to protect lives against the importance of maintaining as much freedom as possible, rather than giving unconditional priority to one of these values.

Perhaps the more plausible interpretation of the idea that life takes precedence over conflicting considerations is that while life does *not* take automatic preference over other considerations, in the case of the COVID-19 pandemic even a cursory glance at the costs and benefits of lockdowns made it clear that lockdowns were justified. Thus, the argument goes that we do not need an in-depth investigation of the benefits and costs of lockdowns to conclude that, at least in this particular instance, they were justified. It is true that we often and inevitably make intuitive judgements that involve striking a balance between competing considerations.[16] Perhaps the balance between the pros and cons of lockdowns was so clearly on the side of lockdowns during the relevant stages of the COVID-19 pandemic that there simply was no question about their justifiability.

But this argument does not strike me as convincing, either. While it is certainly true that the COVID-19 pandemic posed a risk to the health and/or life of many people and that the number of people falling ill and dying was presumably considerably reduced by the lockdowns, it is also clear, first, that lockdowns are extremely severe restrictions on freedom – as evidenced by the fact that, presumably for most of us, even those who were not in a position of particular vulnerability, they were by far the most severe restrictions on freedom that we have experienced in our lifetimes – and, second, that they affected literally everyone. So both in terms of the quality of the restriction and in terms of the quantity of people affected, they stand out as extreme. In light of this, we simply cannot make the judgement that they are justified unless we have some grasp of their consequences for people's ability to live their lives, and then engage in a proper balancing exercise.

To make the point in a different way, it may have seemed that the prospect of many more people dying of COVID-19 than absolutely necessary was so awful that this situation simply had to be avoided. I agree that this outlook was awful, but proportionality as well as common sense instruct us to assess whether the cure might be worse than the disease. The sad truth is that the COVID-19 pandemic presented us with a moral dilemma, in that there was no "good" option available to states. All possible courses of action, ranging from letting the virus rip through society to the strictest of lockdowns, would have resulted in grave harm. The task for states in this position was to balance the relevant considerations and find the solution which led to the least harm overall, whereas what seems to have happened is that faced with the possibility of large additional numbers of people dying, public and political discourse decided to largely ignore the harms of lockdowns in their deliberations.

The second argument relied on by states in justifying lockdowns is that it was necessary to prevent the healthcare system from being overburdened. The best interpretation of this idea seems to me to be that protecting life does not necessarily trump all other considerations, but that the balance between life and freedom must be struck such that it is ensured that medical treatment will be available for everyone who needs it.

But this argument is unconvincing. First, and more as a preliminary point, it seems plausible to assume that for economic reasons, hospital capacities are designed such that hospitals will regularly – say, during winter, when more people fall ill – be near or at capacity. This means that even a relatively small increase in admissions (for example because of a pandemic) could overburden the health service; under the approach examined here, this would then justify drastic lockdowns, irrespective of their possibly very severe side effects. This cannot be right.

Second, it is not clear why the protection of the health service should be given priority over all other considerations. The idea is certainly psychologically understandable to some extent: it is comforting to know that if one catches the virus and becomes severely ill, treatment will be available. Surely the mere thought of being severely ill and being denied treatment that could save one's life is terrifying. But apart from appealing to an anxiety that many will share, the harsh reality is that there are many other terrible things that can and do happen to people, in normal times and even more so during pandemics and lockdowns. It is simply not clear why the avoidance of this particular evil (hospitals being overburdened) should be prioritised over all others, including, for example, the avoidance of the evil of inflicting considerable developmental damage or trauma on children that will presumably burden many of them for the rest of their lives.

The argument regarding the need to prevent the health services from being overburdened and the argument regarding giving preference to protecting lives over other considerations both suffer from the same flaw. They elevate one (certainly relevant and important) consideration from a principle that has to be balanced with all other principles to the status of an absolute rule.[17] Thus, these approaches do not do what proportionality and common sense instruct us to do, namely to balance all relevant considerations, taking into account both the importance of the values at stake and the number of people affected. Rather, they unjustifiably give preference to just one of the many relevant considerations.

It seems, then, that the existing arguments about striking the balance were flawed. How should the balance have been struck? I do not know the answer to that difficult question. My goal in this paper is not primarily to make new proposals about how to deal with pandemics but more to assess the plausibility of the arguments relied on in the public and political discourse about lockdowns. There is no doubt that striking the appropriate balance between saving lives and maintaining a state of normal freedom is extremely difficult. Resolving it requires much more than one academic coming up with a proposal; namely a collaborative effort that is best carried out by way of open public debate among politicians, the media, academic experts in a broad range of disciplines, and the citizenry at large. My criticism of the existing discourse is that the one-sidedness and narrowness of the existing debates did not allow for the potential of such a discourse to be realised.

Conclusion

The fact that after one and a half years of intense focus on the COVID-19 pandemic, this paper and its author reach the conclusion that it is not yet possible to answer the question about the proportionality of the recent lockdowns is, if correct, itself a cause for concern. Remember that proportionality is not a technical legal doctrine that has little bearing on important issues in the real world. On the contrary, proportionality is a structure that guides judges through the process of reasoning whether repressive state measures are justifiable. The considerations that judges rely on when applying proportionality are, by and large, the same as those that citizens, journalists, and politicians rely on when assessing the morality or appropriateness of such measures. The question of the proportionality of lockdowns is at the very core of the assessment of their moral, legal, and constitutional legitimacy. After a long period of time in which the pandemic dominated the media, public and political discourse, and virtually everyone's thinking to an unprecedented extent, the fact that we still have no answers to some of the basic, crucial questions concerning the legitimacy of the course of action chosen by large parts of the world points to a weakness in our democratic culture.

One can certainly regret the political polarisation in the United States, with its hysterical shouting, absence of genuine argument[18] as well as the willingness to compromise, and the presence of (usually two) conflicting narratives even in situations where all proponents of democracy should agree on one interpretation of the world or one course of action. But with regard to the COVID-19 pandemic, Europe – or at least the United Kingdom and Germany (as the two countries whose public and political discourse I have followed closely) – has suffered from the opposite problem. It cannot be right that on a question as new, difficult, and unresolved as the question about the proper response to the COVID-19 pandemic, and in a situation that is novel, fluctuating, and unpredictable, only one course of action – lockdown – is admitted to the realm of respectable public discourse. A mature democracy will actively discuss more than just one course of action in such circumstances. To be fair, the respective ideas whose far-reaching absence in public discourse I bemoan in this chapter – thinking more about the costs of lockdowns to freedom, questioning the relevance of the average age of the people dying of COVID-19, and questioning the preference given to the protection of life over other considerations – were all at some point considered and discussed. But they were rejected too quickly and eradicated from the realm of respectability too fiercely, leaving the lockdown-endorsing strategy as the only acceptable one and pushing the discussion of alternatives into the private sphere. Citizens in a mature democracy have to insist that alternative strategies to the one chosen by their leaders are openly and comprehensively discussed, even in the face of the anxiety and hysteria which a pandemic with a new, invisible, and in many cases lethal threat brings about. In the present context, this is not primarily a matter of free speech but rather of instrumental value for reaching proportionate and therefore justifiable and constitutionally legitimate policies. If that necessary discourse had happened, as it should have in mature democracies, we would now have better answers to the question of the proportionality of lockdowns.

Notes

1 I would like to thank Mattias Kumm, Jo Murkens, Yossi Nehushtan, Peter Ramsay, and Paul Yowell for helpful discussions and valuable comments on previous drafts.

2 Kai Möller, *The Global Model of Constitutional Rights* (Oxford Oxford University Press, 2015), 13–14.

3 Moshe Cohen-Eliya and Iddo Porat, *Proportionality and Constitutional Culture* (Cambridge: Cambridge University Press, 2013), ch. 2.

4 Etinenne Mureinik, "A Bridge to Where? Introducing the Interim Bill of Rights", *South African Journal on Human Rights* 10 (1) (1994): 31, 32; Cohen-Eliya and Porat, *Proportionality and Constitutional Culture*, ch. 6; Kai Möller, "Justifying the Culture of Justification", *International Journal of Constitutional Law* 17 (4) (2019): 1078.

5 Mattias Kumm, "The Idea of Socratic Contestation and the Right to Justification: The Point of Rights-Based Proportionality Review," *Law & Ethics of Human Rights* 3 (2) (2010): 141.

6 "Great Barrington Declaration and Petition", 2020, *Great Barrington Declaration*, https://gbdeclaration.org/

7 David Bilchitz, "Necessity and Proportionality: Towards a Balanced Approach", in *Reasoning Rights: Comparative Judicial Engagement*, eds. Liora Lazarus, Christopher McCrudden, and Nigel Bowles, (London: Hart Publishing, 2016), ch. 3.

8 Robert Alexy, *A Theory of Constitutional Rights* (Oxford: Oxford University Press, 2002), 401.

9 Article 2 (1) of the German Basic Law begins: "Everyone has the right to freely develop his personality". The Universal Declaration of Human Rights mentions the idea of the (free) development of one's personality three times (in Articles 22, 26, and 29). The idea is also often referred to by the European Court of Human Rights, particularly in the context of Article 8 of the European Convention on Human Rights (the right to respect for private and family life).

10 Helen Pidd and Georgina Quach, "Revealed: England's pandemic crisis of child abuse, neglect and poverty".. *Guardian*, 11 August 2021, www.theguardian.com/society/2021/aug/11/revealed-englands-pandemic-crisis-of-child-abuse-neglect-and-poverty

11 Tirion Havard, "Domestic Abuse and COVID-19: A Year into the Pandemic".. *House of Commons Library*, last modified 11 May 2021, https://commonslibrary.parliament.uk/domestic-abuse-and-covid-19-a-year-into-the-pandemic/

12 Jeremy Waldron, *Torture, Terror, and Trade-Offs: Philosophy for the White House* (Oxford: Oxford University Press, 2010), 308: "Treatment may be described as inhuman if it fails in sensitivity to the most basic needs and rhythms of a human life: the need to sleep, to defecate or urinate, the need for daylight and exercise, and perhaps even the need for human company".

13 Yossi Nehushtan, "The British Lockdown is Disproportionate", *IACL-AIDC Blog* (blog), 9 April 2020, https://blog-iacl-aidc.org/2020-posts/2020/4/9/the-british-lockdown-is-disproportionate; Jonathan Sumption, "Government by decree: COVID-19 and the Constitution", (lecture, Cambridge Freshfields Annual Law Lecture, Cambridge, 27 October 2020), https://resources.law.cam.ac.uk/privatelaw/Freshfields_Lecture_2020_Government_by_Decree.pdf, 13.

14 In Germany, the issue was raised by the well-known mayor of Tübingen, Boris Palmer (Green party), who commented in a TV interview in April 2020: "I will just state it brutally. In Germany, we are possibly saving people who would be dead in half a year anyway – because of their age or their pre-existing conditions" (my translation); Der Tagesspiegel, "Wir retten möglicherweise Menschen, die in einem halben Jahr sowieso tot wären", *Der Tagesspiegel*, last modified 28 April 2020, www.tagesspiegel.de/politik/boris-palmer-provoziert-in-coronavirus-krise-wir-retten-moeglicherweise-menschen-die-in-einem-halben-jahr-sowieso-tot-waeren/25782926.html; While Palmer's

language is insensitive, his comment could, however, have been the beginning of an important conversation. Instead, it turned out to be its end.

15 Nehushtan, "The British Lockdown is Disproportionate".

16 Kai Möller, "Proportionality: Challenging the Critics", *International Journal of Constitutional Law* 10 (3) (2012): 709, 728–730.

17 On the distinction between principles ("optimisation requirements") and rules ("fixed points"), see Alexy, *A Theory of Constitutional Rights*, ch. 3.

18 As bemoaned, for example, by Ronald Dworkin in *Is Democracy Possible Here? Principles for a New Political Debate* (Princeton: Princeton University Press, 2006), 4–5, with regard to the 2004 presidential election: "I mean 'argument' in the old-fashioned sense in which people who share some common ground in very basic political principles debate about which concrete policies better reflect these shared principles. There was none of that argument in the formal election rhetoric of the last presidential election".

References

Alexy, Robert. 2002. *A Theory of Constitutional Rights*. Oxford: Oxford University Press.

Bilchitz, David. 2016. "Necessity and Proportionality: Towards a Balanced Approach". In *Reasoning Rights: Comparative Judicial Engagement*, edited by Liora Lazarus, Christopher McCrudden, and Nigel Bowles. London: Hart Publishing: 41–62.

Cohen-Eliya, Moshe and Iddo Porat. 2013. *Proportionality and Constitutional Culture*. Cambridge: Cambridge University Press.

Der Tagesspiegel. 2020. "Wir retten möglicherweise Menschen, die in einem halben Jahr sowieso tot wären". *Der Tagesspiegel*, 28 April, www.tagesspiegel.de/politik/boris-palmer-provoziert-in-coronavirus-krise-wir-retten-moeglicherweise-menschen-die-in-einem-halben-jahr-sowieso-tot-waeren/25782926.html.

Dworkin, Ronald. 2006. *Is Democracy Possible Here? Principles for a New Political Debate*. Princeton: Princeton University Press.

Great Barrington Declaration. 2020. "Great Barrington Declaration and Petition". *Great Barrington Declaration*, 4 October, https://gbdeclaration.org/

Havard, Tirion. 2021. "Domestic Abuse and COVID-19: A Year into the Pandemic". *House of Commons Library*, 11 May, https://commonslibrary.parliament.uk/domestic-abuse-and-covid-19-a-year-into-the-pandemic/

Kumm, Mattias. 2010. "The Idea of Socratic Contestation and the Right to Justification: The Point of Rights-Based Proportionality Review". *Law & Ethics of Human Rights* 4 (2): 142–175. doi:10.2202/1938-2545.1047.

Möller, Kai. 2012. "Proportionality: Challenging the Critics". *International Journal of Constitutional Law* 10 (3): 709–731. doi:10.1093/icon/mos024.

Möller, Kai. 2015. *The Global Model of Constitutional Rights*. Oxford: Oxford University Press.

Möller, Kai. 2019. "Justifying the Culture of Justification". *International Journal of Constitutional Law* 17 (4): 1078–1097. doi:10.1093/icon/moz086.

Mureinik, Etienne. 1994. "A Bridge to Where? Introducing the Interim Bill of Rights". *South African Journal on Human Rights* 10 (1): 31–48. doi:10.1080/02587203.1994.11827527.

Nehushtan, Yossi. 2020. "The British Lockdown is Disproprotionate". *IACL-AIDC Blog*, 9 April, https://blog-iacl-aidc.org/2020-posts/2020/4/9/the-british-lockdown-is-dispr oportionate

Pidd, Helen and Georgina Quach. 2021. "Revealed: England's pandemic crisis of child abuse, neglect and poverty". *Guardian*, 11 August. www.theguardian.com/society/2021/aug/11/revealed-englands-pandemic-crisis-of-child-abuse-neglect-and-poverty

Sumption, Jonathan. 2020. "Government by decree: Covid-19 and the Constitution". Lecture, Cambridge Freshfields Annual Law Lecture, Cambridge, 27 October 2020, https://resour ces.law.cam.ac.uk/privatelaw/Freshfields_Lecture_2020_Government_by_Decree.pdf

Waldron, Jeremy. 2010. *Torture, Terror, and Trade-Offs: Philosophy for the White House.* Oxford: Oxford University Press.

12

LOCKDOWNS AND INTERGENERATIONAL JUSTICE

Yossi Nehushtan[1]

Introduction

Since early 2020, the UK's government has been struggling to find the proportionate and just way of responding to the pandemic. Its response thus far has been criticised from different, at times opposite, points of view. Within the context of equality, it has been noted that the common UK (and global) response to the pandemic – that is, imposing blanket lockdowns, strict limitations on freedom of movement, and strict social-distancing rules – has increased inequalities between the well-off and the poor, or more generally, between the powerful and the powerless or vulnerable. Here, "vulnerable" does not only refer to those who are vulnerable regarding the virus, but also to those who are vulnerable regarding the harms caused by lockdowns, and most notably, the poor, women, those who need mental or physical care or treatment, those who live with abusive family members, and so forth. Existing inequalities have been increased as a result of lockdowns, both nationally and internationally, and thus between individuals, but also between countries, or in particular, between the West – or the Global North – and the Global South or "global poor" (Green, 2021). Here, however, a mostly neglected aspect of the UK's response to the pandemic will be highlighted: its systematic discriminatory nature regarding younger generations. Even though the focus will be on the UK, most of the arguments are applicable to other countries that applied similar COVID-19 policies.

In deciding its response to COVID-19, the UK government has made a policy decision to sacrifice both the short-term and long-term well-being of young people in the UK in order to shortly prolong the life of the elderly. The UK's policy regarding the pandemic has discriminated against younger generations by imposing blanket regional and national lockdowns and strict social-distancing rules on the entire population, regardless of whether certain age groups are likely to be

DOI: 10.4324/9781003259336-16

affected by COVID-19, and while ignoring the completely different impact that the policy had on different age groups' current and future well-being. As of early 2022, the current UK's policy, post-lockdown and post-social-distancing, continues to discriminate against younger generations, as they are the ones who will pay the cost of lockdowns – for decades to come, and without being compensated for the sacrifices they were forced to make.

While blanket lockdowns and strict social-distancing rules discriminated against younger generations, isolating only the elderly and vulnerable was both necessary and not discriminatory. Such a policy is supported by scientific evidence, complies with the moral duties that are imposed by the concept of intergenerational justice, and can also be justified behind a Rawlsian "veil of ignorance", the latter being an intellectual exercise the purpose of which is to guide us in formulating morally sound public policies, also in cases of uncertainty. Isolating the elderly and the vulnerable should, however, have been advisory rather than compulsory.

This chapter starts by presenting the relevant facts regarding the harm that was caused by COVID-19, continues to describe the harm that was caused by lockdowns – especially to younger generations – and concludes by explaining why the principle of equality, the concept of intergenerational justice, and John Rawls' philosophical argument about the veil of ignorance all support the anti-lockdown argument and the argument for voluntary self-isolation of the elderly and vulnerable.

COVID-19, lockdowns, and the age factor: The facts

Before setting out the arguments about how COVID-19-related public policies discriminated against younger generations, a few non-disputable, yet disturbingly overlooked facts should be re-examined. These facts are:

(1) Lockdowns have been normalised – and may be imposed again

In the UK and elsewhere, lockdowns or restrictions short of lockdown were an anomaly or exception to normality when they were first imposed, but they have now been normalised, a clear example of an exception that becomes the rule or the norm (Agamben, 2021). They may be imposed again. In November 2021, almost two years after the beginning of the pandemic, they were imposed again in Austria and the Netherlands. The fear that lockdowns may be imposed again is also based on the huge popular support previous lockdowns received, with 90 percent of the public in the UK supporting the first lockdown in March 2000 and 85 percent supporting the second lockdown in January 2021 (YouGove). Even though more-recent findings, from September 2021, found that only 32 percent supported a third lockdown in case of a rise in cases and hospitalisations (YouGov), it is hard to predict how public opinion may change when circumstances change and when moral panic or mass hysteria strike again.

The emergence of the Omicron variant in December 2021 had scientific advisers to the UK government refusing to rule out lockdowns as a possible response (*Independent*, 2022). The popular media constantly asked whether a third lockdown may be necessary, with some newspapers, most notably the *Guardian*, openly propagating views that supported a new lockdown. This shows that lockdown, the most extreme, draconian, scientifically controversial, and morally suspicious measure, which had never been applied before 2020 – not in its COVID-version anyway – has been fully normalised and is now being considered by some as a legitimate tool for merely reducing hospitalisations and not overwhelming the health services; the same health services, that, in some states, including the UK, are repeatedly overwhelmed, especially during the winter, because of non-COVID-related reasons. In the UK, for example, 94 percent of hospital beds and 81 percent of critical-care beds were already full by mid-December 2021, before the start of the Omicron surge (*The Guardian*, 2021). Jeremy Hunt, chairman of the Commons Health and Social Care Committee, added that there are permanent staffing shortfalls in every major specialism within the National Health Service (NHS) that go beyond the problems caused by the Omicron variant (UK Parliament – Committees, News Article, 2022). Lockdown, therefore, became a substitute for providing adequate health services that can cope with both expected and unexpected increases in hospitalisations.

(2) The ongoing failure to measure the harm caused by lockdowns

Imposing periodical blanket lockdowns or strict social-distancing rules for more than a few weeks at a time, or at all, is an extreme measure that was always likely to result in immense harm. In the UK, it already resulted in almost unprecedented harm to the financial, social, and mental well-being of millions, leading the UK into its worst-ever recession, dwarfing the 2008 financial crash. Both recession and poverty are silent killers whose long-term harm could possibly exceed the harm caused by the virus itself. Quite shockingly, the British government had not initially tried to measure the harm caused by lockdowns. No such attempt was recorded before the imposition of the first lockdown in March 2020. It was not until later, on 30 November 2020, that an impact assessment was released – giving MPs just two days to read it before the tier system, or regional lockdown, was introduced to the UK. In that impact assessment, there was no real attempt to weigh the benefits of imposing lockdowns against the harm that is likely to be caused by them. The British government openly admitted that since this impact-assessment process is "too complex", they were not even going to try to measure the harms that are caused by lockdowns. The impact assessment from 2020 did refer to the question of how lockdowns may affect the economy, yet it concluded that "given the unprecedented nature of both the virus and the restrictions that have been required to mitigate it, it is not possible to assess the balance of these effects". (HM Government, 2020). Thus, the most draconian measures were imposed, including unprecedented harsh measures that had clear potential for inflicting immense harm on millions and on society as a whole, without any real effort to assess the harm that they may cause.

Others, however, have attempted to answer this question and found that the harm that lockdowns inflicted in Canada, for example, was ten times greater than their benefits – in terms of loss of life and quality of life (Joffe, 2021). As for the UK, it has been found that

> the economic costs of the lockdown…is far larger than [the] annual total expenditure on the UK national health service…[and] the benefits of that level of resources applied to health…would be expected to generate far more lives saved than is plausibly attributable to the lockdown in the UK…. The cost per QALY [quality-adjusted life year] saved of the lockdown looks to be far in excess…(often by a factor of 10 and more) of that considered acceptable for health treatments in the UK.
>
> *Miles, Steadman, and Heald, 2020*

Beyond the narrow context of the cost-benefit analysis of lockdowns regarding saving lives only, it should have been clear from the very beginning that long blanket lockdowns may result in immense emotional, mental, financial, and physical harm to millions, and the collapse of multiple sectors of the economy, the fabric of society, and perhaps also public order – as objections to strict COVID-19 policies may become more violent. Lockdowns also diminished democracy itself, as introducing extreme COVID-19 policies and enforcing them disproportionately violated a long list of political and social rights and freedoms, disrupted democratic procedures, and shifted powers from parliaments to governments.

Lockdowns, especially long ones, should have never been an option worth considering, not before fully evaluating their impact. Indeed, before first being imposed in non-democratic China in 2020, they were never seriously considered as an anti-pandemic measure. As to short-term, intermediate lockdowns, they will not result in zero infections (Kissler et al., 2020), so it is very likely that the virus will spread again shortly after the lockdown ends, as indeed happened, more than once, around the globe. Lockdowns, therefore, may bring temporary relief (or the appearance of it) but cause long-lasting harm. There were well-informed views, completely ignored by decision makers, according to which lockdowns may be counter-productive even within the narrow context of fighting the pandemic – that is, they may result in an even greater number of COVID-19-related deaths and hospitalisations (Rice et al., 2020). More generally, it has been shown that the mental and emotional effects of social isolation, unemployment, uncertainty, loss of autonomy, and so forth – all direct results of lockdowns – increase the likelihood of one's falling ill when exposed to a virus (Pressman et al., 2005).

Regarding the efficacy of lockdowns, one comprehensive study found "no clear association between lockdown policies and mortality development" (Bjornskov, 2021). Another study found that "well-timed lockdowns" do not directly save lives but rather "can split the peak of hospitalizations into two smaller distant peaks while extending the overall pandemic duration" (Oraby et al., 2021). There are many more findings that throw doubt on the efficacy of lockdowns (AIER staff, 2020; Pandata, n.d.). A meta-analysis of the effects of lockdowns, reviewing 24 studies, found that lockdowns reduced deaths by only 0.2 percent. The review further concludes that stay-at-home orders reduced deaths by 2.9 percent. No clear evidence was found that any individual NPI (non-pharmaceutical interference) had a noticeable effect on mortality (Herby et al., 2022). A broader perception of what "health" means and entails – most notably, being together in the world, living life, and getting involved – will add to the argument against the efficacy of lockdowns (Murphy, 2022).

There are also, of course, some who will argue for the opposite. The problem is that the UK's government, like almost all others, did not seriously attempt to engage with the conflicting scientific evidence, did not attempt to weigh the benefits of lockdowns against their downsides, rushed into the first lockdown in 2020, and even worse, rushed into the second lockdown in 2021 without fully appreciating the efficacy of the first.

Western democracies in fact adopted a cruel, totalitarian approach similar to that of the Chinese government, one that pays little attention to the general welfare of citizens and to transparency, accountability, and open debate. Professor Neil Ferguson, one of the architects of British lockdowns, admitted that when the scientists who advise the UK government observed the Chinese lockdown, they initially presumed it would not be an available option in a liberal Western democracy. He said that "we couldn't get away with it in Europe, we thought... and then Italy did it. And we realised we could", and that "if China had not done it, the year would have been very different". (*The Times*, 2020). It was China that made lockdowns a possibility in the West. The same non-democratic China that is responsible for gross human-rights violations – and which, two years after its first lockdown, in October 2021, locked down a city of four million people after six COVID-19 cases were detected – on 23 December 2021 locked down 13 million people in Xi'an after detecting 127 COVID-19 cases, and in January 2022 locked down a city of 1.2 million people after three COVID-19 cases were detected. Non-democratic, totalitarian China was in fact the role model for not properly balancing a health-related public interest with all other rights and interests that human beings have and the general interest of living in a free and democratic society.

(3) Covid in context

How does COVID-19 compare to other causes of death in UK? The following data is taken from the ONS (Office for National Statistics) website: from March 2020 to March 2022, there were 163,000 cases of deaths *with* COVID-19 (that is, deaths due to whatever reason, occurring within 28 days of a positive COVID-19 test), so 81,500 deaths *with* COVID-19 per year. It is estimated that in 2020, around 50,000 people died *due to* COVID-19. Also in the UK, there are 106,000 deaths *with* influenza and pneumonia per year (24,500 more than COVID-19), of which 30,000 are deaths *due to* influenza and pneumonia. In 2020, deaths due to influenza and pneumonia were consistently lower, by up to 30 percent, than the five-year average. It is safe to assume that many of those who would have died from influenza and pneumonia in 2020, died from COVID-19 instead.

Still in the UK, the number of deaths due to air pollution is 28,000–36,000 a year, of which half could be avoided if the UK had followed World Health Organisation recommendations. The number of alcohol-specific deaths is 8974 a year, and that of domestic second-hand smoking deaths is 10,000 a year, including 40 cases of cot death a year (and 9500 children admitted to hospital). No panic has ever been recorded in light of these numbers. No lockdowns were ever suggested to reduce the number of deaths from air pollution, and no ban on alcohol was ever suggested and no ban on cigarettes has been implemented.

When we put COVID-19 in context, we can appreciate that even though it did pose a real health risk, more severe than that of influenza and pneumonia, and one that also caused distinctive harms other than death, it appears that the magnitude of the health risk was exaggerated, presumably also due to its uniqueness and novelty. This, it turn, puts in question the proportionality of the response to COVID-19, especially when we compare it to other causes of death – and when the efficacy of lockdowns was never scientifically proven.

(4) The risk of dying from/with COVID-19

The real risk from COVID-19 had been known even before the UK imposed its first lockdown in March 2020. By early 2020, it was already known that persons aged 85 years and above accounted for 41 percent of deaths, persons aged 75 and above accounted for 74 percent of deaths, and those aged 65 and above accounted for 89 percent of deaths (Office for National Statistics, 2020b). Age is, therefore (and by far), the most important risk factor. This has not changed, as more-recent data shows that 99 percent of COVID-19 deaths were in people age 50 and over, 74 percent were in people aged 75 and over, and more than 40 percent of deaths were in people 85 and over (Office for National Statistics, 2021d). The risk of dying from (*or with*) COVID-19 – or more accurately, the probability of dying *if* infected by the virus (the case fatality rate) – is 1.5 percent for 60-year-olds, 0.4 percent for 50-year-olds, 0.2 percent for 40-year-olds, and less than 0.1 percent for 30-year-olds (The Economist, 2021). By way of comparison, the US seasonal flu has a case fatality rate of approximately 0.1 percent to 0.2 percent (US Centers for Disease Control and Prevention, 2021).

(5) The general health of those who died from/with Covid

At the start of the pandemic, 90.9 percent of those who died in March, April, and May 2020 either from the virus or *with* the virus had at least one pre-existing condition. On average, those who died between the ages of 60 and 69 years had 2.1 pre-existing conditions, and those over the age of 70 had 2.3 pre-existing conditions (Office for National Statistics, 2021e). From the second quarter of 2021, those with a pre-existing condition accounted for 81.2 percent of deaths in England and Wales from COVID.

(6) The median age of those who died from/with COVID-19

In the UK, the median age of death for males is 82.3, and for females it's 85.8 (Office for National Statistics, 2021f). The median age of those who died due to or with COVID-19 between March 2020 and August 2021 was 82 (Office for National Statistics, 20201g-August 2021). From the start of the pandemic, even the most radical scientist supporters of lockdowns and strict social-distancing rules predicted that the proportion of COVID-19 victims who would have died in the near future anyway, even if COVID-19 never existed, could be as many as half or two-thirds (Knapton, 2020).

(7) COVID and care homes.

As to care homes in Europe, the WHO estimated that "up to half of those who have died from COVID-19 were resident in long-term care facilities" (Kluge, 2020). A more up-to-date estimate from the UK suggests that deaths in care homes accounted for around a third of fatalities from the pandemic (Booth and McIntyre, 2021). The median life expectancy for people admitted to nursing beds in England is 418 days – and for residential beds it's 665 days (Forder and Fernandez, 2011). Thus, care-home residents who died from or with COVID-19, had an average life expectancy of no more than one to two years.

COVID-19: The meaning of the above facts

Points 4–7 above show that that the risk from COVID-19 to healthy people under the age of 65 is minimal, and from a broad social perspective, negligible. They show why COVID-19 was, from the very beginning, a highly discriminatory virus, in the sense that it posed a serious health risk almost exclusively to older people with pre-existing conditions.

Points 4–7 above also highlight a neglected fact: describing the aim of lockdowns as being that of "saving lives" is misleading. Life has an expiry date. Therefore, it can never be "saved" but rather prolonged; death cannot be avoided, only postponed. This is important for two reasons.

First, when we talk about "saving lives", it may imply that all lives are of equal worth when we decide whether the cost of "saving" them is reasonable. However, when we use the more accurate concept of "prolonging life", it forces us to ask (a) for how long a certain life can be prolonged, and (b) whether the cost of prolonging lives for X amount of time is reasonable. In a world where resources are limited, the question of cost is inevitable, because prolonging the life of some comes at a cost to the quality of life – and at times to the lives themselves – of others.

Second, the hard reality is that COVID-19 kills mostly old people with severe underlying health conditions who would likely have died in the near future anyway. For healthy people under 65, the virus is not significantly more dangerous or deadly than many other illnesses. For younger people, the risk is negligible. The number of deaths among people who would have not died anyway in the near future is relatively low, and certainly not meaningful enough to justify the horrendous and long-lasting harms that have been inflicted on them by imposing long lockdowns and strict social distancing rules.

The case against blanket lockdowns and for isolating the elderly and vulnerable

With no vaccine that is likely to be effective against all variants of the virus – or against some variants for more than six months to a year, the likely devastating results of achieving herd immunity without implementing precautionary measures to protect the elderly and vulnerable, the non-sustainability of long-term blanket lockdowns or strict social-distancing rules, the inefficiency of short-term lockdowns, and the elderly being accountable for the vast majority of deaths and hospitalisations, it seems that isolating only the elderly and vulnerable (and those who live with them or care for them), and allowing everyone else to continue with life almost as normal, was always the only viable, just, and compassionate response to the virus.

This is not an argument that is made with the wisdom of hindsight. I expressed these views as early as April 2020, at the beginning of the first UK lockdown (Nehushtan, 2020). Toby Green wrote his seminal book on *The Covid Consensus* in 2021, in which he described in detail the devastating harms that lockdowns are causing and likely to cause during these times (Green, 2021). In a recently published book, Mark Woolhouse OBE, a professor of infectious disease epidemiology at the University of Edinburgh, reveals the views that he held and desperately tried to convey to politicians from the beginning of the pandemic, according to which (in light of the highly discriminatory nature of COVID-19, which affects almost only the elderly) imposing lockdowns was an act of panic and nothing less than political and scientific madness (Woolhouse, 2022). And there were many others – with the "Great Barrington Declaration" probably being one of the most prominent and clearest anti-lockdown voices – that were systematically ignored by almost all governments.

As early as October 2020, in between the first and second British lockdowns, the "Great Barrington Declaration" had been published (Kullforff, Bhattacharya, and Gupta, 2020). The declaration, which was written by three world-leading epidemiologists from Harvard, Oxford, and Stanford, and which was signed by nearly 60,000 medical and public-health scientists and practitioners, asserted that the most compassionate approach that balances the risks and benefits of reaching herd immunity, is to allow those who are at minimal risk of death to live their lives normally to build up immunity to the virus through natural infection, while better protecting those who are at highest risk.

The declaration emphasised the need for "focused protection", that is, protecting the old and vulnerable in any way possible until they are vaccinated or herd immunity is achieved. Adding to the declaration itself, its authors said that

> the premise of the Declaration lies on two scientific facts. First, while anyone can get infected, there is more than a thousand-fold difference in COVID-19 mortality between the oldest and youngest. Children have lower mortality from COVID-19 than from the annual influenza. For people under the age of 70, the infection survival rate is 99.95% … we know that among common conditions, age is the single most important risk factor. Second, the harms of the lockdown are manifold and devastating.

For a detailed account of the harms of lockdowns, see in the declaration website.

Quite surprisingly, however, almost no government acted on the common-sense and fact-based advice regarding focused protection, with almost all European countries and many others, with the exception of relatively few (e.g., Sweden and South Korea – to name the most successful), imposing blanket lockdowns of various kinds (Yang, 2020). In the UK, shortly before the nationwide lockdown was imposed on 23 March 2020, the government's plan was to advise or impose isolation on people aged 70 and above "for a long period of time" (BBC, 2020), while allowing all others to continue with life as normal. Later that year, in May 2020, towards the end of the first lockdown, the idea came up again, this time supported by the "segmenting and shielding" strategy (Van Bunnik et al., 2021), but it was inexplicably dismissed (Sample and Mason, 2020).

The UK never implemented the reasonable focused-protection policy, opting for periodical, long, blanket lockdowns instead. The reasons for this were never clear and were never explicitly disclosed by the government. One possible reason was the concern that the NHS would not be able to treat large number of patients during a relatively short period of time. As far as that was the reason for not applying a focused-protection approach, it reflects what has been the true pandemic from 2020 to 2022: tunnel-vision decision-making, whereby the one and only concern was to "save lives" (from COVID-19 only), while completely ignoring the harm that may be caused to the financial, social, and mental well-being of millions as a result. Even if the concern regarding overwhelming the NHS was not misguided, it should not have been used as a trump card that automatically justifies blanket lockdowns (Moller, 2022). Not burdening the NHS was in fact used as a trump card, and avoiding the possibility of ill people not being treated well or at all became the main justification for lockdowns (most notably in the UK). It is ironic that now, post-lockdowns, we find that the same lockdowns and overcautious COVID-19 protocols at hospitals, result in longer-than-ever waiting lists for medical treatment and significant delays to medical diagnoses that will inevitably result in what lockdowns were meant to prevent: ill people not being treated well or at all, and thus dying prematurely or having a compromised quality of life. The only difference is that the deaths of those whose treatment or diagnosis was cancelled or delayed will not appear on any scary daily statistics of COVID-19 deaths. They will also not cause moral panic and will not prompt any rushed and extreme change in public policies, whereas the possibility of COVID-19 patients dying because the NHS may be overwhelmed resulted in exactly that.

The second possible reason for not applying a focused-protection policy was probably the fear that it might be perceived as discriminatory or ageist (Lawrence and Harris, 2021). This reflected the opinion of several well-known figures in the UK (Parveen, 2020). In the age of paralysing political correctness, the government did not dare to apply a policy that would have been perceived as an unjust discrimination against the elderly and vulnerable. By not doing so, the government betrayed its duty to act on reason and instead acted on irrational sentiments. A careful consideration of the principle of equality in our case would have led to a different policy.

Blanket lockdowns as discrimination against the younger generations: The argument from equality

One way to answer the concern about discrimination could have been to not impose isolation on the elderly but rather to advise the elderly and the vulnerable and those who live with them to self-isolate, while providing full care and generous financial support for them. The state would have had to support them in any possible way – mentally, socially, and financially – until herd immunity was achieved, or if herd immunity was not plausible, until a vaccine was taken by a sufficient number of people. Had the elderly and vulnerable chosen to not self-isolate, they would have done so at their own risk. After all, the state does not act in similar paternalistic ways prohibiting the elderly and vulnerable, or anyone else, from committing acts of self-destruction such as smoking, drinking heavily, having a non-healthy diet, and so on, even when these self-destructive ways of life burden the health services and therefore put others at risk. To take one example: in London, alcohol-related harm accounts for 35 percent of all A&E (accidents and emergency) attendances at hospitals, and up to 70 percent of all attendances at peak times over weekends (Mayor of London, n.d.). In the UK in 2018, 1.3 million people were admitted to hospital because of alcohol-related reasons, a figure that represents 7.4 percent of all hospital admissions across the country (News Medical, 2020). Yet no serious attempt, certainly not one that violates people's liberties and autonomy, has been made to protect the NHS from being overwhelmed by these hospital admissions, even though this could have reduced waiting times for those who suffer from illnesses and injuries which are not related to their self-destructive lifestyle, if they have any. There was never any prevailing reason for the state to act in a paternalistic way here by forcing the elderly to protect themselves from the virus if they preferred to socialise with friends and family during their last years.

A different way of answering the alleged discrimination problem, and under the assumption that compulsory isolation of the elderly was necessary to protect the NHS, is to argue that the discriminatory isolation is in fact justified. Equality means treating like cases alike and different cases differently. The differences between comparable cases should be relevant to the different treatments we wish to apply. That is clearly the case here. If, for example, a deadly virus affects only or mostly pregnant women, or members of an ethnic minority group, it would be highly unreasonable to impose a blanket national lockdown to tackle such a focused health threat. Regarding COVID-19, people aged 70 and above are – by far – more likely to be hospitalised, need intensive care, or die if they contract the virus. Within this context, they are therefore different from younger people. That difference is relevant to the treatment they should get, and it justifies treating them differently.

The elderly might have felt stigmatised or even humiliated by this discriminatory policy, but as much as these sentiments could be genuine and understandable, they cannot affect public policy, simply because these sentiments would be irrational. The elderly have been self-isolating anyway during the best part of 2020 and early 2021, either because of lockdowns or voluntarily. Isolating only the elderly, preferably by advising them to do so, would not have made them significantly worse off – or worse off at all. It could have, however, made everyone else significantly better off.

Not limiting the self-isolation policy to the elderly in the name of equality demonstrates one of the main problems with the principle of equality: the "levelling down" problem. If "formal" equality, whereby everyone is treated the same regardless of the relevant differences between them, is our only concern, and if the only claim here is that isolating only the elderly stigmatises them, and if relaxing all freedom-of-movement limitations may cause the health services to collapse, then the only option left is to "level down" the treatment to affect everyone – and to continue with blanket lockdowns. This, as argued above, is the worst option of all. Treating everyone equally, regardless of their age and vulnerability, by imposing a blanket lockdown or strict social-distancing rules, resulted in the greatest harm to the greatest number. And that greatest harm has not been distributed equally. The younger generations have suffered the most – and will be the ones that will suffer the most, for decades.

Blanket lockdowns as discrimination against the younger generations: The argument from intergenerational justice

The last point leads us to the argument from intergenerational justice. The concept of intergenerational justice is often used to describe the moral duties that present generations owe to past and future people, and at times to the descendants of victims of past injustices (Thompson, 1999; Gosseries and Meyer, 2009). Here, the concept will be used mostly to describe the moral duties that different living generations owe to each other, yet the rationale of the following arguments also applies, at least in part, to the duties that the present generation owes to future people.

In just states, the concept of intergenerational justice reflects the social contract between citizens – and between them and the state. Generally, the state – and younger generations – have a duty of care toward older generations. This duty normally entails providing adequate medical and social care for the elderly, paying the pensions of those who retired from work (as the pension financial model is based on current working generations paying for the pensions of retired generations), not unjustly discriminating against the elderly, and so on. The state – and older generations – also have a duty of care toward younger generations – and this point was almost completely overlooked since the start of pandemic. One of the manifestations of this duty is leaving younger generations a liveable world and not severely harming their prospects of having a life in which they can maintain a satisfactory level of well-being, self-actualisation, security, autonomy, and so forth.

Isolating only the elderly until wide immunity is achieved, either by vaccination or naturally, or advising them to self-isolate while everyone else is continuing with life almost as normal, and providing appropriate care and support for them, meet the moral duty of younger generations towards older ones. Blanket lockdowns, however, and the imposition of strict social-distancing rules on everyone equally, were acts of injustice towards younger generations. In the vast majority of cases, it only slightly prolonged the life of those who would have died soon anyway from old age or non-COVID-related health issues. Yet it will have a devastating financial, social, mental-health, and physical-health impact that is likely to inflict severe burdens on a large number of members of younger generations for decades – as is shown below. This makes such a policy an act of extreme intergenerational injustice.

It is reasonable and just to expect younger generations to care for the elderly and to prolong their life at the expense of their own well-being, as long as the sacrifice that is required from younger generations is in itself reasonable. That principle has always guided public policy in the UK, where the NHS and the government were never expected to do whatever it takes and spend however much it takes to shortly prolong the lives of those with extremely short life expectancy. When resources are limited, and they always are, doing so would have unreasonably compromised the legitimate and long-term interests of younger generations – and would not have been sustainable in the long run anyway. But the COVID-19 policies, especially that of lockdowns, did exactly this. Younger generations were forced or manipulated to significantly sacrifice their current and future financial, social, physical, and mental well-being just to shortly prolong the lives of the elderly. This policy was both uncompassionate and unjust. It was in fact cruel. Younger people who opposed lockdowns were forced to comply and to make unreasonable sacrifices to shortly prolong the lives of the elderly. Those who supported lockdowns were sometimes manipulated by not being told the truth about the huge price they will pay for decades as a result of lockdowns, by not being exposed to reliable information or any information at all about the discriminatory nature of COVID-19, by being told by the authorities that COVID-19 "affects everyone", and by being led to believe that the virus is much more dangerous than it actually is – at least for people under the age of 50.

Imposing lockdowns and strict social-distancing rules slightly prolonged the lives mostly of those with a relatively short life expectancy. Those who were sacrificed in order for the elderly to live slightly longer were mainly the poor and young. In the UK, according to the Financial Conduct Authority's report from 2020, the number of financially vulnerable adults rose during the pandemic by 3.7 million (or 15 percent) to 27.7 million. For those aged 18–34, the rise is 40 percent, while it has actually decreased among retirees (Financial Conduct Authority, 2021). Millions of younger people lost their jobs and career prospects by the end of 2020 (Office for National Statistics, 2020a), while retired people did not. Young people under 25 accounted for nearly two-thirds of job losses between February 2020 and February 2021 (Henehan, 2021). It has been estimated that the UK now "faces decades of financial risk as £370bn pandemic bill mounts" (*The Guardian*, 2021), and it is quite clear which generations are going to pay said bill. It has been predicted by the Institute for Fiscal Studies that the UK's budget for 2022 will leave the average worker almost £13,000 a year worse off by the mid-2020s as a result of inflation and tax increases – both the result of lockdowns (*The Guardian*, 2021). In terms of taxes alone that must be raised to fund the astronomical costs of lockdowns and the British furlough scheme, the Resolution Foundation, a British think tank, published an analysis showing that households would on average be paying £3,000 more each year in taxes by 2024–25 (Financial Times, 2021). Lower incomes and greater job insecurity will result in millions of younger people seeing their pensions shrink, while those of retired people are untouchable.

Millions of younger people lost at least a year's worth of knowledge and social-isation in schools and got inferior online university education and no university experience, none of which affected the retired. Children's lives have been severely disrupted during the pandemic due to long school closures, exam cancellations, and a ban on socialising – all during a crucial time for their mental and social development. There is already growing evidence that social intelligence and brain development are being affected by lockdowns (Sahakian et al., 2021), and it is not at all clear whether the harm caused could ever be remedied or remedied equally among children from different backgrounds. It is clear, however, and not at all surprising, that "disadvantaged pupils in England lag behind in Covid learning catch-up" (*The Guardian*, 2021), being members of the most vulnerable group regarding lockdowns – the young and the poor.

Younger people were exposed to abuse at home, anti-social behaviour, and experiences that will affect their mental health for years, perhaps decades, long after those whose lives were "saved" – in fact shortly prolonged – will no longer be with us. In more detail: there was a 29 percent rise in referrals for first suspected episodes of psychosis between April 2019 and April 2021 (*The Guardian*, 2021). Children's NHS mental-health referrals have doubled during the pandemic (*The*

Guardian, 2021). In 2020, between April and December, 372,438 under-18s were referred for mental-health help, the highest number recorded and 28 percent more than the 292,212 referred in the same period in 2019. Under-18s received 3.58 million sessions of treatment in those nine months, 20 percent up on the year before. The number of children and young people needing emergency care because they were in a mental-health crisis rose by 20 percent to 18,269. And all the while, the number of adults referred for help from April to December 2020 was slightly down on the year before (*The Guardian*, 2021). The number of children admitted to hospital for eating disorders has surged by 70 percent since the pandemic started, with psychiatrists warning they are unable to keep up with numbers needing help (*Telegraph*, 2022). Children and teenagers who are anxious, depressed, or self-harming are now being denied help from swamped NHS child and adolescent mental health services (CAMHS), and in some areas it now takes children and teenagers two years after being referred by their general practitioner to start receiving help. Experts note that the inability to access CAMHS care is leading to children's already fragile mental health deteriorating even further, and to them self-harming, dropping out of school, feeling uncared for, and having to seek help at hospital emergency services (*The Guardian*, 2022). The full list of harms that have been caused and are still being caused to younger generations as a result of lockdowns is just too long to be described in full here.

More generally, one of the main things that many of us lost during and because of lockdowns is life experiences – and life opportunities or possibilities (Ratcliffe, 2022). Whereas the elderly and the young have lost life experiences, at times meaningful ones, almost equally, it is mostly the younger generation that lost life opportunities. As Ratcliffe rightly points out, "A human life is not something that can simply be put on standby for an extended duration and then switched back on without consequence; there is much that cannot be recovered" (Ratcliffe, 2022). This is, of course, a serious concern regarding mostly younger generations – and much less so regarding those with relatively short life expectancy.

There is another aspect of lockdowns and strict social-distancing rules that harmed mostly the younger generations in a way that was almost completely ignored. During the best part of 2020, and again in 2021, strict social-distancing rules prevented many people from being with their loved ones before they died (mostly regarding care-home residents) and from having proper funerals and sharing their experiences of grief with others after their loved ones died. As Ratcliffe noted, "To be cut off from someone shortly before and as they die, to be denied a proper funeral, to be prevented from participating in other established rituals, to be unable to grieve together – all of this can impede the ability to integrate bereavement into the ongoing structure of one's life" (Ratcliffe, 2022). Bearing in mind that persons aged 75 and above accounted for 74 percent of COVID-19 deaths (and people aged 85 and over for 40 percent), that the median age of those who died due to or with COVID-19 between March 2020 and August 2021 was 82 (Office for National Statistics, March 2020-August 2021g), and that the proportion of COVID-19 victims who would have died in the near future anyway, even if COVID-19 never existed, could be as many as half or two-thirds, it becomes clear that those who will suffer from long-term harm as a result of being separated from their loved ones are not those who died but rather their younger family members. Those who died from or with COVID-19 had a terrible end-of-life experience that sometimes lasted for many months, whereby they were not able to see their loved ones and say goodbye to them before they died. That experience affected their quality of life and probably mental health as well, for either days, weeks, or more than a few sad months. The younger family members suffered from a similar bad experience – not being able to spend time with a loved one before they died – but it is them and not those who died who will also suffer from long-term mental harm as a result of being deprived of the opportunity to spend time with a loved one before they died, say goodbye to them, and grieve properly after they died.

Sacrificing the younger generations was not inevitable. To take one example, the evidence regarding the risk of keeping schools open has been dubious at best from the very beginning of the pandemic. As early as April 2020, a study from University College London found that school closures are likely to have a relatively small impact on the spread of COVID-19 and should be weighed against their profound economic and social consequences, particularly for the most-vulnerable children. The research found that recent modelling studies of COVID-19 predict that school closures alone would prevent only 2–4 percent of deaths (Viner et al., 2020). A few months later, in August 2020, the European Centre for Disease Prevention and Control found that

> a small proportion (<5%) of overall COVID-19 cases reported in the EU/ EEA and the UK are among children (those aged 18 years and under).... Children are more likely to have a mild or asymptomatic infection…it is unknown how infectious asymptomatic children are…very few significant outbreaks of COVID-19 in schools have been documented.... Investigations of cases identified in school settings suggest that child to child transmission in schools is uncommon and not the primary cause of SARS-CoV-2 infection in children whose onset of infection coincides with the period during which they are attending school, particularly in preschools and primary schools.... There is conflicting published evidence on the impact of school closure/ re-opening on community transmission levels, although the evidence from contact tracing in schools, and observational data from a number of EU countries suggest that re-opening schools has not been associated with sig-nificant increases in community transmission.
>
> *ECDC, 2020*

Later on, in June 2021, a study from Warwick University found no evidence that schools are playing a significant role in driving the spread of COVID-19 in the community (Southall et al., 2021). Yet despite the lack of conclusive evidence about the health benefits of closing schools during the pandemic – and the obvious, cer-tain, immense, and partly irreversible harm that is caused to children as a result of both closing schools and enforcing lockdowns and strict social-distancing rules – the UK, like many other countries, decided to sacrifice the short-term and long-term well-being of its youngest generations, in order to achieve a speculative goal of slightly prolonging the lives of the elderly. This policy did not follow "the science", was not based on reason, and did not apply any valid moral principles. This policy was a moral crime of the state against its youngest and voiceless.

Blanket lockdowns, discrimination against younger generations, and the veil of ignorance

Some of the arguments made here are likely to encounter harsh criticism, that will be probably focus on their alleged ageism, lack of compassion toward the elderly, and failure to accord proper weight to the sanctity of life. Such criticism will be misplaced and misguided. That is so because every rational person, whether old or young, must see the merits of the above arguments if they put themselves behind a Rawlsian veil of ignorance (Rawls, 1971).

The idea of the veil of ignorance was developed by John Rawls in order to explain why a society, in order for it to be just, must comply with certain principles of justice and must have certain institutions that will apply these principles. Behind the hypothetical veil of ignorance, we are required to decide about the principles of justice that will exist in a certain future society, without knowing who we will be in that society. We are designing a future society in which we will find ourselves – but we do not know anything about ourselves in that future society. We do not know our fortune in the distribution of natural assets and abilities. We do not know what our intelligence, strengths, and weaknesses will be. We do not know what our sex, sexual orientation, ethnic origin, or age will be. We do not know which conceptions of the good we will hold, or what our special psychological propensities, place in society, and class position or social status will be. All we know is that we will find ourselves in a certain society that will be governed by the principles of justice that are decided by us behind that veil of ignorance. We also know that behind the veil of ignorance, we are rational persons concerned with furthering our own interests, but obviously without knowing in full what these specific interests may be.

The idea of the veil ignorance is meant to allow us to formulate fairly general principles of justice that will govern the state, yet it is equally effective in guiding us towards defining and implementing more specific policies – and even specific decisions. Being inspired by the idea of the veil of ignorance, we need to always put ourselves in that position in order to decide which moral principles should guide our behaviour. Every time a specific moral question arises, a specific question about the way in which we should treat others, we should distance ourselves from the specific case and imagine ourselves in a position where we need to provide a moral answer to the moral question without knowing which "player" we are or will end up being within that specific case.

Within the context of the pandemic, the idea of the veil of ignorance requires us to decide how to respond to it without knowing if, as people who will be subject to that response, we will end up being poor or well off; part of the Global North or the Global South; parents to young children who need our constant care or childless; being able to continue working and being fully paid, or furloughed, or being unemployed with no safety net; living in a spacious house with a garden or in a tiny flat; spending lockdown with a supportive family/partner or with an abusive one; and being old and vulnerable or young and healthy. All we know is that after providing the moral answer to the moral question of how to reply to the pandemic, we could find ourselves as any of the "players" in that case. And we also know that when answering that moral question – that is, when deciding the state's response to COVID-19 – we are acting as rational people. We know that any public policy on which we decide behind a veil of ignorance may benefit some and harm others. Alternatively, we know that any policy may harm most people or even all of those who will be subjected to that policy, but not to the same extent. And most importantly, we also know that under any chosen policy, we might find ourselves as the worst off, as the ones who will most adversely affected by the policy. Rational people behind a veil of ignorance, according to Rawls, will then choose the policy that will cause them the least amount of harm if they are the ones who are most adversely affected by it. A self-interested, rational person behind a veil of ignorance will always opt for the public policy that would leave her less worse off compared to other policies, under the assumption that she may find herself in the worst-off position regarding every policy that could be applied.

One may wonder whether decision makers would have rushed into lockdowns, more than once, if as a result they had to stay at home with young children and no help, lose their job or part of their income, lose their career or life prospects, lose access to non-COVID-related health services, and so forth. It is not far-fetched to assert that lockdowns were so easily imposed because they had relatively little effect on those who decided to impose them, and precisely because they did not put themselves behind a veil of ignorance while making that decision.

Returning to the "generational" aspect of COVID-19 and lockdowns: Which response to COVID-19 will we then choose behind the veil of ignorance? If we choose the policy according to which we should advise the elderly and the vulnerable to self-isolate – and generously and fully support them while they do that – while allowing all others to live a life with minimal social-distancing rules, then the worst-case scenario is that we will be old or vulnerable, have a relatively poor quality of life for a long while, and self-isolate (if we so choose) until we die from either old age or COVID-19. The main loss for the elderly, in the worst possible case, is therefore either a slightly premature death or the loss of time and meaningful life experiences at an age where compensating for this loss may be particularly difficult or plainly impossible. This is not a happy situation, but worst-case scenarios are almost never mood-lifting. The question is whether this worst-case scenario is in fact worse than the one that younger generations will face under lockdown.

If we choose the policy of periodical, long, blanket lockdowns and strict social-distancing rules, one of the worst scenarios is that we will be relatively young, pushed into a lifetime of poverty – with all of its devastating physical health and mental-health implications; suffering from long-term severe health problems or dying at a young age because a life-saving or quality-of-life-improving diagnosis or treatment has been cancelled or postponed by the COVID-consumed NHS; suffering from severe mental-health issues that may adversely affect our life for years or decades; or simply living for decades in a country that mortgaged its future for the fight against COVID-19 and now decides to pay that mortgage back not by taxing big corporations and the well off but rather by cutting social services, raising taxes, and imposing never-ending austerity because "we are all in this together".

It is clear that a rational, self-interested person behind a veil of ignorance, who wishes to avoid the worst consequences if they find themselves the least well off as a result of a COVID-19 policy, will choose to be the worse-off elderly person under the former policy rather than the worse-off young person under the latter. Any rational person would prefer to self-isolate at a very old age, even for a long while (especially if the alternative is for everyone else to also self-isolate), or even to die from COVID-19 a bit prematurely at a relatively old age, than to suffer as a young person during long lockdowns, and to continue suffering from decades of poverty, misery, pain, and loss of income and opportunities – or to die prematurely at a young age due to compromised health services while the NHS is busy slightly prolonging the lives of the elderly. The intellectual exercise of putting ourselves behind a veil of ignorance frees us from irrational sentiments and paralysing political correctness that presents themselves as compassionate and humane but which are in fact unjust and cruel. It allows us to make moral decisions that will be coherent, consistent, and acceptable to all rational persons who are not affected by biases, irrational sentiments, or irrelevant considerations. As such, it provides what is probably the most persuasive argument against lockdowns.

Conclusion

This chapter started by illustrating the true harm that was caused by COVID-19, its highly discriminatory nature, and some of the multiple harms that were caused by lockdowns, especially to younger generations. That is a first step towards the crucial need to strike a balance between the benefits of lockdown and its downsides, a step that, quite astonishingly, was never taken by almost any government that imposed strict and long lockdowns in 2020 and 2021.

It is a sad fact that too many scientists around the globe influenced and encouraged governments to impose lockdowns, and then to prolong them, while demonstrating tunnel-vision decision-making that focused on one factor only (reducing COVID-19 cases, hospitalisations, and deaths) while being completely blind to the immense harm that their suggested lockdowns will cause. Woolhouse, while criticising the UK's response to COVID-19 and his fellow scientists' pro-lockdown approach, argues that "we were mesmerised by the once-in-a-century scale of the emergency and succeeded only in making a crisis even worse. In short, we panicked. This was an epidemic crying out for a precision public health approach and it got the opposite". (*The Guardian*, 2022). Yet panic does not fully explain this colossal failure of public policy. The over-reliance on "science" and scientists; the exclusion of scholars in the social sciences and humanities from the decision-making process; the silencing of voices of doubt, scepticism, and criticism; and the lack of willingness to have a proper public and academic debate about the response to COVID-19 also contributed to transforming a severe but short-term and treatable health crisis into a multifaceted, long-term disaster. While deciding on public policies as a response to COVID-19, too many scientists and governments sidelined all areas of knowledge and all aspects of human life, focusing only on minimising the harm that may be caused by COVID-19.

It is perhaps easier for scholars from the social sciences or humanities to think about public policies holistically, to put together different sources of data and knowledge, and to analyse them from different angles while appreciating the problem to its full complexity, as was demonstrated nicely by Green, a historian who identified the global harms caused by lockdowns in real time (Green, 2021), while leading scientists were busy playing with pointless models and scenarios that, according to their own admission, contributed very little to the quality of political decision-making (The Spectator, 2021).

Addressing the pandemic from an intradisciplinary point of view – one that does not ignore the harm that is caused by the virus but adds to it well-informed social and moral considerations – leads to the conclusion that isolation for the elderly and vulnerable only, preferably by giving advice rather than by imposing it, while allowing others to continue with life almost as normal, was necessary, not discriminatory – and was morally just. It was and still is the only response that will minimise the harm that may be caused by the pandemic – while also minimising the harm that will be caused to every one of us, including the elderly who will survive the virus. Not applying that policy and instead applying blanket lockdowns and strict social-distancing rules was discriminatory against younger generations – and a moral crime against young people in the UK and beyond.

Note

1 My Thanks are due to Kai Möller for extremely valuable comments on an earlier draft; to Joseph Raz, John Adenitire, Faye Thomas, and Isobel Horsley for insightful discussions on this topic; and to Grace Higgins and Megan Alexander for their truly exceptional research assistance. I benefitted from comments from participants in the Bonavero Institute of Human Rights "Perspectives" seminar at Oxford University, the "Work-in-progress" seminar at the School of Law, Keele University, and the faculty seminar at St. Gallen University, Switzerland.

Bibliography

Agamben, G. 2021. *Where Are We Now? The Epidemic as Politics*. London: Eris.
AIER Staff. 2020. "Lockdowns Do Not Control the Coronavirus: The Evidence". American Institute for Economic Research, December, www.aier.org/article/lockdowns-do-not-control-the-coronavirus-the-evidence/

Andrew Gregory 2021. Children's NHS mental health referrals double in pandemic. *The Guardian* 23.9.2021. www.theguardian.com/society/2021/sep/23/childrens-nhs-men tal-health-referrals-double-in-pandemic

BBC. 2020. "Coronavirus: Isolation for over-70s 'within weeks'". *BBC,* March 15, www.bbc. co.uk/news/uk-51895873

Bjornskov, C. 2021. "Did Lockdown Work? An Economist's Cross-Country Comparison". *CESifo Economic Studies* 67 (3): 318–331.

Booth, R., and McIntyre, N. 2021. "Covid-related deaths in care homes in England jump by 46%". *The Guardian*, 19 January, www.theguardian.com/world/2021/jan/19/covid-rela ted-deaths-in-care-homes-in-england-jump

Campbell, Denis. 2021. "Extent of mental health crisis in England at 'terrifying' level". *The Guardian*, 9 April, www.theguardian.com/uk-news/2021/apr/09/extent-of-mental-hea lth-crisis-in-england-at-terrifying-level

Campbell, Denis. 2022. "Swamped NHS mental health services turning away children, say GPs". *The Guardian*, 3 April, www.theguardian.com/society/2022/apr/03/swamped-nhs-mental-health-services-turning-away-children-say-doctors

Delphine Strauss. 2021. Budget will leave millions worse off next year, studies find. *Financial Times* 28.10.2021. www.ft.com/content/676c58d3-aa7a-4209-a2fe-0cc8fb145a80

ECDC, 2020. *COVID-19 in children and the role of school settings in COVID-19 transmission.* Stockholm: ECDC.

Financial Conduct Authority. 2021. "Financial Lives 2020 survey: the impact of coronavirus". *Financial Conduct Authority,* 11 February, www.fca.org.uk/publications/research/financial-lives-2020-survey-impact-coronavirus

Forder, J. and J.L. Fernandez. 2011. "Length of stay in care homes". Report commissioned by Bupa Care Services. PSSRU Discussion Paper 2769.

Fraser Nelson. 2021. My Twitter conversation with the chairman of the Sage Covid modelling committee. *The Spectator*, 18/12/2021. www.spectator.co.uk/article/my-twitter-conversation-with-the-chairman-of-the-sage-covid-modelling-committee

Gosseries, A., and Lukas H. Meyer. 2009. *Intergenerational Justice.* Oxford: Oxford Scholarship Online.

Green, T. 2021. *The Covid Consensus.* London: C. Hurst and Co Publishers.

Gregory, Andrew. 2021. "Children's NHS mental health referrals double in pandemic". *The Guardian*, 23 September, www.theguardian.com/society/2021/sep/23/childrens-nhs-mental-health-referrals-double-in-pandemic

Helm, Toby. 2021. "Britain faces 'decades of financial risk' as £370bn pandemic bill mounts". *The Guardian*, 25 July, www.theguardian.com/world/2021/jul/25/britain-faces-decades-of-financial-risk-as-370bn-pandemic-bill-mounts

Henehan, K. 2021. "Uneven steps: Changes in youth unemployment and study since the onset of COVID-19". Resolution Foundation Briefing. www.resolutionfoundation.org/app/uploads/2021/04/Uneven-steps.pdf

Herby, Jonas, Lars Jonung, and Steve H. Hanke, 'A Literature Review and Meta-analysis of the Effects of Lockdowns on COVID-19 Mortality'. *Studies in Applied Economics,* January. https://sites.krieger.jhu.edu/iae/files/2022/01/A-Literature-Review-and-Meta-Analy sis-of-the-Effects-of-Lockdowns-on-COVID-19-Mortality.pdf

HM Government. 2020. "Analysis of the health, economic and social effects of COVID-19 and the approach to tiering". *HM Government*, 30 November, https://assets.publish ing.service.gov.uk/government/uploads/system/uploads/attachment_data/file/944823/ Analysis_of_the_health_economic_and_social_effects_of_COVID-19_and_the_approac h_to_tiering_FINAL_-_accessible_v2.pdf

Joffe, A.R. 2021. "COVID-19: Rethinking the Lockdown Groupthink". *Frontiers in Public Health* 9.

Kissler, S.M., C. Tedijanto, E. Goldstein, Y.H. Grad, and M. Lipsitch. 2020. "Projecting the transmission dynamics of SARS-CoV-2 through the postpandemic period". *Science*, 368 (6493): 860–868.

Kluge, H.H.P. 2020. "Statement – Invest in the overlooked and unsung: build sustainable people-centred long-term care in the wake of COVID-19". *WHO*. www.who.int/eur ope/news/item/23-04-2020-statement-invest-in-the-overlooked-and-unsung-build-sustainable-people-centred-long-term-care-in-the-wake-of-covid-19

Knapton, S. 2020. "Two thirds of coronavirus victims may have died this year anyway, government adviser says". *The Telegraph*, 25 March, www.telegraph.co.uk/news/2020/03/25/two-thirds-patients-die-coronavirus-would-have-died-year-anyway/

Kullforff, M., J. Bhattacharya, and S. Gupta. 2020. "The Great Barrington Declaration". *Great Barrington Declaration*, https://gbdeclaration.org/

Laura Donnelli 2022. Number of children admitted to hospital for eating disorders surges 70 per cent since pandemic. *The Telegraph* 4/1/2022. www.telegraph.co.uk/news/2022/01/04/number-children-admitted-hospital-eating-disorders-surges-70/

Lawrence, D.R and J. Harris. 2021. "Red herrings, circuit-breakers and ageism in the COVID-19 debate". *Journal of Medical Ethics* 47(9): 645–646.

Mayor of London. n.d. *London*, www.london.gov.uk/what-we-do/health/tackling-alcohol-misuse-london

Miles, D., M. Stedman and A. Heald. 2020. "Living With COVID-19: Balancing Costs Against Benefits in The Face of The Virus". *National Institute Economic Review* 253: 60–76.

Moller, K. 2022. "The Proportionality of Lockdowns". In *Pandemic Response and the Cost of Lockdowns: Global Debates from Humanities and Social Sciences,* edited by P. Sutoris, S. Murphy, Y. Nehushtan, and A. Mendes Borges. Abingdon: Routledge.

Murphy, S. 2022. "Stopping the Spread of Health". In *Pandemic Response and the Cost of Lockdowns: Global Debates from Humanities and Social Sciences,* edited by P. Sutoris, S. Murphy, Y. Nehushtan and A. Mendes Borges. Abingdon: Routledge.

Nehushtan, Yossi. 2020. "The British Lockdown is Disproportionate" *IACL-IADC* [Blog], 9 April, https://blog-iacl-aidc.org/2020-posts/2020/4/9/the-british-lockdown-is-dispr oportionate

New Medical. 2020. "NHS reveals record-breaking number of alcohol-related hospital admissions". *New Medical*, 5 February, www.news-medical.net/news/20200205/NHS-reveals-record-breaking-number-of-alcohol-related-hospital-admissions.aspx

Office for National Statistics. 2020a. "Employment in the UK: December 2020". *Office for National Statistics*, 15 December, www.ons.gov.uk/employmentandlabourmarket/peopl einwork/employmentandemployeetypes/bulletins/employmentintheuk/december2020

Office for National Statistics. 2020b. "Deaths involving COVID-19, England and Wales: deaths occurring in May 2020". *Office for National Statistics*, 15 May, www.ons.gov.uk/peoplepop ulationandcommunity/birthsdeathsandmarriages/deaths/bulletins/deathsinvolvingcov id19englandandwales/deathsoccurringinapril2020

Office for National Statistics. 2020c. "Deaths involving COVID-19, England and Wales: deaths occurring in May 2020". *Office for National Statistics* 23 June, https://cy.ons.gov.uk/peopl epopulationandcommunity/birthsdeathsandmarriages/deaths/bulletins/deathsinvolvin gcovid19englandandwales/deathsoccurringinmay2020

Office for National Statistics. 2020d. "GDP monthly estimate, UK: April 2020". *Office for National Statistics*, 12 June, www.ons.gov.uk/economy/grossdomesticproductgdp/bullet ins/gdpmonthlyestimateuk/april2020

Office for National Statistics. 2021a. "GDP first quarterly estimate, UK: October to December 2020". *Office for National Statistics*, 12 February, www.ons.gov.uk/economy/grossdomesti cproductgdp/bulletins/gdpfirstquarterlyestimateuk/octobertodecember2020

Office for National Statistics. 2021b. "International comparisons of GDP during the corona-virus (COVID-19) pandemic". *Office for National Statistics*, 1 February, www.ons.gov.uk/ economy/grossdomesticproductgdp/articles/internationalcomparisonsofgdpduringth ecoronaviruscovid19pandemic/2021-02-01

Office for National Statistics. 2021c. "GDP monthly estimate, UK: July 2021". *Office for National Statistics*, 10 September, www.ons.gov.uk/economy/grossdomesticproductgdp/ bulletins/gdpmonthlyestimateuk/july2021

Office for National Statistics. 2021d. "Deaths registered weekly in England and Wales, provi-sional: week ending 15 January 2021". *Office for National Statistics*, 26 January, www.ons. gov.uk/peoplepopulationandcommunity/birthsdeathsandmarriages/deaths/bulletins/ deathsregisteredweeklyinenglandandwalesprovisional/weekending15january2021#dea ths-registered-by-age-group

Office for National Statistics. 2021e. "Pre-existing conditions of people who died due to COVID-19, England and Wales". *Office for National Statistics*, 23 November, www.ons. gov.uk/peoplepopulationandcommunity/birthsdeathsandmarriages/deaths/datasets/pre existingconditionsofpeoplewhodiedduetocovid19englandandwales

Office for National Statistics. 2021f. "National life tables – life expectancy in the UK: 2018 to 2020". *Office for National Statistics*, 23 September, www.ons.gov.uk/peoplepopulationa ndcommunity/birthsdeathsandmarriages/lifeexpectancies/bulletins/nationallifetablesun itedkingdom/2018to2020

Office for National Statistics. 2021g. "Average age of death (median and mean) of per-sons whose death was due to COVID-19 or involved COVID-19, by sex, deaths registered in March 2020 to August 2021, England and Wales". *Office for National Statistics*, 10 September, www.ons.gov.uk/peoplepopulationandcommunity/birthsdeathsandma rriages/deaths/adhocs/13691averageageofdeathmedianandmeanofpersonswhosedeathw asduetocovid19orinvolvedcovid19bysexdeathsregisteredinmarch2020toaugust2021engl andandwales

Oraby, T., Michael G. Tyshenko, Jose Campo Maldonado, Kristina Vatcheva, Susie Elsaadany, Walid Q. Alali, Joseph C. Longenecker and Mustafa Al-Zoughool. 2021. "Modelling the effect of lockdown timing as a COVID-19 control measure in countries with differing social contacts". *Scientific Reports* 11: 3354.

Osama T., B. Pankhania, A. Majeed. 2020. "Protecting older people from COVID-19: should the United Kingdom start at age 60?" *Journal of the Royal Society of Medicine* 113 (5): 169–170.

Pandata. n.d. "Infobank – Lockdowns". *Pandata*, www.pandata.org/infobank-lockdowns/

Partington, R. and Elliott, L. 2021. Wage squeeze will leave average worker almost £13,000 worse off, Sunak warned. *The Guardian* 28.10.21.

Parveen, N. 2020. "Elderly must not be left out of lockdown easing, says Michael Palin". *The Guardian*, 3 May, www.theguardian.com/society/2020/may/03/elderly-must-not-be-left-out-of-lockdown-easing-says-michael-palin

Pidd, Helen. 2021. "Psychosis cases rise in England as pandemic hits mental health". *The Guardian*, 18 October, www.theguardian.com/society/2021/oct/18/psychosis-cases-soar-in-england-as-pandemic-hits-mental-health

Pressman S.D., S. Cohen, G.E. Miller, A. Barkin, B.S. Rabin, and J.J. Treanor. 2005. "Loneliness, Social Network Size, and Immune Response to Influenza Vaccination in College Freshmen". *Health Psychology*, 24 (3): 297–306.

Ratcliffe, M. 2022. "What We Lost in Lockdown". In *Pandemic Response and the Cost of Lockdowns: Global Debates from Humanities and Social Sciences,* edited by P. Sutoris, S. Murphy, Y. Nehushtan, and A. Mendes Borges. Abingdon: Routledge.

Rawls, J. 1971. *A Theory of Justice.* Cambridge: Belknap Press.

Richard Adams. 2021. Disadvantaged pupils in England lag behind in Covid learning catch-up. *The Guardian*, 29.10.2021. www. theguardian.com/education/2021/oct/29/disadvantaged-pupils-in-england-lag-behind-in-covid-learning-catch-up

Robin McKie. 2022. Britain got it wrong on Covid: long lockdown did more harm than good, says scientist. *The Guardian*, 2 January 2022. www.theguardian.com/world/2022/jan/02/britain-got-it-wrong-on-covid-long-lockdown-did-more-harm-than-good-says-scientist

Sahakian, Barbara Jacquelyn, Christelle Langley, Fei Li, and Jianfeng Feng. 2021. "How the pandemic may damage children's social intelligence". *The Conversation*, 12 February, https://theconversation.com/how-the-pandemic-may-damage-childrens-social-intelligence-154975?utm_medium=email&utm_campaign=Latest%20from%20The%20Conversation%20for%20February%2015%202021%20%201863418166&utm_content=Latest%20from%20The%20Conversation%20for%20February%2015%202021%20-%201863418166+CID_a1732fee940d733a51dd581ba713f417&utm_source=campaign_monitor_uk&utm_term=how%20important%20this%20kind%20of%20development%20is%20to%20childrens%20growing%20brains

Sample, I., and R. Mason. 2020. "UK could relax lockdown for millions if over-70s are shielded, say scientists". *The Guardian*, 5 May, www.theguardian.com/society/2020/may/05/longer-lockdown-for-over-70s-would-allow-fewer-restrictions-for-rest-of-uk-scientists-suggest

Singer B.J., R.N. Thompson, and M.B. Bonsall. 2021. "The Effect of the Definition of 'Pandemic' on Quantitative Assessments of Infectious Disease Outbreak Risk". *Scientific Reports* 11.

Southall E., A. Holmes, Edward M. Hill, Benjamin D. Atkins, Trystan Leng, Robin N. Thompson, Louise Dyson, Matt J. Keeling, and Michael J. Tildesley. 2021. "An analysis of school absences in England during the COVID-19 pandemic". *BioMed Central Medicine*, 19 (137).

The Economist. 2021. "See how age and illnesses change the risk of dying from COVID-19". *The Economist*, 11 March, www.economist.com/graphic-detail/covid-pandemic-mortality-risk-estimator

Thompson, J. 1999. *Intergenerational Justice: Right and responsibilities in an intergenerational polity.* Abingdon: Routledge.

UK Parliament - Committees, News Article, 6 January 2022. https://committees.parliament.uk/committee/81/health-and-social-care-committee/news/160095/omicron-and-emergency-care-crisis-could-derail-plans-to-tackle-backlog-warn-mps/

US Centers for Disease Control and Prevention. 2021. "Estimated Flu-Related Illnesses, Medical visits, Hospitalizations, and Deaths in the United States — 2018–2019 Flu Season". *Centers for Disease Control and Prevention*, 29 September, www.cdc.gov/flu/about/burden/2018-2019.html

Van Bunnik, Bram A.D., Alex L. K. Morgan, Paul R. Bessell, Giles Calder-Gerver, Feifei Zhang, Samuel Haynes, Jordan Ashworth, et al. 2021. "Segmentation and shielding of the most vulnerable members of the population as elements of an exit strategy from COVID-19 lockdown". *Philosophical transactions of the Royal Society of London B, Biological Sciences* 376.

Viner, R.M., Simon J. Russell, Helen Croker, Jessica Packer, Joseph Ward, Claire Stansfield, Oliver Mytton, Chris Bonell and Robert Booy. 2020. "School closure and management practices during coronavirus outbreaks including COVID-19: a rapid systematic review". *The Lancet Child and Adolescent Health* 4(5): 397–404.

Weale, S. 2020. "School closures likely to have little impact on spread of coronavirus, review finds". *The Guardian*, 7 April, www.theguardian.com/education/2020/apr/06/school-closures-have-little-impact-on-spread-of-coronavirus-study

Whipple, T. 2020, 25 December. "Professor Neil Ferguson: People don't agree with lockdown and try to undermine the scientists", *The Times*. www.thetimes.co.uk/article/peo ple-don-t-agree-with-lockdown-and-try-to-undermine-the-scientists-gnms7mp98

Woodcock, A. 2020. "Coronavirus: Government paper offers no assessment of economic impact of restrictions on areas in different tiers". *Independent*, 30 November, www.inde pendent.co.uk/news/uk/politics/coronavirus-tiers-economy-impact-covid-b1764 060.html

Woolhouse, Mark. 2022. *Year the World Went Mad: A Scientific Memoir from the Pandemic.* London: Sandstone Press Ltd.

Yang, E. 2020. "Experience From Other Countries Show Lockdowns Don't Work". *American Institute for Economic Research*, 9 August, www.aier.org/article/experience-from-other-countries-show-lockdowns-dont-work/

13

LOCKDOWN LIVED EXPERIENCE, ILLNESS, POWER, AND EPISTEMIC INJUSTICE[1]

Roxana Baiasu

Introduction

This paper offers a contribution to recent discussions concerning the marginalisation or exclusion of the humanities from pandemic-related decision-making processes which have shaped important lockdown policies. More specifically, I focus on certain contributions that philosophy and, in particular, certain interactions between phenomenology, genealogical analysis, and social epistemology can make to this topic.

The phenomenological analysis draws attention to basic aspects of the lived experience of individuals in lockdown situations that might involve unfair power relations. The critical, genealogical investigation is concerned with some of these power relations; it examines and challenges models of dominant decision-making processes concerning lockdown which employ top-down views formed from privileged positions of power and are conducive to the marginalisation of certain groups, the neglect of their needs, and thus to their being wronged and harmed – hence to certain forms of injustice. I focus on two forms of injustice related to lockdown decision-making processes and, more specifically, two forms of what Miranda Fricker calls "epistemic injustice": testimonial injustice and hermeneutical injustice. Testimonial injustice occurs when individuals' relevant testimonies concerning, for example, the serious negative impact certain lockdown regulations have on their lives are not (sufficiently) taken into account due to a deficit in the credibility assigned to these individuals. Hermeneutical injustice occurs, for example, when decision-making processes fail to make sense of the experiences of individuals and of their attempts to express them due to the use (or rather misuse) of a limited quantitative model or utilitarian conceptual framework. I suggest that by using a social epistemological conceptual framework and certain phenomenological and genealogical tools it is possible to shed more light on wrongs and injustices

DOI: 10.4324/9781003259336-17

produced by a certain misuse of power. Insofar as these philosophical investigations reveal them, these injustices can be adequately examined and addressed both theoretically and practically.

Living in the state of pandemic and lockdown

This section offers an analysis of some basic aspects of what it is like to live in lockdown in order to contribute to an understanding of the complex ways the lockdown negatively affects our lives. A phenomenological approach to the lockdown starts from individuals' lived experience and how their ways of making sense of the world and their place in it have been impacted by the COVID-19 pandemic. The phenomenological analysis I offer here intersects with an approach which draws on Foucault's genealogical discussion of the formation of meaning, knowledge, and power in the "state of plague" and disciplinary societies (Foucault, 2020).

It could be said that lived experiences of the lockdown include some positive aspects (some people were content to spend more time with their children and family, to pursue certain activities, or develop news skills or knowledge that otherwise they would not have had time to devote to, and so on). I do not intend to contest or discuss positive aspects of the lived experience of lockdown. The issue I am concerned with here is how the lockdown negatively impacts the everyday lives of individuals.

The "Panopticism" chapter of Foucault's *Discipline and Punish* begins with a description of typical measures taken at the end of the seventeenth century when a plague affected a town (Foucault, 2020: 195 f.). One might think that twenty-first-century lockdown measures taken during the COVID-19 pandemic are very different from the measures taken in Europe in the seventeenth century. Indeed, one cannot contest significant differences between them, differences related, for example, to the advance of technology or of economic and governmental systems; however, it can be argued that some basic schemes of social control and life seem to be quite similar.

Let us begin with a consideration of certain spatial features of the surrounding world. There are spatial features of what Foucault calls "the state of plague" that appear to be manifest in what I suggest can be called "the state of pandemic". During a plague, Foucault notes, strict "spatial partitioning" is one of the main measures taken to tackle it (Foucault, 2020: 195). Similarly, a core feature of the lockdown during the COVID-19 pandemic is a spatial partitioning that sets apart individuals or social "bubbles" (the latter might be, for example, constituted by households, care homes' residents and staff, or groups of pupils in schools). Spatial locations are no longer open and fluid but are delimited by rigid boundaries strictly set by governmental regulations. Spatial partitioning is constituted, for example, through people's seclusion in their homes and their very limited movement outdoors. In lockdown, social space is partitioned not only by walls but also by distancing rules, face masks, visors, and other PPE items (compare Carel, Ratcliffe and Froese, 2020).

The risk of contagion or the threat of punishment motivates compliance in relation to the partitioning of space and isolation measures. The fluidity of everyday social space suddenly disappears. In lockdown, individuals live in a frozen space which blocks agency and social interactions. The "public" space is no longer shared. It is partitioned by strict boundaries, limitations, and restrictions. The closing of most public spaces, the rigid delimitations of portions of space through distancing rules, the limiting of the number of people in indoor areas, and the cleaning and disinfection of public spaces are just a few manifestations of the loss of the shareability of space which corresponds to the fragmentation of space and the isolation that individuals experience in the pandemic mode of "inhabiting" space.

This distorted mode of "inhabiting" space turns out to be a mode of dis-inhabiting space: one no longer feels at home in a world in which most things are in some way or another distanced, severed, and no longer readily available or reachable. The world becomes uncanny and threatening – difficult to make sense of. Meaning mechanisms previously available are broken down. Manifestations of the dysfunctions of meaning mechanisms include impaired well-being and the increase of mental health issues (I shall say more about these matters later).

The dis-inhabiting of space in lockdown is also characterised by an impoverished sense of the corporeality of worldly encounters or even a loss of the embodied sense of lived space and social interactions. In lockdown, touching, stroking, caressing, hugging, or even meeting friends or relatives are in most cases prohibited outside the household or one's small social bubble. This kind of situation is especially difficult for those who live alone, and even more so when they are vulnerable due to mental or somatic illness or age. The company of friends or relatives, hospital visits, being by the bedside of loved ones who are severely ill or dying are possibilities which are banned in the lockdown world. During the COVID-19 lockdown, most social encounters took place in a virtual, two-dimensional, technological space. This is a very constricted space which is delimited by laptop, phone, tablet, or computer screens. Possibilities of touching or of just seeing others are significantly curtailed or even in some cases, where there is no access to the necessary technology, completely inexistent.

It could then be said that in lockdown the "social" world shrinks. It is characterised by a reduced visibility of others: one does not see other people much; one can only see them from a distance which severs one from the others; or one is not able to see the loved ones at all, often for an unpredictable amount of time.

Let us now turn our attention briefly to time, and to some aspects of time experience in lockdown. Corresponding to the lived experience of spatial partitioning and isolation, time is experienced as frozen. The passing of time might seem to be suspended due to the appearance of time as repetitive, uniform, and homogenous. The "time for..." or "time to..." schemas of pre-pandemic times and everyday social practices (enacted, for example, by the time to go to work, the time to go out and meet some friends, the time to visit one's relatives living further away, and so on) appear to break down. These time schemas, which are constitutive of everyday meaningful situations, become dysfunctional: the scope of the enactment of these time schemas is severely truncated. Furthermore, there is a loss of the shareability of time: everyday time loses a great deal of its public, social character. In lockdown, individuals no longer spend much time with others, and when they do so, in most cases it is via the medium of a partitioned space or virtual space; similarly to an obscure or frosted-glass wall or a fog, this distancing reduces visibility and blurs the sense of being with other people.

Space and time can be understood as constituents of our everyday existence and of our ways of making sense of the world, ourselves, and other people. In lockdown, for the most part, these are severely disrupted. Meaning mechanisms and schemas which were previously taken for granted break down in lockdown. It could be said that the experience of the lockdown is a distinctive experience of vulnerability which involves a crisis or breakdown of meaning. In its turn this breakdown of meaning has a major impact on individuals' well-being (Baiasu, 2020, 2021). In lockdown, possibilities of resilient coping are very limited and often have not been supported by governments that have used a particular kind of approach to lockdown – to which I now turn.

Panoptic power

As I mentioned earlier, in *Discipline and Punish* Foucault discusses what he calls the state of plague. I would like to note here how the state of pandemic can be understood as a critical situation which, although it shares some features with the state of plague, involves, however, certain distinctive characteristics and radical modes of a breakdown of meaning.

The state of plague is localised. It also has a simple structure, which is shaped by certain basic possibilities: life, death, or punishment (Foucault, 2020: 195). A main goal in the state of plague is life preservation. One is constantly under threat: the threat of death due to the plague, or of punishment if one does not conform to state regulations. Some of the structural aspects of the state of plague are shared by the state of pandemic. However, the state of pandemic is much more complex due to various disciplinary mechanisms used to keep it under control, some of which will be discussed below. So two important differences between the state of plague and the pandemic can be noted here: the former is local and rather simple, while the latter is global and very complex.

Foucault notes a distinction between the state of nature, in relation to which the source of laws and rights can be accounted for, and the state of plague, which, he argues, constitutes the origin of discipline (Foucault, 2020: 199). Discipline appears to be required in the state of plague or of the pandemic to tackle individual and social dysfunctions and all sorts of potential danger, threats, disorder, and abuse. As Foucault puts it, "Discipline fixes" (Foucault, 2020: 219). Discipline can be used to fix dysfunctions and to combat evil across society and its institutions (including family, the workplace, the school, hospital, prison, and so on).

Life in lockdown involves a crisis of meaning and values in many communities and individual lives; for the most part, mechanisms of meaning and value are broken down in lockdown. Discipline is meant to fix these broken-down mechanisms of meaning, knowledge, and social existence.

The state of plague, Foucault argues, constitutes the origin of disciplinary power, which is implemented through mechanisms of subtle coercion. Disciplinary, coercive practices brand individuals, producing labels and binary divisions which are used to categorise subjects (Foucault, 2020: 199). In their turn, such binary divisions and categories are used in the service of normalisation and control practices. It could be said that the pandemic functions as a state propitious for the development of disciplinary systems and the swarming of disciplinary practices. Spatial partitioning can serve the goal of subordinating individuals and subjecting them to disciplinary practices of control: individuals can be ruled and controlled more efficiently if they occupy a partitioned space divided by strict boundaries, and even more so if they internalise the disciplinary schemes that shape their behaviour.

I would like now to focus on a form of power enacted by the design and implementation of a certain model of lockdown: I call this form of power and model of lockdown "panoptic". I draw on Foucault's analysis of panopticism in *Discipline and Punish*, and apply and develop it to investigate the nature of panoptic power in lockdown. I do not wish to claim that all forms of power and lockdown are panoptic. It could be argued, however, that many are. But this is not what I am concerned with here. The focus on the panoptic model is rather meant to shed light on certain forms of injustice.

In the "Panopticism" chapter, Foucault describes the organisation and structure of Jeremy Bentham's panopticon. One of Bentham's proposals for social reform shaped by the utility principle includes penal reform. More specifically, Bentham designed a prison model, the panopticon, which he thought would be more humane. The panopticon is the model of a circular prison, the space of which is partitioned in such a way that it can accommodate separate cells for each prisoner that are viewable by a guard from a central tower. The prisoners are kept separate; they cannot see each other and cannot communicate with one another. They also cannot see the guard who can potentially watch them at any point in time; they do not know when the guard watches them. Bentham thought the panopticon was a more efficient model of prison which would no longer use physical punishment.

Foucault points out that panopticism can be understood as a general power scheme which is salient in the case of the prison site designed by Bentham but is more or less explicitly enacted by the structures of other institutions such as schools or hospitals. Foucault develops a detailed analysis of panopticism as a distinctive form and exercise of power which involves a complex hierarchical system of channels of power (Foucault, 2020: 216, 205). The network of power, he notes, develops through the surveillance of individuals and groups, and through the observation, reporting, and recording of their behaviour and agency. Panopticism is not just a form and enactment of power but also a form of knowledge (Foucault, 2020: 208). In the panoptic space, everyone but the observer in the central tower can be potentially seen and observed. Foucault points out that panopticism is manifest not only in the prison model. It is a form of power which has been disseminated during industrialisation and pervades our time's core structures and the institutions of the modern world: it is enacted in schools, hospitals, families, and other areas of everyday life and politics (Foucault, 2020: 205). I shall come back to this point shortly, but would like to note here that, in the context of the lockdown, the possibility of panopticism is related to the possibility of one's being constantly observed. In lockdown, surveillance and observation are implemented through a number of channels and mechanisms of power, which include, for example, CCTV cameras, police patrols, helicopters surveying neighbourhoods, and so on. Furthermore, in lockdown people vigilantly watch each other and are often ready to report cases in which lockdown rules are breached.

The panoptic viewpoint of power is located at the "centre" of the observed space. This point of view is also positioned at a higher level: it is a view "from above". The metaphor of vision used in this context, which is that of a centralising, highly positioned viewpoint, stands for a certain model of knowledge. According to this model, knowledge is understood as knowledge from above, that is, from a privileged location in the epistemic hierarchy. The privileged knowledge from above is allegedly an objective, all-encompassing form of comprehension which is able to penetrate all relevant details concerning the things that fall under its purview. Panoptic knowledge can survey the entire partitioned space and transcends all locations within it. It can thus be contrasted with a limited, partial knowledge which is formed from marginal locations within a partitioned, peripheral space. The observer in the central "tower" is not seen, but can potentially see all subjects entrapped in the panoptic space. The panoptic model of knowledge thus involves an asymmetrical epistemic relation which, I suggest in the next section, constitutes a form of injustice.

The observer cannot be seen and is anonymous (Foucault, 2020: 200). As Foucault notes, they can be anyone who gets access (possibly in a democratic way) to the location or standpoint of panoptic power. Panoptic knowledge begins with a "faceless gaze" (Foucault, 2020: 214) directed upon its objects, namely the individuals that are observed and thus kept under control. It develops through a naturalistic approach which employs an empiricist "toolkit" including observation, experimenting, and reporting. Panoptic knowledge is formed in a "lab of power" (Foucault, 2020: 204). In this "scientific" lab, individuals' behaviour and states are examined and controlled through surveillance and punishment. The panoptic lab of power is a site of experiments carried out on humans.

The numerous victims of the panoptic lab of power and its experimentalism during the pandemic include individuals who are subjected to this power as well as individuals who exert it. Incompetent leaders who fail to master knowledge that would easily be available to them might be among the first victims of the pandemic (compare Foucault, 2020: 208). I say more about some aspects of this failure of knowledge in the next section.

An example of a large-scale experiment of the panoptic power lab during the pandemic concerns the *full* closure of schools in lockdown. This is a difficult case of a lockdown procedure which has been harder to assess than other cases since the impact of COVID-19 on children has been much less severe and direct than on adults. School-closure policies have been much debated in certain contexts. This difficult case of lockdown procedure can illustrate, perhaps better than other measures, how panoptic power is problematic and fails to deal with certain challenging cases.

The full (or nearly full) closure of schools for long periods of time is achieved through children's spatial severing from their peers and teachers, as well as from support staff who are concerned with their safety and well-being and can intervene when needed. This lockdown policy has had an impact on certain groups of children and their mental health. For example, a recent study on "Child mental health in England before and during the Covid 19 lockdown" mentioned the negative impact of the lockdown on the well-being of a number of children; more specifically, it showed 'that the increase in probable mental health problems reported in adults also affected in 5–16 [sic] year olds in England with the incidence rising from 10.8% in 2017 to 16.0% in July 2020 across age, gender, and ethnic groups'; for example, 'more than a quarter of children (aged 5–16 years) and young people (aged 17–22) reported disrupted sleep'. Another study of a group of 168 children noted an increase in depressive symptoms. Findings also revealed a lack of support and very limited access to mental-health services (Newlove-Delgado, McManus, et al. 2021).

However, there have been so far few studies on the effect of COVID-19 and lockdowns on children's mental health, and the results sometimes conflict, depending perhaps on the socioeconomic, ethnic, and cultural factors as well as other circumstances of the studies' participants. In contrast to the studies mentioned above, other research found no impact of lockdown on the children considered by this research, or even identified a positive impact on some of them. For example, one study's initial results from a school survey (of 1000 children aged 13–14) in England indicates that "mental health in those who were struggling in October 2019 improved on all three measures in Spring 2020' (Newlove-Delgado, McManus, et al. 2021).

It could be said that the *full* reopening of schools – including compulsory attendance – affected some vulnerable families, such as, for example, families with clinically vulnerable children. These families found themselves under the threat of either state penalties or COVID-19 infection potentially resulting in severe, life-threatening illness affecting the children. However, there seems to be a consensus that 'school closures might have a detrimental effect on children', and '*should be applied only cautiously* and in combination with other measures' (Otte Im Kampe, Ann-Sophie Lehfeld, et al. 2020, my emphasis) and perhaps should be 'used as a last resort' (Viner et al., 2020). The reopening of schools should also be applied cautiously. Schools reopening without accommodating the needs of vulnerable children (without allowing them, for example, to stay at home when needed with or without providing access to distant learning) might also have a detrimental effect on the health of these children.

The cases of *full* closure and reopening of schools mentioned above can be used to illustrate a panoptic exercise of power which employs typical mechanisms of experimenting, observation, reporting, and coercion. This exercise of panoptic power is informed by a top-down knowledge formed from a central location and a point of view from above. Although the results of the medical studies mentioned above appear to conflict, these studies seem to agree that school closure and reopening must be applied very *cautiously*. The panoptic exercise of power fails to do so: it fails to take into account the lived experience of vulnerable children, their needs or rights; they can thus become victims of panoptic experimentalism. This failure is partly due to an objectification of these individuals and to other epistemic harms, some of which I discuss in the remainder of the paper.

Panoptic knowledge takes individuals as *mere objects*, as physical bodies that can be considered parts of socioeconomic systems (Foucault, 2020: 208). The panoptic "gaze" objectifies individuals (Foucault, 2020: 220). Their objectification is part of the process of their subjection to a disciplinary system. The disciplinary exercise of power can be motivated and driven by values of utility and economic efficiency.

Taken as mere bodies, individuals constitute utility units or resources that are understood and assessed in terms of productivity, efficiency, and the consequences and impact their behaviour and condition have on society. Panoptic decision and policymaking that are fundamentally shaped by utilitarian and economic values and principles neglect other more "humanistic", person-based values (such as well-being, caring, and quality of life).

These phenomena of panopticism mentioned above are more visible during lockdown. Let us consider, for example, a panoptic policy concerning the protection of the chronically ill, and the elderly in care homes. From this perspective, the complete isolation of these populations during lockdown would be the result of a utilitarian decision-making process which seeks to prevent the outcome that "bodies pile high" and disrupt the whole socioeconomic system. The well-being and nurturing of these individuals or the issue of how the quality of their life could be improved are not taken seriously into consideration.

The implementation of the panoptic schema is assessed by criteria such as utility, production increase, cost, time, and so on – that is, in terms of economic principles of efficiency. These principles motivate the need for centralised knowledge and disciplinary power to conrol the implementation of the panoptic schema.

Foucault stresses that panopticism can be understood as a general schema of power and knowledge which pervades everyday life and the organisation and running of social institutions such as schools, hospitals, prisons, the workplace, and so on (Foucault, 2020: 205). At the same time, panopticism informs very subtle forms of coercion which are rather implicit and invisible when social life unfolds smoothly. A pandemic lockdown, however, can make visible the panoptic epistemic schema of power shaping the joints of the social world. Disciplinary practices of control become salient in the context of the disruption of everyday existence in lockdown and, more generally, in a pandemic. The goal of what has been often called "the new normal" is pursued through practices of normalisation. The slogan "Learn to live with Covid", often reiterated by certain political leaders, is unclear and ambiguous. This ambiguity is used to serve the implementation of normalisation regulations and practices which stabilise an acceptance of the status quo shaped by panoptic power.

The exercise of disciplinary power might be well intended and guided by goals such as the combatting of evil or the neutralising of dangers (Foucault, 2020: 209). For example, spatial partitioning and distancing in the case of an epidemic or pandemic is one of the first measures that can be taken to prevent the spread of the infection. Foucault points out that disciplinary power is dangerous when it is misused and is shaped primarily or solely by values of efficiency or productivity. If so, the scope of values is curtailed; it is for the most part reduced to the increase of utility. This misuse of power might be facilitated by an expansion of the disciplinary network which enhances state control, centralised police, and surveillance. In the pandemic, multiple mechanisms and practices of normalisation which are employed to enact the "new normal" fabricate new modes of existence which can be subjected to economical systems. Panopticism's "fabrication of individuals" has an ontological impact on individuals' existence and the social world.

Let us sum up a few important points concerning the Foucauldian notion of panopticism that are particularly relevant in connection to the reflections on lockdown pursued in this paper. Panoptic knowledge 'from above' is essentially related to power, which is exercised in order to control and discipline: it employs mechanisms of subjection which are designed to bring about order and the subject's compliance. Panoptic power is not exercised for the sake of power itself but for the sake of utility, productivity, and efficiency. An analysis which draws on this conceptual framework can shed light on certain ways in which dominant, primarily quantitative decision- and policymaking processes concerning lockdown issues as well as top-down views from privileged positions of power are conducive to the marginalisation of certain individuals and groups, the neglect of their needs and lived experiences, and thus to their being wronged and harmed (ontologically, socially, mentally, or physically) – hence to certain forms of injustice. Panoptic knowledge and power are based on, and enact injustice. In the next section, I investigate certain elements of panoptic injustice. More specifically, I suggest that panoptic knowledge involves what Miranda Fricker calls epistemic injustice.

Panoptic epistemic injustice

In this section I am concerned with the following question: How are marginalised groups or individuals wronged and harmed by panoptic knowledge and power in lockdown? I focus on a form of epistemic harm, namely epistemic injustice, in lockdown contexts shaped by panoptic power.

In her book *Epistemic Injustice: Power and the Ethics of Knowing* and other texts, Miranda Fricker develops the notion of epistemic injustice; this is understood as a dysfunction of knowledge and power. As Fricker notes, it is sometimes helpful to investigate such dysfunctions in order to better grasp how social knowledge can be adequately produced and how power can be exercised fairly. In her work on epistemic injustice, Fricker notes that this is a form of injustice which produces harm and wrongs the subject in their capacity as a knower, and which discriminates against the subject as an epistemic agent. The dysfunction of knowledge which constitutes epistemic injustice is not simply a failure of knowledge or a matter of error but is an unfair way of relating to the subject that produces a certain knowledge content. Fricker distinguishes between two forms of epistemic injustice: testimonial injustice and hermeneutical injustice. Let us consider first testimonial injustice.

Testimony is considered to be an important source of knowledge; it is a central topic in recent epistemology, and there are numerous discussions concerning testimonial knowledge. I do not intend to engage with these here but would like to briefly note some general characteristics of this form of knowledge. Testimonial knowledge is knowledge that we gain, for example, by reading books, by listening to other people's discourses and reports, learning from teachers and educators, or from the media. Testimony can be spoken or written, but it can also be communicated through behaviour or other forms of expression, such as, for example, music or dance.

Testimonial injustice involves an error in judgement concerning the speaker's credibility (Fricker, 2010, 2008). Their credibility is misjudged; this misjudgement is due to prejudice or bias. When this is the case, the communicator, who is wronged in their capacity as a knower due to prejudice, is downgraded, marginalised, or neglected. Fricker points out that this is due to an unjust deficit of credibility assigned to them. For example, if a woman reports sexual abuse and she is not taken seriously, and her case is not investigated properly, she is a victim of testimonial injustice. The woman is assigned a diminished level of credibility due to certain prejudices – in this case, gender prejudices. Or, for example, if a patient seeks to recount their experience and they are not given proper attention, are not listened to because they are considered to lack medical expertise in relation to their condition, they are assigned a diminished level of credibility and are wronged in their capacity as knowers of the illness they experience (Fricker, 2017), and might be subjected to practices of silencing (compare Dotson, 2011).

In lockdown, testimonial injustice occurs, for example, when the testimonies, pleas, or claims for consideration and support of certain vulnerable groups or sections of the population (such as people with serious, chronic illness or mental illness) are ignored at the level of governmental policies that have an impact on these people. In some cases, they are deprived of a platform on which they could make their claims for support and help – and thus they are silenced. The study mentioned earlier concerning child and adolescent mental health in England notes certain findings indicating that during the lockdown in 2020

> 44·6% of 17–22 year olds with probable mental health problems reported not seeking help because of the pandemic. Clinicians have raised similar concerns about timely access to services, and a sharp decrease in Child and

Adolescent Mental Health Services referrals has been observed.... 21·6% of children and 29·0% of young people with probable mental health problems reported having no adult at school or work to whom they could turn during lockdown.

Newlove-Delgado, McManus, et al., 2021: 353

Members of such vulnerable populations are not seen and not heard in lockdown; they are neglected and marginalised. This testimonial blindness is a complex form of harm and wrong: the individuals are wronged as knowers whose testimonies could play an important role in the shaping of policies concerning public health and, more specifically, mental health. They are morally wronged insofar as their right to health is breached (see Wolff, 2012). The study points out that it is anticipated that "the cumulative effects of not intervening will result in *widening health and education inequalities*" (Newlove-Delgado, McManus, et al., 2021: 353, my emphasis).

Panoptic exercises of power discount the knowledge, lived experiences, and testimonies of vulnerable sections of the populations that are directly affected by these policies. Panoptic policies wrong and harm them epistemically and morally, and can have a negative, long-lasting impact on their lives.

Let us now turn our attention to hermeneutical injustice. It might be useful to note very briefly some aspects of the historical and conceptual background of this notion. Broadly understood, hermeneutics is concerned with interpretation, understanding, and meaning. In the so-called "European" philosophical tradition, the method of hermeneutics has been developed in connection to phenomenology. Philosophers like Martin Heidegger or Hans-Georg Gadamer employed hermeneutical phenomenology to offer interpretations of lived experiences, interpretations which make explicit implicit modes of understanding and implicit meanings. I propose an approach which links hermeneutic phenomenology to political and ethical issues such as justice and power. I explore some aspects of this link by drawing on Fricker's and other philosophers' work on hermeneutical injustice and Foucault's analysis of panoptic power, and point to some new directions of inquiry in order to apply this approach to a critical analysis of certain features of the lockdown during the COVID-19 pandemic.

Fricker takes the notion of hermeneutical injustice to designate a failure of interpretation which wrongs and harms people (Fricker, 2010). As Fricker points out, hermeneutical injustice consists in an individual's or group's failure to make sense of an experience due to a gap in social understanding and interpretative resources for social meaning. The failure to render intelligible a social experience is due to a lack of language and concepts which could express the experiences of powerless groups. A "poverty of intelligibility", as Fricker puts it, produces a form of inequality and marginalisation of the powerless. This involves what Elizabeth Anderson and Fricker call a "background hermeneutical marginalisation", which, they argue, constitutes a form of discrimination, and more specifically, a discrimination which concerns language and the interpretation of individuals' experiences.

(Anderson, 2012; Fricker, 2017. See also Medina, 2012). This form of injustice is manifest in communicative, testimonial exchanges.

In a number of cases that Fricker has in mind, the communicator encounters almost insurmountable difficulties when they attempt to share their experiences, which are due to a lack of the right words and adequate conceptual framework that could enable them to express their experiences. For example, women who had experienced sexual intimidation or abuse prior to the conceptual invention and stabilisation of the term "sexual harassment" were not able to adequately express the injustice and harm that they were being subjected to. The term "sexual harassment", which was coined to describe the complex situation in which most women find themselves at some point in their life, was simply lacking.

However, in a number of other cases, relevant conceptual resources exist as part of a general social, conceptual reservoir of meanings. In these cases, I suggest, hermeneutical injustice is not due to the sheer inexistence of adequate meaning schemes or a useful conceptual framework but is due to the exclusion or marginalisation of potentially relevant conceptual resources and forms of discourse. Practices which privilege the discourse and meaning schemes of powerful groups and resist the integration of conceptual schemes that vulnerable groups employ to make sense of their experiences produce hermeneutical discrimination. It could also be said that this is the result of what Pohlhaus calls "wilful ignorance" or what Medina calls "active ignorance" (Pohlhaus, 2012; Medina, 2013; see also Mills, 2007, 2015).

Often, young people with mental health problems and other patients with mental disorders had difficulties expressing and communicating their lived experiences and their need for support. Some of them only got this support when their situation became highly critical and they accessed hospital emergency services; it could be said that in such contexts some of their symptoms expressed their lived experience of suffering and cry for help and support. Chronically ill patients or patients with serious conditions who had their medical treatments suspended in lockdown tried to voice their lived experiences of illness, isolation, neglect, and the breach of their right to health and healthcare but often did not have any impact on decision- and policymaking processes.

Hermeneutic injustice occurs when such difficulties in communication are due to, or enhanced by, certain power structures' resistance to, and lack of recognition of, the forms of expression and discourse of vulnerable people – such as the ones mentioned above, who attempt to communicate in some way or another their *lived* experiences, their pleas for support, and claim to healthcare. Panoptic structures of power employ an objectifying interpretative framework – allegedly objective and allegedly the most relevant for policymaking and decision-making processes – which is produced from a top-down perspective. In virtue of its nature, this conceptual framework excludes or marginalises sense-making schemes and meaning resources of vulnerable groups which enable them to express their lived experiences, needs, values, and rights claims. This hermeneutical marginalisation is harmful for vulnerable populations, such as children and young people with mental health problems or people who are chronically ill: they are thus harmed epistemically and wronged morally. They are also harmed practically insofar as their access to healthcare is very limited.

Hermeneutical justice can be promoted if policies and decision-making processes concerning public health enrich the collective repertoire of meanings to develop more inclusive interpretative resources which make it possible to integrate, and respond adequately to, the needs and rights claims of vulnerable people. This form of hermeneutical openness to marginalised sense-making schemes can facilitate and promote adequate and just policies concerning public health.

Conclusion

The investigation carried out in this paper has been concerned with the "dark side" of lockdown (arguably, there is also a "bright side", and it could be said that there are positive aspects of the lockdown and corresponding legitimate forms of power, but these have not been my concern here). The inquiry has been primarily motivated by two interrelated questions. First, how does the lockdown negatively impact individuals and their lives? And second, what sort of exercise of power harms and wrongs them in this context?

This paper offers a contribution to the inquiry into these complex issues. In relation to the first question, the analysis has focused on certain basic aspects of the lived experience of the lockdown world and what can be called the state of pandemic, which include the following features: the isolating partitioning of space, the restricted shareability of public space, time, and the world, and their frozen structures. These are basic aspects of the crisis of meaning and the breakdown of our ways of life. They are core features of the dysfunctions of meaning-making mechanisms and of social life, and are constitutive of the conditions that enable the development of certain power forces.

Concerning the second question, I have looked at a form of power that allegedly "fixes" things but which, at a deeper level, wrongs and harms people. I have called this form of power panopticism (borrowing this concept from Michel Foucault). Panoptic power "fixes" things through order and disciplinary mechanisms which are governed by efficiency goals and are informed by top-down knowledge gained from a privileged viewpoint 'from above'. This is a location from which the objectifying surveillance of subjects who occupy marginal locations is potentially all-pervasive. New meaning mechanisms, new ways of life of the "new normal", are generated which are often regulated by norms that are primarily shaped by economic principles and political interests. I do not intend to say that there are no legitimate forms of political power implementing lockdown or exercised during the lockdown; however, the power that is panoptic is a form of power that wrongs and harms people. How does it wrong people? It wrongs people in many ways, but here I have focused on one important aspect of panoptic injustice, namely a corresponding form of epistemic injustice. I have pointed out that marginalised, vulnerable individuals or groups are degraded and discriminated against in two ways. First, as a result of the exercise of panoptic epistemic power they are demeaned and discriminated against as knowers of their vulnerable situations during lockdown; their expression of their needs, concerns, and claims is neglected or silenced by certain lockdown policies and regulations (this is a case of what Fricker calls testimonial injustice). Second, I have indicated that panoptic discourse, which is fundamentally informed by values of efficiency and utility and misguided ideals of objectivity, marginalises forms of discourse and meaning schemes which are primarily shaped by other values such as, for example, well-being, the right to health, compassion, or care (this kind of injustice, I suggested, is a form of hermeneutical injustice).

What is the point of this theoretical discussion? How can it contribute to a critical reflection on practical issues concerning decision-making, the design, and implementation of fair policies, including public health policies, in pandemic times? The analysis offered in this paper sheds more light on certain injustices which are a result of a misuse of power – the panoptic power – in the state of pandemic. If such injustices are exposed, they can be better addressed by adequate policies and processes of decision-making. They can become a clear target of ameliorative approaches that can be developed by integrating bottom-up knowledges from the point of view of disadvantaged individuals and groups – approaches that can thus pursue justice with respect to lockdown decision-making processes and the design of policies, including public health policies.

Note

1 I am very grateful to Yossi Nehushtan for his very helpful suggestions. I would also like to thank Sinead Murphy, Ian James Kidd and Peter Sutoris for their comments on my paper.

Bibliography

Anderson, Elizabeth. 2012. "Epistemic Justice as a Virtue of Social Institutions". *Social epistemology* 26 (2): 163–173.

Baiasu, Roxana. 2020. "The openness of vulnerability and resilience". *Angelaki* 25 (1–2): 254–264.

Baiasu, Roxana. 2021. "Phenomenology of Illness, Resilience and Wellbeing". In *Phenomenology of Bioethics*, edited by Susi Ferrarello. New York: Springer.

Carel, Havi. 2016. *Phenomenology of illness*. Oxford: Oxford University Press.

Carel, Havi, Matthew Ratcliffe, and Tom Froese. 2020. "Reflecting on experiences of social distancing". *The Lancet* 396: 87–88.

Dotson, Kristie. 2011. "Tracking Epistemic Violence, Tracking Practices of Silencing". *Hypatia* 26 (2): 236–257.

Fricker, Miranda. 2010. *Epistemic Injustice: Power and the Ethics of Knowing*. Oxford: Oxford University Press.

Fricker, Miranda. 2017. "Evolving Concepts of Epistemic Injustice". In *The Routledge handbook of epistemic injustice*, edited by Ian James Kidd and José Medina. London; New York: Routledge, pp. 53–60.

Fricker, Miranda and Katharine Jenkins. 2017. "Epistemic Injustice, Ignorance, and Trans Experiences". *The Routledge companion to feminist philosophy* edted by Ann Garry, Serene. J. Khader, and Alison Stones. New York; London: Routledge, pp. 268–278.

Foucault, Michel. 2020. *Discipline and Punish: The Birth of the Prison.* London: Penguin Books.

Medina, José. 2012. "Hermeneutical Injustice and Polyphonic Contextualism: Social Silences and Shared Hermeneutical Responsibilities". *Social Epistemology* 26(2): 201–220.

Medina, José. 2013 *Epistemologies of Resistance: Gender and Racial Oppression, Epistemic Injustice, and Resistant Imaginations.* Oxford: Oxford University Press.

Mills, Charles. 2007. "White Ignorance". In *Race and Epistemologies of Ignorance.* Edited by Shannon Sullivan and Nancy Tuana. Albany, New York: SUNY Press, 11–38.

Mills, Charles. 2015. "Global White Ignorance". In *Routledge International Handbook of Ignorance Studies.* Edited by Matthias Gross and Linsey McGoey. London/New York: Routledge, 217–227.

Newlove-Delgado, Tamsin; McManus, Sally; Sadler, Katharine; Thandi, Sharon; Vizard, Tim, Cartwright, Cher; Ford, Tamsin, "Child mental health in England before and during the COVID-19 lockdown", *Lancet Psychiatry*, 2021 May; 8(5): 353–354.

Otte Im Kampe, E., A-S. Lehfeld, S. Buda, U. Buchholz., and W. Haas. "Surveillance of COVID-19 school outbreaks, Germany, March to August 2020". *Euro Surveill* 25 (38).

Pohlhaus Jr., Gaile. 2012. "Relational Knowing and Epistemic Injustice: Toward a Theory of Willful Hermeneutical Ignorance". *Hypatia* 27(4): 715–735.

Viner, R.M., Simon J. Russell, et al. 2020. "School closure and management practices during coronavirus outbreaks including COVID-19: a rapid systematic review". *Lancet Child Adolesc Health* 4: 397-404.

Wolff, J. 2012, The Human Right to Health. London/New York: W.W. Norton & Company.

14

WHAT WE LOST IN LOCKDOWN

Matthew Ratcliffe

A life of possibilities

During the COVID-19 pandemic, extreme social restrictions have been accompanied by frequent talk of delaying things, putting life on hold for a little longer, and maintaining self-discipline for now so that we can eventually get back to normal. As the days, weeks, and months of "lockdown" (by which I mean combinations of stay-at-home and work-from-home orders, school-closures, and closure of non-essential retail and hospitality) stretched out ever longer, talk of mere delay and of being able to *do it all again* became increasingly removed from the realities of many people's situations. A human life is not something that can simply be put on standby for an extended duration and then switched back on without consequence; there is much that cannot be recovered.

It is debatable whether lockdowns will ultimately have saved or cost lives, and what applies to some countries, states, and regions will not apply to all. However, in deciding whether to implement such measures, and later in evaluating their impact, it is at least clear that the costs of lockdowns need to be made explicit alongside any anticipated benefits. In doing so, it is also important to consider the global situation, rather than adopting an exclusively national perspective. Even if one or more lockdowns are judged to have succeeded in their local aims, it is arguable that their combined impact on the world's poorest people have been and will continue to be devastating (Green, 2021).

In what follows, I will draw attention to an important cost of lockdowns that has not, in my view, been adequately acknowledged: what I will refer to as the *loss of life possibilities*. The nature of this kind of loss is not fully captured by references to more specific, concrete losses, thus rendering it difficult to articulate. It is also difficult to incorporate into a cost-benefit analysis, given that (a) it cannot be measured in a straightforward way, and (b) it has involved the undermining of deeply held values

DOI: 10.4324/9781003259336-18

that would ordinarily be presupposed by such assessments. I conclude by offering a tentative account of how this undermining has occurred, suggesting that intensive, monothematic messaging has gripped us in such a way that measures taken to slow the spread of SARS-CoV-2 have been evaluated in isolation from wider concerns.

When attempting to convey the kind of privation that I am concerned with here, it is easy to go awry. For example, following a televised debate that took place in the UK in January 2021, Lord Sumption received widespread criticism for maintaining that all lives are *not* of "equal value" and that the needs of the young should be prioritised over those of older people. One reason his point was met with disapproval is that it was also taken to encompass younger people with serious health conditions (although Sumption subsequently made clear that this was not what he had intended at all). But others "shuddered" at the more general claim that not all lives are equal.[1] I suspect, though, that the point Sumption was trying to make can be conveyed in a different way. If we consider a human life as something that resides wholly in the present, it is at least morally uncomfortable to maintain that Person A at this moment is of less value than Person B at this moment in light of A's being significantly older. However, in addressing whose needs ought to be prioritised, we could think of a human life as a temporally extended process stretching from birth to death, rather than a present snapshot. A life course has a temporally organised structure which ordinarily involves pursuing projects and pastimes, sustaining commitments, and building upon one's achievements. When thinking in terms of the whole, we see that prioritising the needs of Person A over those of Person B can involve denying B certain important opportunities that were available to A, opportunities that may well be of consequence for the overall trajectory of a life. Hence, valuing both lives equally over the long term is consistent with prioritising the needs of B at the present moment over those of A at the present moment.

Of course, the issue only arises in circumstances where B really does stand to lose important opportunities, rather than merely having to put some things on hold for a while and make other minor sacrifices. But many people have indeed suffered such losses. Indeed, if my interpretation of Sumption's remarks is broadly right, they point beyond the issue of what one subset of the population stands to lose compared to another and towards a more general concern that applies to young and old alike. In contemplating the effects of lockdowns, human lives can be thought of as temporally organised, fragile processes. We are not enduring entities that might be stored away for a while like possessions in a drawer, to be retrieved largely unscathed at a later date. Central to the living of a human life, and equally to the *experience of living*, is—for the majority of people—the pursuit and actualisation of significant possibilities that reflect organised arrangements of projects, cares, concerns, commitments, relationships, and pastimes (in short, our values).

The philosopher Jean-Paul Sartre (1943/1989) suggested that there is an important sense in which we *are* our possibilities. Sartre's claim is phenomenological in nature—it concerns how we *experience* ourselves and our surroundings. Ordinarily, we do not start off by surveying a value-free, objective realm, only then proceeding to assign significance to the various things that surround us. Instead, we encounter things as immediately significant to us; they matter to us in a range of ways. For example, as I write these words, the keyboard in front of me, the screen, the paper with notes scribbled on it, and other items of equipment together constitute a practically meaningful whole that reflects the nature of my current project. Insofar as these things appear significant to me, they also captivate my attention and elicit situationally appropriate activities.

Now, the ways in which things appear significant to us and how they engage us practically are not to be accounted for merely in terms of how particular entities look to us in the present and how we respond to them. Rather, we experience our surroundings as a coherent, practically meaningful whole, and we do so in light of enduring habits, expectations, projects, commitments, cares, and concerns. To a large extent, how something currently matters to us is a reflection of our longer-term values. What worries, threatens, saddens, excites, or enthralls us hinges on what we already care about. If someone really did value or care for absolutely nothing, then no situation they encountered would matter to them. In contrast to this, human experience generally involves experiencing and engaging with dynamic arrangements of unfolding possibilities which relate to more stable backgrounds of values.

The relevant aspect of experience is more readily apparent when we reflect on circumstances that involve its erosion or disruption. People with diagnoses of severe psychiatric illness sometimes describe a world devoid of practical significance, which appears strangely distant, somehow unreal. In conjunction with this, they might report feeling profoundly diminished as a person, no longer fully alive. Sometimes, such experiences are described with explicit reference to the loss of types of possibilities that were once taken for granted. Consider, for example, the following first-person descriptions of what it is like to be depressed: "It is impossible to feel that things will ever be different.... I feel like nothing is worth anything"; "The world holds no possibilities for me when I'm depressed; every avenue I consider exploring seems shut off" (Ratcliffe, 2015: 67). Similarly, those who have endured traumatic events sometimes describe a subsequent inability to experience or even contemplate meaningful future possibilities; it is as though the course of their lives has been prematurely cut short (Ratcliffe, Ruddell, and Smith, 2014). Even those of us who have not experienced anything like this can contemplate less pronounced experiential changes that occur during the course of our daily lives – those times when our surroundings seem strangely bereft of significance, somehow distant, or when none of our projects draw us in and we feel disconnected or lacking in direction. The ability to experience and engage with things in meaningful ways that reflect backgrounds of values is thus susceptible to various subtly different and usually transient disturbances.

According to Sartre, there is a way in which we might also be said to *choose* the most fundamental projects and values that constitute who we are, thus also choosing –albeit indirectly – what matters to us and how. However, setting this bold claim aside, it remains plausible to maintain that certain projects, commitments, roles, pastimes, and associated values are partly constitutive of *who we are*, together comprising what Christine Korsgaard (1996) has termed our "practical identity". This can involve our identifying with various roles, such as being a teacher, parent, spouse, religious practitioner, politician, or police officer. Equally integral to this kind of identity, I suggest, are various ongoing projects and relationships to which we are committed.

So, the course of a life does not just involve engaging with possibilities in a generic way, doing what "one does" in various situations. In addition, we experience and engage with distinctive arrangements of meaningful possibilities that reflect and sustain who we are as unique individuals. The sense of "self" or "identity" in question is not fixed over time. Indeed, being who I am now can involve striving to become something that will change me as a person considerably. Even so, in order to experience and engage with coherently organised networks of possibilities, some degree of stability and consistency is also required. Consequently, practical identity is precarious, fragile. The ability to be who we are depends, in various ways, on circumstances outside of our control – on life events, our health, and changing relationships with other people. For example, those who suffer significant bereavements often talk of losing a part of themselves or no longer being quite the same person, given that so much of what they valued and what they did was dependent upon the deceased in one or another way (Ratcliffe, 2022). Similarly, something to be considered in addressing the impacts of lockdowns is the resultant privation of possibilities, many of which were central to people's lives and even to their identities.

Lockdowns and lost possibilities

Of course, all sorts of circumstances and events can impact greatly upon our lives, including the repercussions of political decisions. However, there is little else that compares to the profundity and scale of loss associated with lockdowns. People were deprived of both (a) life structures, consisting of projects, roles, pastimes, and habits, and (b) valued interpersonal relationships and interactions that would otherwise support their efforts to comprehend and navigate life disruption. Now, experiences of lockdown were highly varied; there are no straightforward generalisations to be had concerning how *we* were all affected. But for many of us, lockdowns did involve the loss of important possibilities. Think of life events, such as being there for a grandchild's first birthday and first steps or being with a family member at the end of life. And consider that first term at university. During a recent conversation about the effects of social restrictions on university students, a neighbour of mine told me of how this had been the most important time of his life: so much happened; so many things changed; so many doors opened. It transformed his outlook on the world, shaping the course of his life in unforeseen ways. Then there are all those early-stage relationships that never progressed, all the projects that had to be cast aside, all the career paths and life trajectories that were blocked. Most of us also had wider-ranging experiences of loss and absence as we walked through deserted cities, passing empty schools, closed shops, and taped-up playgrounds. The surrounding world as a whole was permeated with a sense of what "I", "we", and "they" have lost – my empty office; our empty streets; their empty playground. Everything appeared strangely lacking, conspicuously bereft of the significant possibilities more usually attached to it.

Some losses can be couched in more concrete terms – losses of jobs, money, school days, hours of face-to-face university teaching, businesses, and so forth. However, simply enumerating these does not convey their potential significance in the course of a human life. Furthermore, there is so much that cannot be easily itemised – all of those idiosyncratic ways in which things matter in the context of particular people's lives. Nevertheless, what is common to a range of superficially different privations is their amounting to *losses of significant life possibilities*. As such, they are not reducible to concrete, tangible, measurable, generalisable consequences of lockdown, making them difficult to single out and describe.

With colleagues based at universities in the UK and Japan, I conducted a qualitative survey of people's diverse experiences of social restrictions in the early stages of the COVID-19 pandemic (Froese et al., 2021). In addressing their experiences of loss, respondents identified a variety of specific activities and places, such as going to the cinema, the theatre, concerts, museums, pubs, and restaurants, travelling overseas, and seeing friends and relatives. Some also described these privations *as* losses of possibilities involving people, objects, situations, projects, and pastimes. Some such possibilities, they indicated, were irretrievably lost, rather merely transported – otherwise unaltered – to another point in one's life:

> As an older person the loss of time affects me most, and the possibility that opportunities may have been lost and it will not be possible to reinstate them.

> I have felt a sense of loss over missed opportunities, having planned to go on holiday and that not being possible. I have felt a small sense of loss of youth, as often people say your twenties is a time of great adventure, which has been taken from me and many others. And time is not something that can be given back.

> Loss of places where I have been happy that may close down for ever – local pub, cinema, restaurant, concert hall. Most – not being able to cuddle my cheery grandson when he gets tired and can't quite fall asleep, or read to my granddaughter. And grief for time passing as we get older without new experiences and time is running out.

What is it not to have "new experiences"? Clearly, time does not just stop altogether – events still unfold, and different things continue to be experienced. However, those life experiences that matter to us, that stand out from others, usually involve our engaging with new and significant possibilities which reflect what we take to be important and may also affect us in ways that reshape our values. So there is a difference between experiencing change *per se* and experiencing change that *matters*. Some survey respondents further stated that their losses of possibilities amounted to a lost "life" or "world". It is not that they merely experienced a loss of opportunities relative to an established and enduring life structure. Instead, the very fabric of their lives, the framework of values relative to which things mattered, had been eroded:

> Terrible grief and mourning for my lost "life", for the people I probably will never see again because in this time, our lives have changed.

> I have felt loss and grief for my own life. I had been in a good place, emerging from a somewhat darker time in my life and I do feel like I have been pushed back down the hill again. I do feel a sense of loss for my more independent, more confident self.

> Loss of my world, my travel opportunities, my plans for the next years of retirement.[2]

Among those possibilities that can never be recovered are many that involve other people. Most of our lives are bound up in various ways with the lives of others. We experience, make sense of, and engage with the world in ways that are *ours* rather than just *mine* and *yours* (Attig, 2011). Yet, in the UK alone, millions of people were denied the opportunity to visit and spend time with those they loved. For instance, many thousands of care home residents were isolated from spouses and other family members for months on end. Furthermore, many of these residents deteriorated rapidly or died during that period.[3] As we will now see, the privation of important life possibilities is perhaps most evident when we turn to the testimonies of people who were bereaved during the pandemic and unable to be with those who died or spend time with others during the weeks and months that followed.

Grief

In the UK alone, over 600,000 people die in an average year and millions of others grieve for them. Grief is not simply an enduring emotional reaction to the death of someone we love, it is a multi-faceted process. How that process unfolds over time is not attributable solely to one's own internal mental states and processes. Rather, the course of grief is shaped and regulated in a variety of ways by our relations with other people and our engagement with a wider social world, both before and after a death (Ratcliffe, 2022). During the COVID-19 pandemic, social restrictions prevented many people from being with family members and close friends during the days, weeks, and sometimes even months before they died and from subsequently sharing their experiences of grief with others. For some, this has had a considerable impact on the course of grief over time. Losses of possibilities associated with the death of a person (involving possibilities that were "theirs", "mine", and "ours") were experienced against the backdrop of a wider-ranging loss.

To be cut off from someone shortly before and as they die, to be denied a proper funeral, to be prevented from participating in other established rituals, to be unable to grieve together – all of this can impede the ability to integrate bereavement into the ongoing structure of one's life. Consequently, there are numerous reports of a grief that is intense, enduring, and unchanging. Bereft of the dynamism of a social world involving the shared pursuit and realisation of new and meaningful possibilities, grief itself lacks movement.[4] People report struggling with the effects of various restrictions: being unable to see someone before they died or attend the funeral; being deprived of physical touch; being unable to share one's grief; being unable to make sense of what has happened *with* others; being unable to engage with other aspects of life in ways that might otherwise have mitigated the impact of bereavement. To varying degrees, they were deprived of a shared social world, a context *within which* we more usually make sense of and adapt to bereavement.

A number of respondents to the survey that I have drawn upon experienced bereavements during the pandemic. Themes they mentioned include the difficulties of solitary grief, the lack of physical contact with others, a sense of unreality, being deprived of resources for processing grief, and a grief that is unchanging, somehow on hold:

> Brother-in-law died suddenly and unexpectedly, not due to COVID, and it feels like grief was paused as it could not run the usual course of attending funeral, etc. The sense of unreality still persists as have not been able to see family and be aware of the missing person.

> I lost a close friend (not due to COVID) and found it difficult to grieve on my own.

> I was fortunate to be able to attend but whilst at the funeral social distancing had to be observed, so even when I was by my family we were unable to console each other by hugging or touching. This lack of being able to console one another definitely made the grieving process harder.

> I feel unable to let go of the grief as I feel that I am putting it on hold while we wait for this situation to end and we are all, in a sense, fighting for survival.

> We had a Zoom funeral – it was pretty rubbish, and felt more like it was done because you are meant to have funerals than as a way to actually help process grief.

> It feels disconnected and unreal. I guess that it is related to the inability to be there and grieve as usual, with other people by my side.[5]

Another important consideration is how events associated with the end of life can ripple back and influence one's memories of a person, transforming the significance those memories have. How one remembers what happened back then is altered in light of what subsequently occurred and one's current situation (Goldie, 2012). Again, it is important to emphasise how we tend to think of a human life as a cohesively organised process, involving development, transformation, achievement, and disappointment. The significance attaching to specific memories of a person is shaped by a larger sense of their life as a whole and the part one played in it. This can be affected profoundly by the circumstances in which a life, and a relationship, ended. For instance, one might look back on those joyous moments of being and feeling together, only to recall that the person died frightened and alone, that one's commitment never to be apart from them, never to leave them in times of adversity, was irrevocably broken at the end. In this way, being deprived of interpersonal possibilities not only influences a sense of who we are now and where we are heading; it also affects and even transforms the significance of past accomplishments and past relationships. The point is not exclusive to events surrounding the end of life, and extends to the significance of other important life moments as well. Consider, for example, all those women who were required to give birth without the presence of a partner, other family member, or friend, and how a traumatic birth experience might influence one's perspective on the longer-term process of becoming a parent, shaping both the significance of remembered events and a sense of what the future holds.[6]

Evaluating lockdowns

My aim here has not been to answer the general question of whether some or all lockdowns were ultimately justified in light of their consequences. Rather, my point has been that the costs of lockdowns have included something very important, but which is also difficult to make explicit and convey in its fullness: a widespread loss of life possibilities, which has profoundly affected or will profoundly affect the course of many people's lives – who they are and who they will be. In considering the impacts of lockdown, this needs to be integrated into our evaluative perspective, even though it is not something that can be pinned down precisely. And I think that something has gone wrong in this regard. Ordinarily, our evaluations of significant events that impact upon ourselves, others, and society as a whole are informed and to some extent guided by emotional responses. Our emotional experiences of situations and events reflect an organised web of individual and shared values and concerns. Furthermore, they ordinarily do so in ways that are consistent with *who we are*. How things matter to us emotionally reflects an enduring network of interrelated values: moral, political, and religious values; projects and commitments that comprise our life structure; important interpersonal relationships. Hence, a person's emotional responses tell us something about that person, about the unique configuration of values that partly constitutes who they are (Glas, 2017).

However, there are also occasions when emotional evaluations of situations and events become decoupled from our values. Various different scenarios of this general kind might be discerned, involving conflicting values and/or conflicting emotions, but one that seems especially relevant to the current situation is what Thomas Szanto (2017) calls "emotional self-alienation". This involves responding emotionally to situations and events in ways that are not integrated into one's "overall evaluative outlook". Pre-established values lose their grip on us and our emotional experiences of unfolding events float free of them, in ways that diminish those experiences.[7]

We should of course care deeply about preventing as many people as possible from dying due to a viral illness. Even so, judgements as to whether certain specific measures are appropriate should also take into account the consequences for everything else that we, as a society, value. Presumably, this includes seeking to ensure that we do not ultimately cause considerably more global deaths than we are likely to prevent. But there is also the cost to what we regard as of value *in* life, including what we take to be important or even essential for human flourishing. And that, I assume, includes being able to develop and sustain a practical identity. The unwavering confidence with which so many people have endorsed lockdowns and dismissed critical voices suggests an evaluative perspective that has drifted free of such concerns. To be more specific, I suggest that certain salient considerations and associated performances (including various forms of "social distancing") have gripped our emotions in ways that do not take full account of pre-established values.

It is not implausible to suggest that this was an intended effect of UK government strategy, given the extent to which the population has been continually subjected to monothematic messaging, epitomised by "Stay at home; protect the NHS; save lives!" Now, one could respond that it was important to get the point across and that capturing people's emotions in such a way as to motivate compliance was entirely appropriate in such an unprecedented and dangerous situation. That said, virus cases, hospitalisations, deaths, and the dangers posed by the virus were presented day after day, month after month, in abstraction from any wider concern with illness and death. How many, we might ask, died of cancer and heart disease during the same period? How many of these and other deaths were, in principle, preventable too? How many lives could have been saved over the years by directing even a fraction of the resources at other problems? How many lives could be greatly enhanced and extended by increased efforts to reduce poverty and provide opportunities for the most disadvantaged? How many global deaths could have been prevented by doing everything possible to mitigate disruption of established global vaccination programmes during the pandemic – how many children will now die of measles, who would not otherwise have done so?

On top of all this are the losses of possibilities suffered by so many people – loss of the ability to sustain and become who we are, to pursue projects, to follow a particular path through life. In the face of this, uncritical advocacy of lockdowns has involved not only an obliviousness to established and cherished values but evaluations that conflict with some such values. It became acceptable to condemn lonely people who sought the company of friends, to chastise someone who went out for more than one walk per day in order to relieve anxiety, to actively disapprove of children for being in a playground. Along with this came widespread acceptance of the need to deprive people of the right to be with a partner as they die (sometimes after many years of marriage with no prior experience of prolonged separation), to prevent many children from interacting with others their own age for months on end, and to insist that thousands of women give birth without the company and support of partners or others. Especially when combined with bright-siding among the privileged about the joys of baking sourdough bread and of finally listening to the birds singing, unqualified endorsement of lockdowns appears to involve an alienation from much that we, as a society, value in human life. Any balanced evaluation needs to recognise the extent to which lockdowns ran roughshod over certain, deeply engrained values, relative to which costs and benefits would more usually be discerned – the very basis for our evaluations. This requires full acknowledgement of what it is for people to be *denied possibilities* to such an extent that life structures become unsustainable. In the absence of that acknowledgement, the catalogue of what we lost in lockdown will include a loss of connection with our own societal values and perhaps the longer-term erosion of those values.

Notes

1 For subsequent media coverage, see, for example, www.theguardian.com/law/2021/jan/ 17/jonathan-sumption-cancer-patient-life-less-valuable-others

2 The testimonies quoted here were collected during the early stages of the pandemic, in spring and summer 2020, when social restrictions had only been in place for a few months at most. It is likely that the effects of longer-term restrictions on people's abilities to sustain a life-structure will have been even more pronounced and widespread.

3 See, for example, the following news article, which describes an inability to "process" grief, involving a "freezing of the grieving process": www.itv.com/news/wales/2021-08-22/ wife-with-dementia-no-longer-recognises-husband-after-pandemic-separation?fbclid= IwAR2l92WHKnwdMxDxmXs3W-Fb_Oya2SCbWomoAZq10qMHeNa92oClFJdv 314. The UK-based Alzheimer's Society has drawn attention to the shocking deterioration undergone by many dementia sufferers during the pandemic, exacerbated by isolation, loneliness, and lack of familiar routines: www.alzheimers.org.uk/news/2020-07-30/ lockdown-isolation-causes-shocking-levels-decline-people-dementia-who-are-rapi dly#:~:text=Involving%20almost%202%2C000%20respondents%20affected,in%20peo ple%20with%20dementia%27s%20symptoms

4 See www.telegraph.co.uk/family/relationships/need-grieve-mum-pandemic-has-taken-away/. For several other discussions of grief and lockdown, see: www.griefyork.com/ covid-19.html

5 For an account of how and why social restrictions affect the course of grief, see Ratcliffe (in press). For a detailed discussion of how grief is regulated by interpersonal and social relations, see Ratcliffe (2022).

6 See, for example, the following newspaper article, which provides a detailed account of one woman's birth experience during lockdown: www.independent.co.uk/news/uk/ home-news/not-a-single-soul-who-cared-forgotten-new-mothers-recall-trauma-of-giv ing-birth-in-pandemic-b1774500.html

7 Szanto (2017:273–274) offers the examples of a pacifist who develops a passion for weapons that is at odds with a value system the person continues to endorse, and a flight attendant who brings home charming smiles that do not reflect an actual family situation.

References

Attig, T. 2011. *How We Grieve: Relearning the World* (revised edn.). Oxford: Oxford University Press.

Froese, T., M. Broome, H. Carel, C. Humpston, A. Malpass, T. Mori, M. Ratcliffe, J. Rodrigues, and F. Sangati. 2021. "The Pandemic Experience: A Corpus of Subjective Reports on Life During the First Wave of COVID-19 in the UK, Japan, and Mexico". *Frontiers in Public Health* 9: 1–7.

Glas, G. 2017. "Dimensions of the Self in Emotion and Psychopathology: Consequences for Self-Management in Anxiety and Depression". *Philosophy, Psychiatry, and Psychology* 24: 143–155.

Goldie, P. 2012. *The Mess Inside: Narrative, Emotion, and the Mind*. Oxford: Oxford University Press.

Green, T. 2021. *The COVID Consensus: The New Politics of Global Inequality*. London: Hurst & Company.

Korsgaard, C.M. 1996. *The Sources of Normativity*. Cambridge: Cambridge University Press.

Ratcliffe, M. 2015. *Experiences of Depression: A Study in Phenomenology*. Oxford: Oxford University Press.

Ratcliffe, M. 2022. *Grief Worlds: A Study of Emotional Experience*. Cambridge, MA: MIT Press.

Ratcliffe, M. 2022. (In press). Phenomenological Reflections on Grief during the COVID-19 Pandemic. *Phenomenology and the Cognitive Sciences.*

Ratcliffe, M., M. Ruddell, and B. Smith. 2014. "What is a Sense of Foreshortened Future? A Phenomenological Study of Trauma, Trust and Time". *Frontiers in Psychology* 5: 1–11.

Sartre, J.P. 1943/1989. *Being and Nothingness*. Translated by H.E. Barnes. London: Routledge.

Szanto, T. 2017. "Emotional Self-Alienation". *Midwest Studies in Philosophy* 41: 260–286.

15

DO LOCKDOWNS WORK FOR WOMEN?

The Gendered Impacts of the Pandemic and Policy Responses

Rose Cook and Aleida Mendes Borges

Introduction

The Year 2020 marked the 25th anniversary of the Beijing Platform for Action, a ground-breaking call for action on gender inequality (UN, 2020). Yet, years of progress for women have been reversed in the wake of a pandemic and economic shock expected to be more severe than the 2008 financial crisis (OECD, 2021). Globally, structural inequalities have meant that the poorest and most vulnerable have been disproportionately impacted by the pandemic and associated economic restrictions, and in most cases, women are over-represented in these categories. Furthermore, pre-existing gendered segregation in the labour force has amplified the crisis asymmetrically between men and women (World Economic Forum, 2021). There are also concerns about whether lockdowns have permanently deepened the "second shift" for women due to the intensification of care responsibilities. Others have drawn attention to the "shadow pandemic" of domestic violence taking place under the cover of "stay at home" measures, with the UN estimating that for every three months of lockdown there would be 15 million additional cases of gender-based violence worldwide[1] (UNFPA, 2020), as well as impacts on women's mental health resulting from excessive care demands. As a result of these impacts, the World Economic Forum (2021) has declared that it will now take 135.6 years to close the global gender gap.[2]

Meanwhile, there is an emerging consensus that policy responses to the pandemic have not adequately taken the gendered impacts of the crisis into account (Cook and Grimshaw, 2020; UN Women/UNDP, 2020; Women and Equalities Committee, 2021), with only one in five social-protection and employment policy responses being "gender sensitive" (UNDP/UN Women, 2020).[3] Moreover, policy measures have had uneven impacts, including the presence of gaps in access and

DOI: 10.4324/9781003259336-19

gender-biased implementation which are likely to have compounded the gendered impacts of the crisis (Women and Equalities Committee, 2021).

Chapter outline

This chapter examines emerging global data and literature which highlight the disproportionate impacts of the pandemic and policy responses on women. It starts by explaining how pre-existing asymmetries in the labour force amplified the disproportionate impact of the crisis on women's employment. Subsequently, it considers the unequal division of care work, which led to deepening of the "second shift", and emphasises the importance of taking an intersectional lens to fully appreciate the gendered impacts of the pandemic. Finally, we review a selection of policy responses to the crisis and discuss whether they can be considered gender sensitive, before looking forward to recovery from the pandemic and how to ensure this is shaped through a gendered lens.

Gendered impacts of the COVID-19 crisis

As COVID-19 continues to affect the lives and livelihoods of millions of people around the world, important questions are being asked about the gendered impacts of the pandemic and associated lockdown policies. The gendered impacts are mainly social and economic in nature, extending from worldwide asymmetries in the experience and inclusion of women in society. Across the globe, women hold less-secure jobs, earn less, and save less (UN, 2020). This in turn affects livelihoods, with 25 percent of women aged 25 to 34 estimated to live in extreme poverty (UN, 2020). Lockdown policies led to multiple gendered impacts due to pre-existing gendered labour-market segregation. Gendered impacts of lockdown were also due to the inequitable division of paid and unpaid care work colliding with the closure of schools, childcare, and other formal care facilities.

Impacts due to gendered labour-market segregation

Essential workers

At the beginning of the pandemic, governments published lists of "essential" workers whose jobs were critical to the COVID-19 response. People in these jobs continued to go into workplaces while countries were locked down. The list included doctors and nurses, care jobs including social workers and childcare workers, but also jobs that are typically considered "low-skilled" and are some of the worst-paid and most insecure jobs in the economy, such as supermarket employees and refuse collectors. Essential workers had little choice but to be exposed to the virus, and in most countries, protections were at the discretion of employers.

Analysis of the risks of COVID-19 alongside jobs' gender composition shows that 77 percent of workers with high exposure to the virus[4] are women (Kikuchi and Khurana, 2020); this is mainly due to the high proportion of women in health and social care professions – for instance, women make up 100 percent of nurses in Nepal (as of 2019), 100 percent in Latvia (as of 2018), 98 percent in Czechia (as of 2019), 98 percent in China (as of 2017), 97 percent in Iceland (as of 2019), 97 percent in Algeria, 96 percent in Denmark (as of 2017), and 91 percent in Hungary (as of 2019) (WHO, 2021)[5]. Infection rates among female health workers were disproportionately higher than among their male counterparts. In the USA, 73 percent of female health workers were infected, compared with only 27 percent of male workers. Spain (75.5 percent female vs. 24.5 percent male) and Italy (69 percent female vs. 31 percent male) also reported significantly higher infection rates among female workers (UN Women, 2020a).

In addition to increased virus exposure, female essential workers faced additional economic and health vulnerabilities. A large number of female essential workers' jobs are located in the care sector, which is extremely low paid. A UK analysis shows that the average weekly pay for "high-risk" roles (mainly health and social care jobs) is below the UK median (Kikuchi and Khurana, 2020). Moreover, of those in high-risk roles and being paid "poverty wages", a staggering 98 percent are women (Kikuchi and Khurana, 2020). While they were able to continue working (as opposed to being made unemployed or furloughed), these workers often faced increased workloads for no extra pay.

Closed sectors

In spring 2020, around 2.7 billion workers were affected by lockdown measures, representing approximately 81 percent of the total workforce worldwide (ILO, 2020). The economic impact of lockdown closures has been highly sectoral in nature – sectors involving face-to-face customer contact, social activities, and travel have lost out most. For example, in the UK, the accommodation and food sector had the highest number of at-risk jobs (at risk of redundancy, reduced hours, or being placed on a job-protection scheme) (Allas et al., 2020). These "closed sectors" – defined as not essential and explicitly closed under lockdown measures – are also highly female dominated: for example, in Europe, 56 percent of workers in closed sectors were women, with female shares ranging from 49 percent in Greece to 69 percent in Latvia (Fana et al., 2020). Women's exposure to job loss in hard-hit industries was particularly high in Central America and Southeast Asia (ILO, 2020).

Closed sectors include: hotels, restaurants and accommodation, estate and travel agencies, leisure and recreation services, and personal services, including hairdressing and beauty salons.

The economic risks faced by closed-sector workers are compounded by low pay. Analysis of the socioeconomic composition of closed-sector workers uniformly identifies them as low-paid relative to the economy-wide average (Fana et al., 2020). Low pay also disproportionately affects women since they are over-represented among low-wage workers, meaning many low-paid women have found themselves

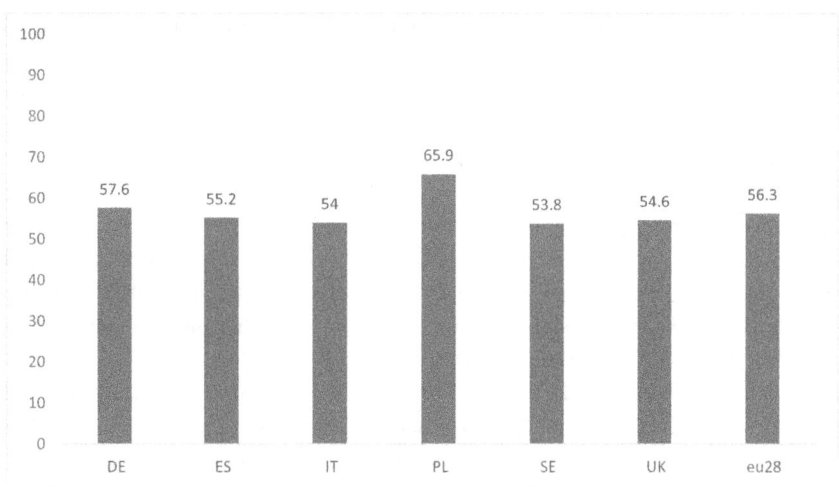

FIGURE 15.1 Proportion of women employees in "closed sectors" in selected countries.
Source: Data from Fana et al. 2020.

unemployed or with reduced working hours, exacerbating their economic vulnerabilities and resulting in broader consequences for families, since female low-earners are increasingly primary breadwinners (Kowalewska and Vitali, 2021).

Informal economy

Informal workers face a higher degree of vulnerability due to not being legally recognised or being insufficiently protected by employment laws and protection. This has been exposed in the current crisis since the closed sectors identified in the previous section employ large numbers of informal workers, who have no safety net. Although informality exists in all countries, regardless of their level of socioeconomic development, it is more prevalent in countries defined as emerging markets and developing economies (EMDEs). The World Bank (2021) estimates that in these nations, informal employment accounts for more than 70 percent of all employment. In Africa, an even larger proportion of the workforce (80 percent) are in the "shadow" of informal labour despite providing vital goods and services (ILO, 2018). South of the Sahara, around a third of households rely on informal food suppliers for critical food security (Resnick et al., 2020). A high proportion of informal-economy workers are women. For example, women are more likely to be informally employed in the majority of countries South of the Sahara (90 percent), in Southern Asia (89 percent), and in Latin America (75 percent) (ILO, 2018). Furthermore, the pandemic has highlighted that in higher-income countries domestic work is an important sector that is female dominated and includes a large share of workers operating informally.

Non-standard employment

Women tend to be over-represented among workers in non-standard employment, including temporary, part-time, and agency work, and in some parts of the growing "gig economy" and self-employment. Many workers in non-standard employment, due to a lack of access to adequate sick pay and unemployment benefits, have continued working during the crisis, risking their health; conversely, they are also more likely to have been made redundant and have poor access to social protection (Spasova et al., 2021). Again, there is a crossover with gendered occupational segregation, since many workers with non-standard contracts are women and work in sectors hard hit by the crisis.

Impacts due to the unequal division of care work

Women are the primary unpaid workers in a system known as "social reproduction" – which includes household labour, physical and emotional caregiving, and other work to meet human needs (Laslett and Brenner, 1989). Women's uncompensated, daily social-reproduction work meets the needs of the people, many of whom are also employees, thus also directly bolstering the paid economy. The "second shift" describes a system in which women do paid work followed by a second shift of unpaid work in the home (Hochschild and Machung, 2012).

Lockdown policies meant that between March and April 2020, there were school closures affecting 84 percent of learners worldwide (UNESCO, 2021), creating an instant need for at-home childcare. Families could not rely on informal care from grandparents and other family due to the need for social distancing. The increased need for childcare has put a strain on working parents of both genders, but overall, due to unequal bargaining power and gendered social norms, mothers have carried a heavier load, placing great pressure on their working lives. This unevenness illustrates how childcare and schools constitute key infrastructure that enables women's effective labour-force participation. The increased burden was not only due to children's needs: the crisis brought additional adult care needs as a result of widespread illness and vulnerability.

Exceptional and unequal care burdens are already reflected in time-use data. In the Asia-Pacific region, on average, 60 percent of women and 54 percent of men reported more unpaid care work, and 63 percent of women and 59 percent of men reported an increase in unpaid domestic work. the gender gap is reflected in the increased intensity of unpaid work as well (with intense work defined as that involving at least three activities): on average, 30 percent of women and 20 percent of men reported increased intensity (UN Women, 2020b). Adams-Prassl et al. (2020) found that, among the population working from home in the USA, UK, and Germany during lockdown, women spent significantly more time on childcare and homeschooling relative to men. This has left women with children susceptible to leaving employment and reduced working hours (Djankov et al., 2021). Women with children have also experienced profound mental health impacts. For example, in the United States, mothers of young children reported high levels of psychological distress (Zamaro and Prados, 2021).

While the overall picture is one of mothers under huge pressure, the gender division of care work during lockdowns seems to depend on the fathers' work situation and family income. Men were more likely to participate in childcare if they worked from home, were furloughed, or unemployed (Andrew et al., 2020). Evidence from Germany shows that men are more likely to become involved in childcare if they are higher earners, meaning also that they are more likely to work from home (Möhring et al., 2020). Mothers mostly continue to do more unpaid work regardless of working arrangements. Some have cautioned that new forms of gender segregation and inequality could emerge post-lockdown if women remain home-based workers while men return to the office (Rubery and Tavora, 2021).

Nonetheless, there are also signs of a shift towards more gender-equitable arrangements. One UK study comparing time-use (Andrew et al., 2020) in April 2020 to data from 2014–15 found that fathers nearly doubled the time they spent on childcare. Such findings have led researchers to predict a more egalitarian division of labour, especially where fathers work from home and mothers work in essential jobs (Hupkau and Petrongolo, 2020).

Intersecting inequalities/vulnerabilities

Along with women, other historically disadvantaged groups have been more exposed to disadvantage by the pandemic, creating intersectional impacts. A recent study found that women, young people, the less educated, and lower earners were more likely to lose their jobs (Soares and Berg, 2021). In the USA, while unemployment increased by 3.6 percent in 2020 for White men and 4 percent for White women, for Black women it increased by 4.9 percent, and for Hispanic and Latino women by 6.2 percent (World Economic Forum, 2021). In Brazil, lockdown policies left more than half the working-age population unemployed and increased the percentage of people living in extreme poverty from 4.5 percent to 12.8 percent. Groups such as women, Black and indigenous people, and those living in rural areas were disproportionately affected such that by the end of 2020, 11 percent of female-headed households and 10 percent of Black households faced hunger, contrasted with 7 percent of White households (Oxfam, 2021).

Gender-sensitivity of the policy response

Policy measures

Given that men and women have been differently affected by COVID-19 and lockdowns, it makes sense to ask whether policy responses have taken this into account. In this section, we focus on selected policy measures which have been put in place to help individuals and families manage lockdown restrictions, providing an initial assessment of their gender-sensitivity. However, we recognise this will provide only a partial account given that, as of May 2021, there have been over three thousand new or adapted social-protection and employment-protection response to the crisis (across 222 countries) (Gentilini et al., 2021).

Job-protection schemes

Since the COVID-19 crisis began, all countries in Europe have implemented some version of a job-protection scheme, intended to help workers retain a salary while they are unable to work. An estimated 50 million workers in Europe were participating in job-protection schemes in April 2020 (Müller and Schulten, 2020). While the schemes have been a lifeline for many, research has also shown that they contained gendered barriers to access and sufficient support, seemingly having been designed with a standard (male) worker in mind. Women's marginal labour-market position – such as for those working in non-standard, low-paid, and vulnerable employment – made them less likely to be eligible for support and to receive support adequate to their needs (Cook and Grimshaw, 2020; Jones and Cook, 2021). For example, schemes in some countries revealed an ingrained assumption that female employment is less essential – in Austria and Germany, "mini-jobs" (part-time, low-paid service-sector jobs mainly done by women) were not eligible for job protection, and in Croatia and Hungary, part-time workers (mostly women) also could not claim. Indeed, Möhring et al. (2021) found that, during the early stages of the crisis, women were less likely to receive job-protection support and more likely to lose employment or be temporarily suspended without pay. Moreover, government support for businesses was more likely to be targeted at male-dominated industries.

Informal economic activity, which includes a high proportion of women workers, has largely been overlooked by government support programmes. This notably includes domestic workers. In countries such as Portugal and Spain, the government provided special measures to address the lack of social security usually afforded to this group of workers. Nonetheless, for the most part these measures reflected the long-standing marginalisation faced by these women and were not considered adequate, exposing the contradiction of their being both essential and expendable (Pandey, 2021).

At present it is unclear whether job-protection schemes were a useful tool to mitigate adverse impacts on women and whether the variations in scheme design were consequential for women's longer-term employment outcomes. While outcomes for women are likely to be better where such schemes existed as compared to where the government offered no support at all, inadequacies in scheme design highlight the need for social security to account for the (gendered) fragmentation and increasing destandardisation of the labour force, adding to growing recognition of the need for more inclusive or universal entitlements (Spasova et al., 2021).

Support for working parents

Many governments have offered support to working parents to account for the additional care and education burden due to the closure of schools and childcare facilities. This includes parental-leave policies and flexible work arrangements. There were a number of approaches to parental leave, including new leave schemes, extensions of existing schemes, or the provision of access to job-protection schemes for childcare purposes. Examples include the Corona Parental Leave scheme in Belgium. In this scheme, paid leave could be granted for 20 percent or 50 percent of working time. Self-employed parents and single parents, however, could apply for a 100 percent work reduction. The rate of pay was 25 percent higher than traditional parental leave and entitlement started when a parent was at least one month employed.

There are two key criteria when assessing the gender sensitivity of COVID-19 parental-leave schemes. The first is the level of pay provided and how this compares to support for those unable to work, such as through job-protection schemes. As Rubery and Tavora (2021: 87) have argued,

> In countries where parental leave is paid at the same or higher level than job [protection] schemes, this could be considered an indicator that the government is not only attaching comparable value to care work but also recognising the importance of both parents' earnings for the family income and the right of both women and men to an independent income.

Austria, Greece, Portugal, and Romania, for example, paid parental leave at the same level as job protection. In other countries (such as Uzbekistan), one parent received full pay to stay home with children for the entire school-closure period. Where parental leave pay is lower than for job protection, this indicates an undervaluing of care; where this is unpaid (as in Spain) or means-tested and very low paid (as in Bulgaria), the result is that women are made economically dependent on other family members.

The gender sensitivity of parental-leave policies is also seen in whether they incentivise a "shared care" model. For example, in Bulgaria employers are only obliged to give parental leave to mothers and single fathers, reinforcing women's role as primary carers. By contrast, parental leave schemes in Belgium and Italy encourage parents to share: in Belgium, parental leave can only be taken on a part-time basis, enabling each employee to reduce working time by up to 50 percent, ensuring full-time care only if both parents take leave; in Italy each parent is entitled to 15 days, with both expected to alternate so that care can be provided for a total of 30 days (Rubery and Tavora, 2021: 87).

Other support for families which will have substantially benefited women includes special provisions for pregnant women (such as in El Salvador, where pregnant women were provided with 30 days of paid sick leave), the continued provision of childcare and education services during lockdowns, as well as elderly and disabled care. The majority of countries in Europe kept childcare services accessible for children of essential workers. In terms of resources, countries around the world provided extra top-ups to child benefit and additional benefits for low-income parents, as well as ad-hoc support payments for carers, often targeted at women.

However, these were often plagued by problems of eligibility and implementation, and could be said to have reinforced women's assumed role as caregivers rather than supporting their economic independence (Holmes and Hunt, 2021).

Outlook

The disproportionate gendered impacts of the pandemic and lockdowns which we have highlighted in this chapter are mainly the result of occupational segregation and of women's disproportionate responsibility for care work. As described by Cohen and Rodgers (2021: 1390), they stem from "the subjugation of women in multiple, fundamental ways having to do with the devaluation of their paid work". The response to the pandemic starkly highlights the higher perceived value of paid work vs. unpaid work and reveals the dependency of the paid economy on social reproduction.

Although the crisis provided an opportunity to acknowledge and address these gendered realities, generally the immediate policy response did not do this, apart from a few positive examples which we have described. This largely gender-blind policy response is likely to have compounded the gendered impacts of the crisis (UN Women/UNDP, 2020; Women and Equalities Committee, 2021). The lack of gender-sensitive policymaking is likely due to women's under-representation in decision-making processes, gendered assumptions about women's participation in paid and unpaid work, and limited use of gender-disaggregated data (Cullen and Murphy, 2020).

The pandemic's impacts will be long lasting, and it may not be too late to implement gender-sensitive measures. Current measures can be adapted in light of guidance for gender-sensitive social protection, such as those issued by Hidrobo et al (2020). Any new measure must recognise the gendered division of paid and unpaid work as integral to our economic system and account for gender segregation in the labour market. Positive examples include the "Economic Recovery Plan for COVID-19" issued by Hawaii's Department of Human Services (Hawaii State Commission on the Status of Women, 2020), which recommends providing paid family leave and paid sick leave, creating universal free childcare and long-term eldercare, boosting pay equity and job creation in education and nursing, and providing marginalised groups with increased access to maternal and child health services. More broadly, King et al. (2020) suggest that COVID-19 is an opportunity to disrupt gender norms and beliefs. To this end, in addition to the types of measures in Hawaii's plan, policies to enable the combination of working and caring should be targeted at both men and women and aimed at normalising men's sharing of caring and household responsibilities.

Notes

1 In this chapter, we focus mainly on gendered employment and economic impacts, as well as those relating to unpaid care work. For research on the "shadow pandemic" see UNDP (2020).

2 The Global Gender Gap Index collated by the WEF. The Global Gender Gap Index benchmarks the evolution of gender-based gaps in four key dimensions (economic participation and opportunity, educational attainment, health and survival, and political empowerment) and tracks progress towards closing these gaps over time.
3 UN Women and UNDP's COVID-19 Global Gender Response Tracker focuses on policy design rather than implementation, and its criteria for gender sensitivity is that a policy either target women's economic security or address the rise in unpaid care work.
4 Based on the degree of close proximity to others and the level exposure to infection involved in performing the job.
5 In countries such as Togo (21 percent as of 2018), Botswana (29 percent as of 2018), Benin (31 percent as of 2018) and East Timor (38 percent as of 2019), the imbalance is towards a male domination of the sector (WHO, 2021).

References

Adams-Prassl, A., T. Boneva, M. Golin, and C. Rauh. 2020. "Inequality in the Impact of the Coronavirus Shock: Evidence from Real Time Survey". *IZA Discussion Papers* 13183.

Allas, T., M. Canal, and V. Hunt. 2020. COVID-19 in the UK: The impact on people and jobs at risk. London: McKinsey.

Andrew, A., S. Cattan, M. Costa Dias , C. Farquharson, L. Kraftman, S. Krutikova, A. Phimister, and A. Sevilla. 2020. "How are Mothers and Fathers Balancing Work and Family under lockdown?". *IFS Briefing Note 290*. London: Institute for Fiscal Studies.

Cohen, J. and Y. van der Meulen Rodgers. 2021. "The Feminist Political Economy of COVID-19: Capitalism, women, and work". Global Public Health *16* (8–9): 1381–1395.

Cook, R. and D. Grimshaw. 2020. "A Gendered Lens on COVID-19 Employment and Social Policies in Europe". European Societies 23 (S1): 215–227.

Cullen, P. and M.P. Murphy.2020. "Responses to the COVID-19 crisis in Ireland: From Feminized to Feminist". Gender, Work & Organization 28 (S2): 348–365.

Djankov, S., P.K. Goldberg, M. Hyland, and E.Y. Zhang. 2021. *The Evolving Gender Gap in Labor Force Participation during COVID-19.* Washington: PIIE.

Fana, M., S. Torrejón Pérez, and E. Fernández-Macías. 2020. "Employment Impact of COVID-19 Crisis: From Short Term Effects to Long Term Prospects". Journal of Industrial and Business Economics 47(3): 391–410.

Gentilini, U., M. Almenfi, I. Orton, and P. Dale. 2021. Social Protection and Jobs Responses to COVID-19: A Real-Time Review of Country Measures. Washington DC: World Bank: https://openknowledge.worldbank.org/handle/10986/33635

Hawaii State Commission on the Status of Women. 2020. Building Bridges, Not Walking on Backs A Feminist Economic Recovery Plan for COVID-19. State of Hawaii: Department of Human Services: https://humanservices.hawaii.gov/wp-content/uploads/2020/04/4.13.20-Final-Cover-D2-Feminist-Economic-Recovery-D1.pdf

Hidrobo, M., N. Kumar, T. Palermo , A. Peterman, and S. Roy. 2020. Gender-sensitive social protection: A critical component of the COVID-19 response in low- and middle-income countries. Washington DC: International Food Policy Research Institute: http://ebrary.ifpri.org/utils/getfile/collection/p15738coll2/id/133701/filename/133912.pdf

Hochschild, A., and A. Machung. 2012. *The Second Shift: Working families and the revolution at home.* London: Penguin.

Holmes, R., and A. Hunt. 2021. Have Social Protection Responses to COVID-19 Undermined or Supported Gender Equality? Emerging Lessons from a Gender Perspective. London: ODI: https://cdn.odi.org/media/documents/ODI_Gender_final.pdf

Hupkau, C. and B. Petrongolo. 2020. *Work, Care and Gender in the Covid 19 Crisis: A CEP COVID-19 Analysis*. London: Centre for Economic Performance, London School of Economics.

ILO. 2018. Women and Men in the Informal Economy: A Statistical Picture. Geneva: International Labour Office: https://www.ilo.org/global/publications/books/WCMS_626831/lang--en/index.htm

ILO. 2020. ILO Monitor: COVID-19 and the World of Work (fifth edn.). Geneva: International Labour Office. https://www.ilo.org/wcmsp5/groups/public/---dgreports/---dcomm/documents/briefingnote/wcms_749399.pdf

Jones, L., and R. Cook. 2021. Does Furlough Work for Women? Gendered Experiences of the Coronavirus Job Retention Scheme in the UK. London: Global Institute for Women's Leadership: https://www.kcl.ac.uk/giwl/assets/does-furlough-work-for-women.pdf

Kikuchi, L. and I. Khurana. 2020. "The Jobs at Risk Index". *Autonomy*, 24 March, https://autonomy.work/portfolio/jari/

King, T., B. Hewitt, B., Crammond, G., Sutherland, H. Maheen, and A. Kavanagh. 2020. "Reordering Gender Systems: Can COVID-19 Lead to Improved Gender Equality and Health?". *The Lancet* 396 (10244): 80–81.

Kowalewska, H., and A. Vitali. 2021. "Breadwinning or on the Breadline? Female Breadwinners' Economic Characteristics Across 20 Welfare States". *Journal of European Social Policy* 31(2): 125–142.

Laslett, B. and J. Brenner. 1989. "Gender and Social reproduction: Historical perspectives". *Annual Review of Sociology* 15(1): 381–404.

Möhring, K., E. Naumann, M. Reifenscheid, A.G. Blom, A. Wenz, T. Rettig, T. Lehrer, et al. 2020. *Die Mannheimer Corona Studie: Schwerpunktbericht zu Erwerbstätigkeit und Kinderbetreuung*. Mannheim: University of Mannheim.

Müller, T. and T. Schulten. 2020. *Ensuring Fair Short-Time Work: A European Overview*. Brussels: ETUI: www.etui.org/sites/default/files/2020-06/Covid-19%2BShort-time%2Bwork%2BM%C3%BCller%2BSchulten%2BPolicy%2BBrief%2B2020.07%281%29.pdf

OECD. 2021. *Coronavirus (COVID-19) Pandemic: Towards A Blue Recovery In Small Island Developing States*. Paris: OECD: www.oecd.org/coronavirus/policy-responses/covid-19-pandemic-towards-a-blue-recovery-in-small-island-developing-states-241271b7/#section-d1e104

Oxfam. 2021. The Hunger Virus Multiplies: Deadly Recipe of Conflict, COVID-19 and Climate Accelerate World Hunger. Oxford: Oxfam GB: https://oi-files-d8-prod.s3.eu-west-2.amazonaws.com/s3fs-public/2021-07/The%20Hunger%20Virus%202.0_media%20brief_EN.pdf

Pandey, K., R. Salazar Parreñas, and G.S. Sabio. 2021. "Essential and Expendable: Migrant Domestic Workers and the COVID-19 Pandemic". *American Behavioral Scientist* 65 (10): 1287–1301.

Resnick, D., E. Spencer, and T. Siwale. 2020. *Informal Traders and COVID-19 in Africa: An Opportunity to Strengthen the Social Contract*. London: International Growth Centre: https://www.theigc.org/wp-content/uploads/2020/08/Resnick-et-al-2020-Policy-Brief.pdf

Rubery, J. and I. Tavora. 2021. *The COVID-19 Crisis and gender equality: Risks and Opportunities*. Brussels: ETUI: https://www.etui.org/sites/default/files/2021-01/06-Chapter4-The%20Covid%E2%80%9919%20crisis%20and%20gender%20equality.pdf

Soares, S. and J. Berg. 2021. "Transitions in the Labour Market under COVID-19: Who Endures, Who Doesn't and the Implications for Inequality". *International Labour Review*.

Spasova, S., D. Ghailani, S. Sabato, S. Coster, B. Fronteddu, and B, Vanhercke. 2021. *Non-Standard Workers and the Self-Employed in the EU: Social Protection During the COVID-19*

Pandemic. Brussels: ETUI: https://www.etui.org/publications/non-standard-workers-and-self-employed-eu

UN. 2020. *Policy Brief: The Impact of COVID-19 on Women*. Geneva: United Nations: https://www.unwomen.org/-/media/headquarters/attachments/sections/library/publications/2020/policy-brief-the-impact-of-covid-19-on-women-en.pdf?la=en&vs=1406

UNDP. 2020. *Gender-Based Violence and COVID-19*. New York: USA: https://www.undp.org/content/undp/en/home/librarypage/womens-empowerment/gender-based-violence-and-covid-19.html

UNESCO. 2021. *Global Monitoring of School Closures*. Paris: UNESCO: https://documents1.worldbank.org/curated/en/618731587147227244/pdf/Gender-Dimensions-of-the-COVID-19-Pandemic.pdf

UNFPA. 2020. *Impact of the COVID-19 Pandemic on Family Planning and Ending Gender-based Violence, Female Genital Mutilation and Child Marriage*. New York: UNFPA: https://www.unfpa.org/resources/impact-covid-19-pandemic-family-planning-and-ending-gender-based-violence-female-genital

UN Women. 2020a *COVID-19: Emerging gender data and why it matters*. Geneva: United Nations: https://data.unwomen.org/resources/covid-19-emerging-gender-data-and-why-it-matters#vaw

UN Women. 2020b. *Unlocking the Lockdown: The Gendered Effects of COVID-19 on Achieving the SDGS in Asia and the Pacific*. Geneva: United Nations: https://data.unwomen.org/publications/unlocking-lockdown-gendered-effects-covid-19-achieving-sdgs-asia-and-pacific

UN Women/UNDP. 2020. *COVID-19 Global Gender Response Tracker: Global Factsheet* (vol. 1). Geneva: United Nations: https://www.undp.org/content/undp/en/home/librarypage/womens-empowerment/COVID-19-Global-Gender-Response-Tracker.html

Women and Equalities Committee. 2021. *Unequal impact? Coronavirus and the gendered economic impact*. London: House of Commons: https://committees.parliament.uk/publications/4597/documents/46478/default/

World Bank. 2021. *As COVID-19 Wreaks Havoc on Service Workers, Is The Informal Sector Increasing Global Inequality? World Bank* [podcast], https://www.worldbank.org/en/news/podcast/2021/05/24/as-covid-19-wreaks-havoc-on-service-workers-is-the-informal-sector-increasing-global-inequality-the-development-podcast

World Economic Forum. 2021. *Global Gender Gap Report 2021*. Geneva: World Economic Forum: www3.weforum.org/docs/WEF_GGGR_2021.pdf

World Health Organisation. 2021. *Global Health Observatory Data Repository: Sex Distribution of Health Workers*. Geneva: World Health Organisation: https://apps.who.int/gho/data/node.main.HWFGRP_BYSEX?lang=en

Zamarro, G. and M.J. Prados. 2021. "Gender Differences in Couples' Division of Childcare, Work and Mental Health During COVID-19". *Review of Economics of the Household* 19 (1): 11–40.

INDEX